Neuroradiology Applications of High-Field MR Imaging

Guest Editor

WINFRIED A. WILLINEK, MD

NEUROIMAGING CLINICS OF NORTH AMERICA

www.neuroimaging.theclinics.com

Consulting Editor
SURESH K. MUKHERJI, MD

May 2012 • Volume 22 • Number 2

SAUNDERS an imprint of ELSEVIER, Inc.

W.B. SAUNDERS COMPANY
A Division of Elsevier Inc.

1600 John F. Kennedy Boulevard • Suite 1800 • Philadelphia, Pennsylvania 19103-2899

http://www.theclinics.com

NEUROIMAGING CLINICS OF NORTH AMERICA Volume 22, Number 2
May 2012 ISSN 1052-5149, ISBN 13: 978-1-4557-3893-9

Editor: Sarah E. Barth
Developmental Editor: Donald Mumford

Neuroimaging Clinics of North America (ISSN 1052-5149) is published quarterly by Elsevier Inc., 360 Park Avenue South, New York, NY 10010-1710. Months of issue are February, May, August, and November. Business and editorial offices: 1600 John F. Kennedy Blvd., Suite 1800, Philadelphia, PA 19103-2899. Business and editorial offices: 6277 Sea Harbor Drive, Orlando, FL 32887-4800. Periodicals postage paid at New York, NY, and additional mailing offices. Subscription prices are USD 342 per year for US individuals, USD 471 per year for US institutions, USD 172 per year for US students and residents, USD 396 per year for Canadian individuals, USD 590 per year for Canadian institutions, USD 502 per year for international individuals, USD 590 per year for international institutions and USD 246 per year for Canadian and foreign students and residents. To receive student/resident rate, orders must be accompanied by name of affiliated institution, date of term, and the *signature* of program/residency coordinator on institution letterhead. Orders will be billed at individual rate until proof of status is received. Foreign air speed delivery is included in all *Clinics* subscription prices. All prices are subject to change without notice. POSTMASTER: Send address changes to *Neuroimaging Clinics of North America*, Elsevier Health Sciences Division, Subscription Customer Service, 3251 Riverport Lane, Maryland Heights, MO 63043. Telephone: 1-800-654-2452 (U.S. and Canada); 314-447-8871 (outside U.S. and Canada). Fax: 314-447-8029. E-mail: journalscustomerservice-usa@elsevier.com (for print support); journalsonlinesupport-usa@elsevier.com (for online support).

Reprints. For copies of 100 or more of articles in this publication, please contact the Commercial Reprints Department, Elsevier Inc., 360 Park Avenue South, New York, NY 10010-1710. Tel.: 212-633-3812; Fax: 212-462-1935; E-mail: reprints@elsevier.com.

Neuroimaging Clinics of North America is covered by *Excerpta Medical/EMBASE*, the RSNA Index of Imaging Literature, *MEDLINE/PubMed (Index Medicus)*, MEDLINE/MEDLARS, SciSearch, Research Alert, and Neuroscience Citation Index.

Printed and bound by CPI Group (UK) Ltd, Croydon, CR0 4YY

Transferred to Digital Print 2012

GOAL STATEMENT

The goal of *Neuroimaging Clinics of North America* is to keep practicing radiologists and radiology residents up to date with current clinical practice in radiology by providing timely articles reviewing the state of the art in patient care.

ACCREDITATION

The *Neuroimaging Clinics of North America* is planned and implemented in accordance with the Essential Areas and Policies of the Accreditation Council for Continuing Medical Education (ACCME) through the joint sponsorship of the University of Virginia School of Medicine and Elsevier. The University of Virginia School of Medicine is accredited by the ACCME to provide continuing medical education for physicians.

The University of Virginia School of Medicine designates this enduring material activity for a maximum of 15 *AMA PRA Category 1 Credit*(s)™ for each issue, 60 credits per year. Physicians should claim only the credit commensurate with the extent of their participation in the activity.

The American Medical Association has determined that physicians not licensed in the US who participate in this CME enduring material activity are eligible for a maximum of 15 *AMA PRA Category 1 Credit*(s)™ for each issue, 60 credits per year.

Credit can be earned by reading the text material, taking the CME examination online at http://www.theclinics.com/home/cme, and completing the evaluation. After taking the test, you will be required to review any and all incorrect answers. Following completion of the test and evaluation, your credit will be awarded and you may print your certificate.

FACULTY DISCLOSURE/CONFLICT OF INTEREST

The University of Virginia School of Medicine, as an ACCME accredited provider, endorses and strives to comply with the Accreditation Council for Continuing Medical Education (ACCME) Standards of Commercial Support, Commonwealth of Virginia statutes, University of Virginia policies and procedures, and associated federal and private regulations and guidelines on the need for disclosure and monitoring of proprietary and financial interests that may affect the scientific integrity and balance of content delivered in continuing medical education activities under our auspices.

The University of Virginia School of Medicine requires that all CME activities accredited through this institution be developed independently and be scientifically rigorous, balanced and objective in the presentation/discussion of its content, theories and practices.

All authors/editors participating in an accredited CME activity are expected to disclose to the readers relevant financial relationships with commercial entities occurring within the past 12 months (such as grants or research support, employee, consultant, stock holder, member of speakers bureau, etc.). The University of Virginia School of Medicine will employ appropriate mechanisms to resolve potential conflicts of interest to maintain the standards of fair and balanced education to the reader. Questions about specific strategies can be directed to the Office of Continuing Medical Education, University of Virginia School of Medicine, Charlottesville, Virginia.

The faculty and staff of the University of Virginia Office of Continuing Medical Education have no financial affiliations to disclose.

The authors/editors listed below have identified no professional/financial affiliations for themselves or their spouse/partner:
Benjamin P. Austin, PhD; Niranjan Balu, PhD; Sarah Barth, (Acquisitions Editor); Wessam Bou-Assaly, MD; Norbert G. Campeau, MD; Hisham M. Dahmoush, MBBCh, FRCR; Wolter L. de Graaf, MSc; Michael Forsting, MD; Thomas A. Gallagher, MD; Sven Haller, MSc, MD; Jeroen Hendrikse, MD, PhD; John Huston III, MD; Iris D. Kilsdonk; Christian La, BA; Seung-Koo Lee, MD, PhD; Peter R. Luijten, PhD; Donald G. McLaren, PhD; Veena A. Nair, PhD; Vitor Mendes Pereira, MSc, MD; Vivek Prabhakaran, MD, PhD; Lubdha M. Shah, MD (Test Author); Ashok Srinivasan, MBBS, MD, DNB; Horst Urbach, MD, PhD; M.A. van Buchem, MD, PhD; J. van der Grond, PhD; Anja G van der Kolk, MD; M.J. Versluis, MSc; Arastoo Vossough, PhD, MD; Mike P. Wattjes, MD; A.G. Webb, PhD; Yijing Wu, PhD; and Guofan Xu, MD, PhD.

The authors listed below have identified the following professional/financial affiliations for themselves or their spouse/partner:
Frederik Barkhof, MD, PhD is a consultant for GE.
William G. Bradley, Jr., MD, PhD is an industry funded research/investigator for GE.
J. Kevin DeMarco, MD is on the Speakers' Bureau for Bracco Diagnostic INC, and is a consultant for GE Medical Systems.
J. Paul Finn, MD is a funded research/investigator for Siemens Medical Solutions, and is on the Speakers' Bureau for Bracco Diagnostics and Lantheus, Inc.
Xavier Golay, PhD is a consultant for Philips Healthcare.
Mark E. Ladd, PhD is an industry funded research/investigator for Siemens Healthcare.
Karl-Olof Lövblad, MD is an industry funded research/investigator for Bayer Schering Pharma.
Suresh K. Mukherji, MD (Consulting Editor) is a consultant for Philips.
Esben Thade Petersen, PhD is a consultant for Philips Healthcare.
Timothy P.L. Roberts, PhD is on the Speakers' Bureau for Siemens, and is a consultant and is on the Advisory Board for Prism.
Howard Rowley, MD is a consultant for GE Healthcare, Bracco, Bayer, Gore, Lundbeck, and Eli Lilly, and receives research support from Guerbet.
Marc Shapiro, MD has a showsite for Siemens' Medical.
Patrick Turski, MD is an industry support research/investigator for GE Healthcare.
Lale Umutlu, MD is a consultant for Bayer Health Care.
P. van Zijl, PhD is an industry funded research/investigator, is on the Speakers' Bureau, and is a patent holder for Philips Healthcare.
Jinnan Wang, PhD is employed by Philips Electronics North America.
Winfried A. Willinek, MD (Guest Editor) is on the Speakers' Bureau for Bracco and Philips Healthcare, and is on the Speakers' Bureau and Advisory Board for Bayer Schering Prarma, Lantheus Medical Imaging, and GE Healthcare.
Chun Yuan, PhD is an industry funded research/investigator for Philips Healthcare and VP Diagnostics, and is a consultant for Imagepace LLC and Bristol Myers Squibb.

Disclosure of Discussion of Non-FDA Approved Uses for Pharmaceutical Products and/or Medical Devices.
The University of Virginia School of Medicine, as an ACCME provider, requires that all faculty presenters identify and disclose any off-label uses for pharmaceutical and medical device products. The University of Virginia School of Medicine recommends that each physician fully review all the available data on new products or procedures prior to clinical use.

TO ENROLL

To enroll in the Neuroimaging Clinics of North America Continuing Medical Education program, call customer service at 1-800-654-2452 or sign up online at http://www.theclinics.com/home/cme. The CME program is available to subscribers for an additional annual fee of USD 196.

NEUROIMAGING CLINICS OF NORTH AMERICA

FORTHCOMING ISSUES

Intracranial Infections
Guarang Shah, MD, *Guest Editor*

Socioeconomics of Neuroimaging
David Yousem, MD, *Guest Editor*

Pediatric Demyelinating Disease and its Mimics
Manohar Shroff, MD, *Guest Editor*

MR Neurography
Avneesh Chhabra, MD, *Guest Editor*

RECENT ISSUES

February 2012
Imaging in Alzheimer's Disease and Other Dementias
Alison D. Murray, MBChB (Hons), FRCP, FRCR, *Guest Editor*

November 2011
Neuroimaging of Tropical Disease
Rakesh K. Gupta, MD, *Guest Editor*

August 2011
Congenital Anomalies of the Brain, Spine, and Neck
Hemant A. Parmar, MD and
Mohannad Ibrahim, MD, *Guest Editors*

RELATED INTEREST

Radiologic Clinics, Vol. 50, No. 1, January 2012
Emergency Radiology
Jorge A. Soto, MD, *Guest Editor*

Contributors

CONSULTING EDITOR

SURESH K. MUKHERJI, MD, FACR
Professor and Chief of Neuroradiology, and
Head and Neck Radiology; Professor of
Radiology, Otolaryngology Head and Neck
Surgery, Radiation Oncology, Periodontics and
Oral Medicine, University of Michigan Health
System, Ann Arbor, Michigan

GUEST EDITOR

WINFRIED A. WILLINEK, MD
Associate Professor of Radiology and Head
of Magnetic Resonance Imaging, Department
of Radiology, University of Bonn, Bonn,
Germany

AUTHORS

BENJAMIN P. AUSTIN, PhD
Postdoctoral Fellow, The UW Cardiovascular
Research Center, Department of Medicine,
University of Wisconsin; Department of
Veterans Affairs, Geriatric Research, Education
and Clinical Center, Madison, Wisconsin

NIRANJAN BALU, PhD
Senior Fellow, Department of Radiology,
University of Washington, Seattle,
Washington

FREDERIK BARKHOF, MD, PhD
Department of Radiology, VU University
Medical Center, Amsterdam, The Netherlands

WESSAM BOU-ASSALY, MD
Clinical Assistant Professor, Department of
Radiology, Neuroradiology Division, University
of Michigan, Ann Arbor VA Hospital, Ann Arbor,
Michigan

WILLIAM G. BRADLEY Jr, MD, PhD, FACR
Professor and Chair, Department of Radiology,
University of California San Diego Medical
Center, San Diego, California

NORBERT G. CAMPEAU, MD
Assistant Professor of Radiology, Division
of Neuroradiology, Mayo Clinic, Rochester,
Minnesota

HISHAM M. DAHMOUSH, MBBCh, FRCR
Neuroradiology Section, Department of
Radiology, Children's Hospital of Philadelphia,
Philadelphia, Pennsylvania

WOLTER L. DE GRAAF, MSc
Department of Radiology, VU University
Medical Center, Amsterdam, The Netherlands

J. KEVIN DEMARCO, MD
Associate Professor of Radiology and Head
of Magnetic Resonance Imaging, Department
of Radiology, Michigan State University, East
Lansing, Michigan

J. PAUL FINN, MD
Professor of Radiology, Medicine and
Biomedical Physics; Chief, Diagnostic
Cardiovascular Imaging; and Director,
Magnetic Resonance Research; Vice Chair,
Imaging Technology, Department of
Radiology, David Geffen School of Medicine
at UCLA, Los Angeles, California

MICHAEL FORSTING, MD
Professor, Department of Diagnostic and
Interventional Radiology and Neuroradiology,
University Hospital Essen, Essen, Germany

THOMAS A. GALLAGHER, MD
Assistant Professor of Radiology, Division
of Neuroradiology, Department of Radiology,
Northwestern Memorial Hospital,
Northwestern University, Chicago, Illinois

XAVIER GOLAY, PhD
Professor and Chair of MR Neurophysics and
Translational Neuroscience, UCL Institute of
Neurology, National Hospital for Neurology &
Neurosurgery, London, United Kingdom

SVEN HALLER, MSc, MD
Médecin Adjoint Agrégé, Division of
Neuroradiology, Department of Imaging and
Medical Informatics, Geneva University
Hospitals HUG, Geneva, Switzerland

JEROEN HENDRIKSE, MD, PhD
Radiologist, Department of Radiology,
University Medical Center Utrecht, Utrecht,
The Netherlands

JOHN HUSTON III, MD
Professor of Radiology, Department
of Radiology, Mayo Clinic, Rochester,
Minnesota

IRIS D. KILSDONK, MD
Department of Radiology, VU University
Medical Center, Amsterdam,
The Netherlands

CHRISTIAN LA, BA
Graduate Student, Neuroscience Training
Program, Wisconsin Institutes for Medical
Research, University of Wisconsin, Madison,
Wisconsin

MARK E. LADD, PhD
Professor, Department of Diagnostic and
Interventional Radiology and Neuroradiology,
University Hospital Essen; Erwin L. Hahn
Institute for Magnetic Resonance Imaging,
University of Duisburg-Essen, UNESCO World
Cultural Heritage Zollverein, Essen, Germany

SEUNG-KOO LEE, MD, PhD
Professor of Radiology and Neurology,
Yonsei University College of Medicine,
Seoul, Korea

KARL-OLOF LÖVBLAD, MD
Professor and Chairman, Division of
Neuroradiology, Department of Imaging and
Medical Informatics, Geneva University
Hospitals HUG, Geneva, Switzerland

PETER R. LUIJTEN, PhD
Department of Radiology, University Medical
Center Utrecht, Utrecht, The Netherlands

DONALD G. MCLAREN, PhD
Research Fellow, Geriatric Research,
Education and Clinical Center, ENRM VA
Medical Center, Bedford, Massachusetts;
Department of Neurology, Massachusetts
General Hospital and Harvard Medical School,
Boston, Massachusetts

SURESH K. MUKHERJI, MD, FACR
Professor and Chief of Neuroradiology, and
Head and Neck Radiology; Professor of
Radiology, Otolaryngology Head and Neck
Surgery, Radiation Oncology, Periodontics and
Oral Medicine, University of Michigan Health
System, Ann Arbor, Michigan

VEENA A. NAIR, PhD
Research Associate, Department of Radiology,
University of Wisconsin, Madison, Wisconsin

VITOR MENDES PEREIRA, MSc, MD
Director of Interventional Neuroradiology,
Division of Neuroradiology, Department of
Imaging and Medical Informatics, Geneva
University Hospitals HUG, Geneva,
Switzerland

ESBEN THADE PETERSEN, PhD
Department of Radiology, University Medical
Center Utrecht, Utrecht, The Netherlands

VIVEK PRABHAKARAN, MD, PhD
Director of Functional Neuroimaging in
Radiology; Assistant Professor of Radiology,
Division of Neuroradiology, Department of
Radiology, University of Wisconsin, Madison,
Wisconsin

TIMOTHY P.L. ROBERTS, PhD
Neuroradiology Section, Department of
Radiology, Children's Hospital of Philadelphia,
Philadelphia, Pennsylvania

HOWARD ROWLEY, MD
Professor of Radiology and Chief, Division of
Neuroradiology, Department of Radiology,
University of Wisconsin, Madison, Wisconsin

MARC SHAPIRO, MD
NeuroImaging Institute of Winter Park, Winter
Park; Department of Diagnostic Radiology,
University of Miami School of Medicine, Miami;
Section of Neuroradiology, University of
Central Florida, Orlando, Florida

ASHOK SRINIVASAN, MBBS, MD, DNB
Clinical Associate Professor, Department of
Radiology, Neuroradiology Division, University
of Michigan, A. Alfred Taubman Health Care
Center, Ann Arbor, Michigan

PATRICK TURSKI, MD
Professor of Radiology, Department of
Radiology, Division of Neuroradiology,
Wisconsin Institutes for Medical Research,
University of Wisconsin, Madison, Wisconsin

LALE UMUTLU, MD
Department of Diagnostic and Interventional
Radiology and Neuroradiology, University
Hospital Essen, Essen, Germany

HORST URBACH, MD, PhD
Department of Radiology/Neuroradiology,
University of Bonn Medical Center, Bonn,
Germany

M.A. VAN BUCHEM, MD, PhD
Department of Radiology, C.J. Gorter Center
for High Field MR, Leiden University Medical
Center, Leiden, The Netherlands

J. VAN DER GROND, PhD
Department of Radiology, C.J. Gorter Center
for High Field MR, Leiden University Medical
Center, Leiden, The Netherlands

ANJA G. VAN DER KOLK, MD
Department of Radiology, University Medical
Center Utrecht, Utrecht, The Netherlands

P. VAN ZIJL, PhD
Department of Radiology and Radiological
Sciences, Johns Hopkins University School of
Medicine; F.M. Kirby Research Center for
Functional Brain Imaging, Kennedy Krieger
Institute, Baltimore, Maryland

M.J. VERSLUIS, MSc
Department of Radiology, C.J. Gorter Center
for High Field MR, Leiden University Medical
Center, Leiden, The Netherlands

ARASTOO VOSSOUGH, PhD, MD
Neuroradiology Section, Department of
Radiology, Children's Hospital of Philadelphia,
Philadelphia, Pennsylvania

JINNAN WANG, PhD
Senior Member Research Staff, Clinical Sites
Research Program, Philips Research North
America, Briarcliff Manor, New York;
Department of Radiology, University of
Washington, Seattle, Washington

MIKE P. WATTJES, MD
Department of Radiology, VU University
Medical Center, Amsterdam, The Netherlands

A.G. WEBB, PhD
Department of Radiology, C.J. Gorter Center
for High Field MR, Leiden University Medical
Center, Leiden, The Netherlands

WINFRIED A. WILLINEK, MD
Associate Professor of Radiology and Head of
Magnetic Resonance Imaging, Department of
Radiology, University of Bonn, Bonn, Germany

YIJING WU, PhD
Postdoctoral Research Fellow, Department of
Medical Physics, Wisconsin Institutes for
Medical Research, University of Wisconsin,
Madison, Wisconsin

GUOFAN XU, MD, PhD
PGY2 Resident, Nuclear Medicine Program,
Nuclear Medicine, UW Hospital and Clinics,
University of Wisconsin, Madison, Wisconsin

CHUN YUAN, PhD
Professor of Radiology, Electrical Engineering,
and Bioengineering, Department of Radiology,
University of Washington, Seattle, Washington

Contents

which are often located at the bottom of a sulcus. 3D-T1-weighted gradient echo sequences are used for multiplanar, curved surface reformations, and voxel-based analyses. 3 T MR imaging is currently the state-of-the-art imaging modality for patients with suspected structural epilepsies in which an epileptogenic lesion has not yet been found.

Diagnostic modalities for the diagnosis of acute stroke have increased in number and quality. Magnetic resonance imaging has increasingly become a central tool for the management of patients with stroke. New sequences, such as diffusion and perfusion, provide insight into the infarcted core and the hypoperfused brain. The use of higher magnetic fields allows us to gain in signal strength, which can be used to improve imaging speed and/or resolution. Recent additional sequences allow perfusion without contrast and susceptibility-weighted imaging can help identify early bleeding. These new techniques should provide more information about the on going ischemic process.

Magnetic resonance angiography (MRA) of the brain obtained at 3 T imaging has made a significant clinical impact. MRA benefits from acquisition at higher magnetic field strength because of higher available signal-to-noise ratio and improved relative background suppression due to magnetic field strength–related T1 lengthening. Parallel imaging techniques are ideally suited for high-field MRA. Many of the developments that have made 3 T MRA of the brain successful can be regarded as enabling technologies that are essential for further development of 7 T MRA, which brings additional challenges.

Recent advances in magnetic resonance (MR) hardware and software have improved the resolution and spatial coverage of head and neck first-pass contrast-enhanced (CE) MR angiography. Despite these improvements, high-quality submillimeter-resolution 1.5 T and 3 T carotid CE MR angiography is not consistently available in the general radiology practice. This article reviews the important imaging parameters and potential pitfalls that affect carotid CE MR angiography image quality, and the dose and timing of the gadolinium-based contrast agent, and summarizes vendor-specific protocols for high-quality submillimeter-resolution carotid CE MR angiography at 1.5 and 3 T.

The introduction of high-field magnetic imaging ($\geq$3 T) has made noninvasive arterial spin labeling (ASL) a realistic clinical option for perfusion assessment in vascular disorders. Combined with the advances provided by territorial imaging of individual intracerebral arteries and the measurement of vascular reactivity, ASL is a powerful tool for evaluating vascular diseases of the brain. This article evaluates its use in chronic cerebrovascular disease, stroke, moyamoya disease, and arteriovenous malformation, but ASL may also find applications in related diseases such as vascular dementia.

Manifestations of atherosclerotic plaque in different arterial beds range from perfusion deficits to overt ischemia such as stroke and myocardial infarction. Atherosclerotic plaque composition is associated with its propensity to rupture and cause vascular events. Magnetic resonance (MR) imaging of atherosclerotic plaque using clinical 1.5 T scanners can detect plaque composition. Plaque MR imaging at higher field strengths offers both opportunities and challenges to improving the high spatial resolution and contrast required for this type of imaging. This article summarizes the technological requirements required for high-field plaque MR imaging and its application in detecting plaque components.

Head and neck imaging has benefited from 1.5 T magnetic resonance (MR) imaging, providing faster sequences, better soft tissue evaluation, and 3-axis imaging, with less radiation and iodine-based contrast injection. The US Food and Drug Administration has approved human MR imaging at high-field strength up to 4 T in clinical practice. 3 T MR imaging has become widely available, with the hope of significant advance in the evaluation of the head and neck region. This article reviews the benefits, disadvantages, and challenges of high-field imaging of the head and neck region, focusing on the imaging of head and neck cancer.

High-field 3 T magnetic resonance (MR) imaging provides greater signal-to-noise ratio (SNR) compared with 1.5 T systems. Various MR imaging clinical applications in children can benefit from improvements resulting from this increased SNR. High-resolution imaging of the brain, arterial spin labeling perfusion imaging, diffusion imaging, MR spectroscopy, and imaging of small anatomic parts are some areas in which these improvements can increase our clinical diagnostic capabilities. However, challenges inherent to 3 T imaging become more relevant in children. The use of 3 T imaging in children has allowed better diagnostic efficacy in neuroimaging, but certain technique modifications may be required for optimal imaging.

Magnetic resonance (MR) imaging at 3 T has proved superior to 1.5 T in the brain for detecting numerous pathologic entities including hemosiderin, tiny metastases, subtle demyelinating plaques, active demyelinating plaques, and some epileptogenic foci, as well as small aneurysms with MR angiography. 3 T is superior to most advanced imaging techniques including diffusion, diffusion tensor imaging, perfusion, spectroscopy and functional MR imaging. The increased signal/noise ratio at 3 T permits higher spatial resolution. Initially spine imaging at 3 T proved more difficult with less successful results. During the past 7 years, technological advances in magnet and surface coil design as well as improved radio frequency transmitters and pulse sequence design in combination with the large body of knowledge accrued by radiologists and physicists during a nine year experience with clinical imaging of the spine with the doubled B0, has resulted in 3 T MRI of the spine achieving a reputation slmilar to that for brain imaging.

In this review, current (clinical) applications and possible future directions of ultrahigh-field ($\geq$7 T) magnetic resonance (MR) imaging in the brain are discussed. Ultrahigh-field MR imaging can provide contrast-rich images of diverse pathologies and can be used for early diagnosis and treatment monitoring of brain disease. These images may provide increased sensitivity and specificity. Several limitations need to be overcome before worldwide clinical implementation can be commenced. Current literature regarding clinically based ultrahigh-field MR imaging is reviewed, and limitations and promises of this technique are discussed, as well as some practical considerations for the implementation in clinical practice.

An increase of the magnetic field strength to ultrahigh-field yields advantageous as well as disadvantageous changes in physical effects. The beneficial increase in signal/noise ratio can be leveraged into higher spatiotemporal resolution, and an exacerbation of artifacts can impede ultrahigh-field imaging. With the successful introduction of intracranial and musculoskeletal imaging at 7 T, recent advances in coil design have created opportunities for further applications of ultrahigh-field magnetic resonance (MR) imaging in other parts of the body. Initial studies in 7 T neck and spine MR imaging have revealed promising insights and new challenges, demanding further research and methodological optimization.

There are several magnetic resonance (MR) imaging techniques that benefit from high-field MR imaging. This article describes a range of novel techniques that are currently being used clinically or will be used in the future for clinical purposes as they gain popularity. These techniques include functional MR imaging, diffusion tensor imaging, cortical thickness assessment, arterial spin labeling perfusion, white matter hyperintensity lesion assessment, and advanced MR angiography.

Foreword
High Field Imaging

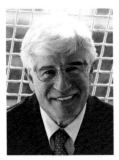

William G. Bradley Jr, MD, PhD

Professor Willinek has done his usual excellent job bringing together top experts for this High Field Imaging Issue of *Neuroimaging Clinics*. This, of course, is not unexpected given his involvement over the past 12 years with the High Field Imaging Symposium at the University of Bonn and his current position as President of the International Magnetic Resonance Angiography Working Group (aka "MR Angio Club").

Professor Willinek has included all the topics in which higher magnetic fields are useful for both clinical and research work, by virtue of either higher spatial resolution, thinner slices, or faster scanning. These topics include high field clinical imaging of brain tumors, epilepsy, inflammation, neurodegeneration, and stroke as well as MR angiography of the brain and neck and plaque imaging. Perfusion imaging at 3 T in the context of stroke and tumor grading is discussed in detail. To round out the other areas of Neuroradiology, there are excellent articles on high field MR imaging of the head and neck, spine, and children. Finally, there are articles on research applications at ultrahigh field MRI and a look into the future of high field imaging.

The contributors are all experts in their subspecialty areas and come from eight different countries, making this truly an international effort well beyond North America. In reading the various contributions to this issue of the *Neuroimaging Clinics*, it is clear that high field MRI has evolved into a very solid clinical modality with many options for future research at high and ultrahigh magnetic fields.

William G. Bradley Jr, MD, PhD
Department of Radiology
University of California San Diego Medical Center
402 Dickinson Street, Suite 454
San Diego, CA 92103-8224, USA

E-mail address:
wgbradley@mail.ucsd.edu

Neuroimag Clin N Am 22 (2012) xiii
doi:10.1016/j.nic.2012.04.001
1052-5149/12/$ – see front matter

Preface

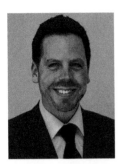

Winfried A. Willinek, MD
Guest Editor

The scope of this issue of *Neuroimaging Clinics* is neuroradiology applications of highfield magnetic resonance (MR) imaging. For more than a decade, highfield MR systems operating at 3 Tesla have been used for imaging worldwide.

The focus of this issue is the clinical application of highfield systems, but it also includes articles on more advanced technology such as MR spectroscopy, diffusion tensor imaging and tractography, arterial spin labeling, and functional MRI. Finally, the current status of 7 Tesla for neuroradiology applications is discussed.

A distinguished group of internationally renowned experts share their knowledge in this issue. All authors provide a diagnostic checklist and recommendations for technical protocols, which I think is particularly helpful for everyday practice.

I would like to thank all the authors for their excellent work and hope that the readers will take advantage of this opportunity to gain valuable knowledge for both research and routine imaging.

Winfried A. Willinek, MD
Department of Radiology
University of Bonn
Sigmund-Freund-Str. 25
D-53105 Bonn, Germany

E-mail address:
Winfried.Willinek@ukb.uni-bonn.de

doi:10.1016/j.nic.2012.03.002

Diffusion Tensor and Perfusion Imaging of Brain Tumors in High-Field MR Imaging

Seung-Koo Lee, MD, PhD

KEYWORDS

- High-field MRI • DT imaging • Perfusion imaging
- Brain • Tumor

Key Points

- High-field MRI provides higher signal-to-noise ratio, shorter scan time and higher resolution images.
- Multiparametric imaging is possible with high-field MRI, which includes diffusion tensor imaging (DTI), perfusion-weighted imaging (PWI), functional MRI, susceptibility-weighted imaging, and MR spectroscopy.
- DTI and PWI are essential diagnostic tools for grading glioma, differentiating glioma from nonglial tumor, and therapeutic monitoring of brain tumors.

Increasing field strength of MRI gives various beneficial effects, such as higher signal-to-noise radio (SNR), better spatial resolution of images, increased chemical shift, and increased T1 relaxation time, resulting in good background suppression in MR angiography.[1] The term *high-field* is comparative concept because 1.5 T MRI was also called *high-field system* in the early 1990s. Although 1.5 T MRI is still regarded as a high-field scanner in an intraoperative system, 3 T MRI is usually considered a clinical high-field system. 7 T or higher human scanners were recently introduced and provide extreme high-quality images, but the term *ultra–high-field* is more proper for them. Practically, 3 T MRI is not less competent to be called *clinical high-field MRI* against 7 T because of its clinical feasibility, system stability, field homogeneity, and whole-body application.

In brain tumor imaging, the multimodality approach is favored for the differential diagnosis of brain tumors and grading of gliomas.[2] Simultaneous acquisition of routine imaging with perfusion, diffusion, functional MRI (fMRI), and MR spectroscopy enables a better diagnostic approach to brain tumors. High-field MRI enables shorter scan time with satisfactory image quality compared with the low-field system, and therefore the high-field system is more suitable for multimodality imaging.

High-field MRI has some disadvantages, such as increased susceptibility artifacts, poorer gray-white matter differentiation on T1-weighted imaging, and increased specific absorption rates. Better blood oxygen level dependent effect in fMRI and susceptibility-weighted imaging is a good example of counterplot to increase susceptibility effect in high-field MRI. Various solutions have been

This work was supported by KRIBB research initiative program.
Department of Radiology, Yonsei University College of Medicine, 50 Yonsei-ro, Seodaemungu, Seoul 120-752, Korea
E-mail address: slee@yuhs.ac

Neuroimag Clin N Am 22 (2012) 123–134
doi:10.1016/j.nic.2012.02.001
1052-5149/12/$ – see front matter © 2012 Elsevier Inc. All rights reserved.

> **Diagnostic Checklist**
>
> - One-stop multiparametric MR protocol is recommended for initial assessment of brain tumors.
> - Clinical usefulness of diffusion tensor imaging (DTI) and perfusion-weighted imaging (PWI) was proven and initial MR protocol should include them.
> - DTI and PWI are reliable biomarkers of glioma grading, differentiation from nonglial tumors, and monitoring of treated glioma.
> - Optional fluid attenuated inversion recovery, permeability imaging, functional MRI, and MR spectroscopy are recommended in specific cases.

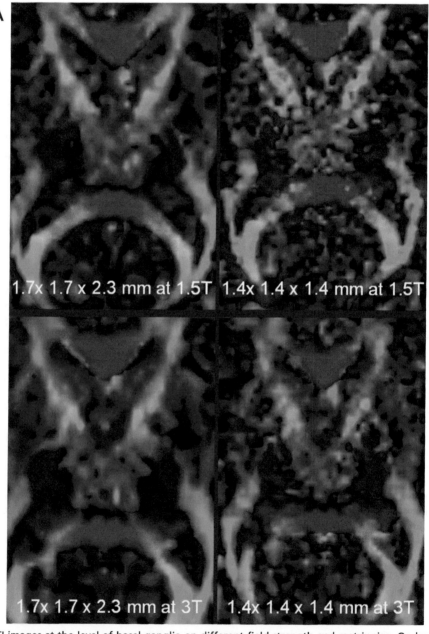

Fig. 1. (*A*) DTI images at the level of basal ganglia on different field strength and matrix size. On large matrix scan (1.7 × 1.7 × 2.3 mm), no significant difference is seen between 1.5 T and 3 T. With high-resolution isovoxel (1.4 × 1.4 × 1.4 mm), 1.5 T shows more noise around internal capsule than 3 T.

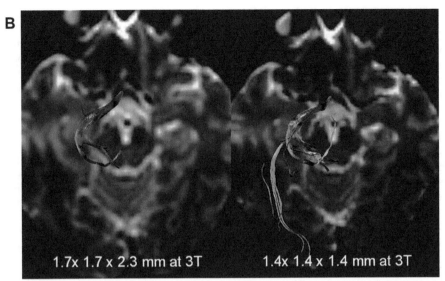

Fig. 1. (*B*) Fiber tracking of optic tract and radiation at 3 T. Regions of interest were placed at optic chiasm, mid-thalamus, and occipital white matter on coronal scan. Large-matrix DTI lost its trajectory, whereas high-resolution isovoxel DTI traces optic radiation until visual cortex.

proposed for apparent T1 contrast of brain tissue and decreasing specific absorption rates during MR examination. With these advantages, high-field MRI is not paralleled by any imaging modality in brain tumor diagnosis. This article describes two advanced imaging techniques performed on clinical 3 T MRI: diffusion tensor imaging (DTI) and perfusion-weighted imaging (PWI).

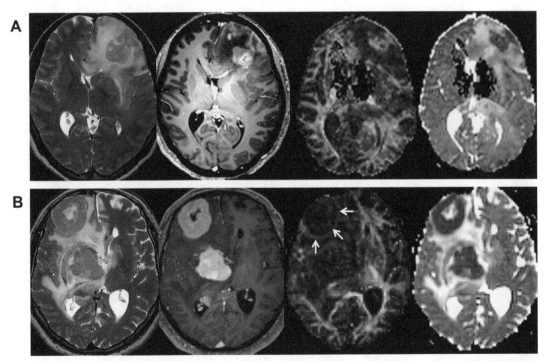

Fig. 2. DTI parameters can differentiate gliomas from nonglial tumors. (*A*) Glioblastoma. Note enhancing lesion at left frontal lobe suggesting malignant focus with underlying gliomatosis infiltrating corpus callosum and temporal lobe. ADC is low and FA is high at enhancing solid portion. (*B*) Lymphoma. Enhancing mass shows low FA and ADC. Surrounding white matter is preserved than glioblastoma with high and linear band on FA map (*arrows*).

DTI OF BRAIN TUMORS IN HIGH-FIELD MRI

As for DTI, its increased resolution provides a lesser partial volume averaging effect and higher SNR, resulting in more accurate fiber tracking.[3-5] Increased matrix size and isovoxel acquisition is much more useful for clinical fiber tracking, especially for identifying complex fibers such as optic radiation (Fig. 1), and for detailed anatomic structures such as brain stem nuclei and gray matter.[3,6] Even though echo planar imaging is extremely susceptible to magnetic field inhomogeneity and image distortion is more apparent with high-field MRI, several solutions have been suggested and implemented to commercial scanners.[7]

DTI provides a quantitative biomarker of brain tissue, fractional anisotropy (FA), and apparent diffusion coefficient (ADC), which are used in the differential diagnosis of brain lesions. White matter fiber tracking is possible based on FA and trajectory of voxels. Two different methods are applied in the calculation of white matter tracts. The first one is a deterministic approach called *fiber assignment by continuous tracking* (FACT).[8] In clinical practice, the FACT method is preferred to probability maps because it is more intuitional and gives direct information to surgeons. However, it has some limitations, such as simple calculation from a seed point, inability to solve fiber-crossing problems, and multiplicity of tracts' connectivity. The probabilistic approach is more scientific, considering multiple fiber connectivity from one region to the others.[9] With any approach, DTI and fiber tracking are essentials tool in preoperative localization of brain tumors and white matter tracts and in determining surgical route for adequate resection.

DTI for Differential Diagnosis and Grading of Brain Tumors

Nontumorous lesions, such as tumefactive multiple sclerosis or demyelinating diseases, should be differentiated from tumors. With the aid of

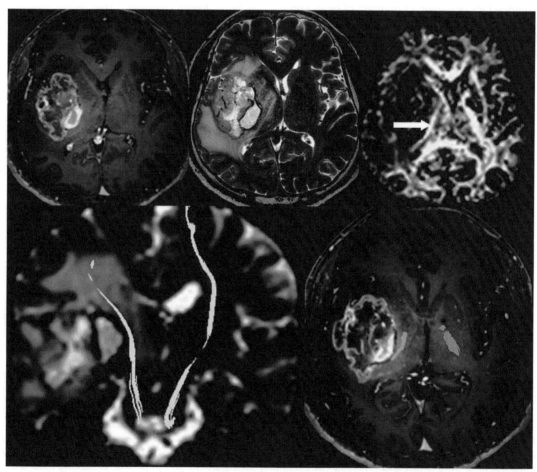

Fig. 3. Preoperative localization of corticospinal tract in glioblastoma. Right corticospinal tract is medially displaced, not invaded by the tumor. FA map also shows compressed but intact high-signal internal capsule (*arrow*).

gadolinium enhancement (open-ring or incomplete-ring sign) and CT, tumor can be differentiated easily in most cases.[10] However, nonenhancing glioma, such as brain stem glioma, in young people is difficult to be differentiated from demyelinating lesions. On DTI, architecture of corticospinal tract is likely to be preserved while demyelinating diseases show disruption of the arrangement of the tracts on fiber tracking.[11]

ADC and FA can be used in differential diagnosis of brain lesions. Integrity of peritumoral white matter is altered in high-grade gliomas, but not in low-grade gliomas or metastasis.[12] FA is significantly lower and ADC is higher in peritumoral edema in cases of brain metastasis.[13] All of these results are related to microscopic infiltration of tumor cells into edematous regions in glioma, whereas only vasogenic edema occurs in metastasis. FA is significantly increased and ADC is decreased in enhancing areas of glioblastoma compared with low-grade gliomas, lymphomas, or metastasis (**Fig. 2**).[14,15] In contrast, another recent study of glioblastoma on 3 T MRI proved that FA of 0.2 or less is well correlated with lower progression-free survival rate.[16] Although FA and other DTI metrics are objective and easily

calculated in most cases of brain tumors, their clinical meaning requires more investigation.

DTI for Preoperative and Postoperative Evaluations

The most powerful aspect of DTI and fiber tracking is preoperative evaluation in space-occupying lesions of brain. Spatial relationships between major white matter tract and brain tumor can be easily identified on DTI.[17–19] In brain tumors, white matter tract can be invaded or displaced by the lesion. Corticospinal tract and arcuate fasciculus are the most frequently studied structures because they are critically related to motor and language function (**Figs. 3** and **4**).

DTI data can now be transferred to a neuronavigation system and used intraoperatively. Geometry of major tract can be shifted from its original position after craniotomy or resection of brain tissue, and this should be taken into account to avoid inevitable injury.[20] In cases of postoperative complication, DTI can be used to assess for injury to white matter tracts and to predict prognosis.

Alteration of brain connectivity after surgery or chemotherapy is related to postoperative changes

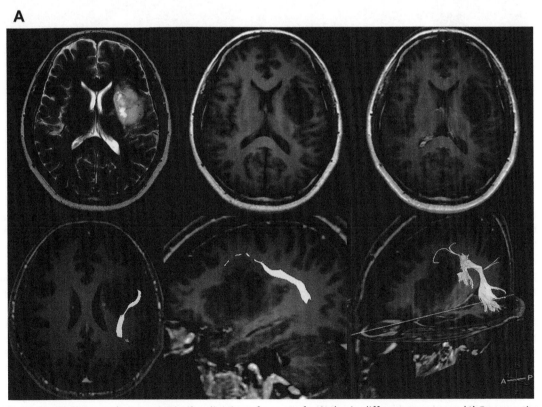

Fig. 4. Preoperative and postoperative localization of arcuate fasciculus in diffuse astrocytoma. (*A*) Preoperative DTI shows arcuate fasciculus displaced by main mass.

B

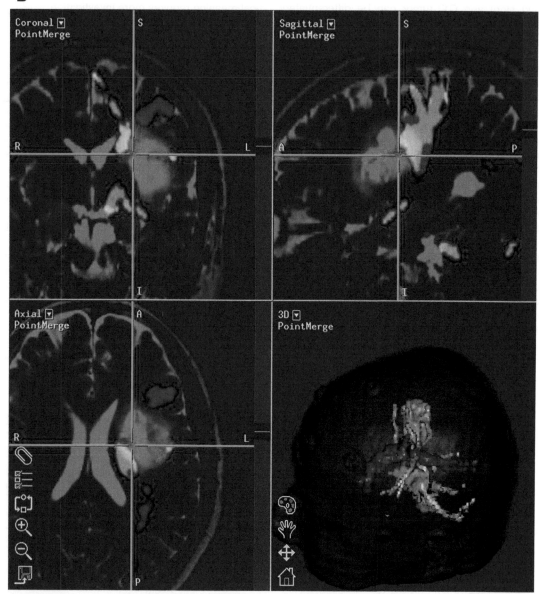

Fig. 4. (*B*) Neuronavigation system during operation depicts red-colored arcuate fasciculus and yellow-colored corticospinal tract. A spatial relationship among tracts and brain tumor can be also seen on multiplanar reconstruction images.

in cognitive function.[21,22] In pediatric posterior fossa tumors, the cerebello-cerebral connection can be altered after surgery. Impairment of cognitive function after cerebellar surgery can be explained through DTI findings describing altered cerebello-cerebral connectivity.

PWI OF BRAIN TUMORS IN HIGH-FIELD MRI

High-field MRI enables multiparametric MR evaluation of brain tumors within a clinically feasible scan time and better image quality. Conventional imaging with gadolinium enhancement is enough in some tumor cases, but advanced studies are mandatory for precise evaluation of tumor infiltration to adjacent white matter, grading of glioma, and differentiation of gliomas from nonglial tumors, because the therapeutic plan is different in those cases.

PWI can be performed three different ways in clinical practice: dynamic susceptibility contrast (DSC) enhanced PWI, arterial spin labeling (ASL)

C

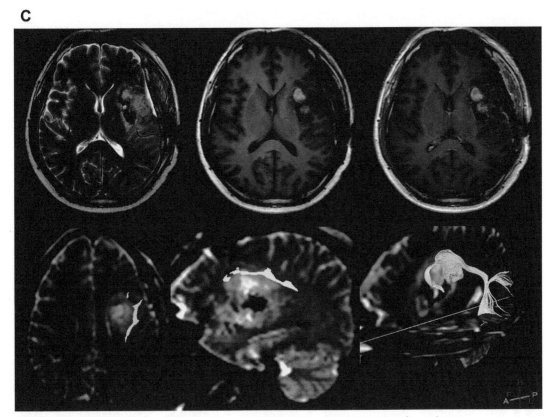

Fig. 4. (*C*) Postoperative DTI shows subtotally removed tumor and intact arcuate fasciculus.

PWI, and dynamic contrast-enhanced (DCE) PWI. With long history and accumulated experiences, DSC PWI is widely accepted as the preferred diagnostic tool in grading of gliomas, differentiation of radiation necrosis, and discrimination of gliomas from metastasis or lymphoma. In contrast with ASL or DCE PWI, calculation of relative changes in cerebral blood volume (rCBV) is simple, and most MRI vendors provide user-friendly image processing tools, although absolute quantification of cerebral blood flow needs a more robust process.

DSC PWI

After injection of bolus gadolinium contrast, perfusion parametrics are obtained based on time-concentration curve and indicator dilution theory. Integration of time-relaxation curve after gamma fitting results in rCBV. Cerebral blood flow is obtained after calculation of arterial input function and mean transit time.

In general, high-grade lesions have larger cerebral blood volume and higher cerebral blood flow.[23] High-grade gliomas have larger rCBV than low-grade gliomas, and lymphomas are likely to

have smaller rCBV than gliomas or metastasis.[24] In peritumoral white matter, rCBV is increased in primary glioma because of microscopic cell infiltration, whereas metastasis shows smaller rCBV from pure vasogenic edema (**Fig. 5**).[25] This finding is similar to FA changes at the peritumoral region on DTI analysis.

Differentiating radiation necrosis from tumor recurrence is critical for follow-up evaluation after surgery or radiation treatment. rCBV is one of the most reliable biomarkers for discriminating viable tumors from radiation necrosis. Increased rCBV at the area of enhancement suggests viable tumors rather than necrosis (**Fig. 6**).[26] Recently, more objective and semiquantitative histogram analysis of perfusion parameters was applied. Peak height position of rCBV histogram can differentiate recurred tumor from radiation necrosis.[27]

PWI can be used for monitoring antiangiogenic therapy or other new anticancer drugs.[28] Caution should be taken during radiation or chemotherapy because pseudo-progression of enhancing lesion can be seen. rCBV also has a differential impact in detecting pseudo-progression, which has lower rCBV than real progression.[29]

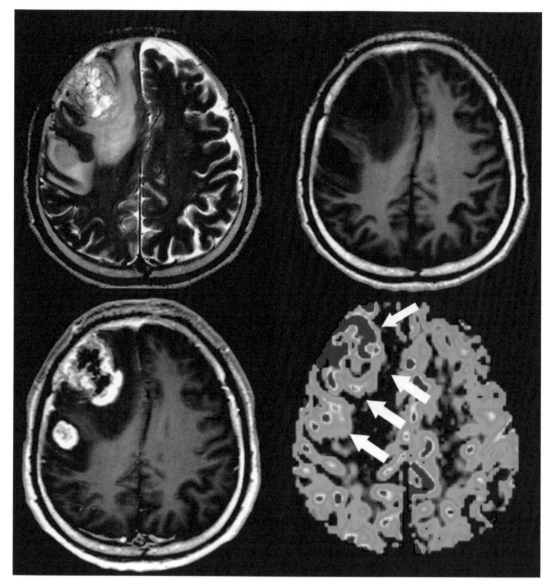

Fig. 5. Pathologically proven multicentric glioblastoma. Initial radiologic report was metastasis because of multiplicity of the lesions. Conventional imaging depicts two enhancing masses in peripheral areas of right frontal lobe with surrounding edema, suggesting metastasis rather than primary brain tumor. Note increased rCBV at peritumoral white matter (*arrows*).

ASL PWI

ASL has not been used in daily practices until recently because of its low SNR at 1.5 T MRI and complicated postprocessing algorithm. However, clinical ASL is now practicable because of the wide distribution of 3 T commercial MRI and user-friendly software for online and offline image processing. ASL uses endogenous arterial water as a diffusible tracer. There is continuous exchange of water between blood and brain tissue, and therefore proximal spine labeling results in the changes of total magnetization of brain tissue in an imaging slice. Tagged and nontagged images are obtained and absolute cerebral blood flow is calculated. Different ASL techniques have been proposed, namely continuous ASL (CASL), pulsed ASL (PASL) and pseudo-CASL.[30–32] CASL has higher SNR and image quality than PASL, whereas PASL has benefits in tagging efficiency with different flow velocities. Pseudo-CASL has advantages of both CASL and PASL. Regardless of spin labeling technique, clinical ASL should be simply obtained from the latest commercial high-field MRI, instantly

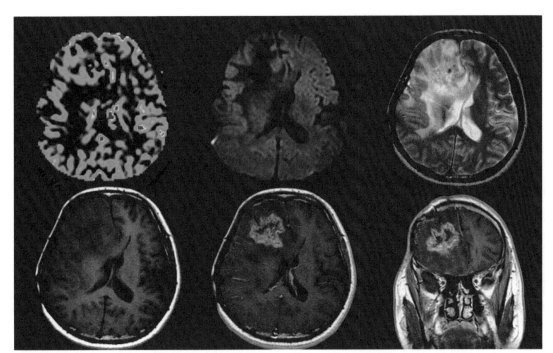

Fig. 6. Radiation necrosis 1 year after operation and radiotherapy. Note soap bubble–like enhancement of right frontal lesion with marked mass effect. Decompressive resection was performed and no tumor cells were found on pathologic examination.

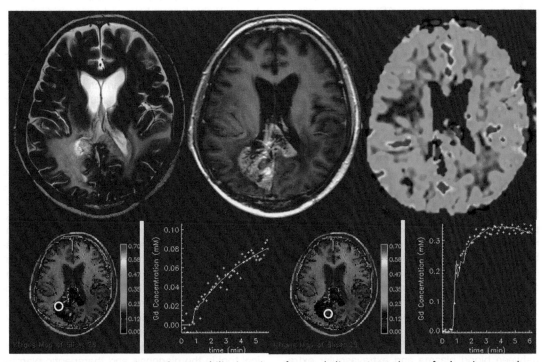

Fig. 7. Dynamic contrast-enhanced permeability imaging of treated glioma. Lateral part of enhancing area shows slow increase of T1 signal on dynamic scan. The rCBV of this area is not increased as much as the posteromedial part of enhancing lesion. Posteromedial area of enhancing lesion shows early rapid rising of T1 signal on dynamic scan, suggesting vascular phase of viable tumor. In treated glioma, a mixture of radiation necrosis and viable tumor is common and can be explored with DSC and DCE PWI.

Table 1
Recommended one-stop intra-axial tumor preoperative protocol on 3 T MRI

Sequence	Thickness/Gap (mm)	Matrix	Remarks	Scan Time (min:s)
Survey	10/10	256	Reference scan for parallel imaging included	0:35
DTI	2/0	128	b = 600 mm/s, 32 diffusion direction	5:46
FLAIR	5/2	352	FLAIR can be performed after gadolinium injection	2:56
T2 axial	4/0	400	Thin section and high resolution	2:42
T1 axial	5/2	256	Precontrast T1, thick-slice scan	3:36
DCE PWI	Reconstructed to 6 mm	192	3D multishot gradient-echo T1 Single-dose 1.0 M gadobutrol injection	0:47 Prescan 6:17 Dynamic
3D T1 Postcontrast	Reconstructed to 1 mm	256	Multiplanar reconstruction to axial, sagittal, and coronal images	7:41 with 220 slices
DSC PWI	Reconstructed to 4 mm	128	3D multishot gradient echo T2* Single-dose 1.0 M gadobutrol injection	1:44

Note: Field of view (FOV) is usually 23 cm for Asian people, but detailed parameter can be varied according to head size. Total scan time: 32:04 or more.

processed on operating console or offline, and must provide absolute quantification data for more active clinical application.

3 T MRI is superior to 1.5 T in ASL quality and can be implemented as a routine procedure in brain tumor imaging.[33,34] ASL provides direct quantification of cerebral blood flow in contrast with DSC PWI, which needs a complicated algorithm for absolute quantification. Territorial ASL, which was more recently introduced, is a novel technique that identifies a different proximal flow. Because territorial ASL can separately analyze anterior and posterior circulation flow, it can be applied in stroke imaging or vascular variants in normal brain, and its further application in brain tumor imaging is expected.[35,36]

DCE PWI: Permeability Imaging

Postcontrast T1 or FLAIR imaging is a qualitative permeability imaging technique because gadolinium enhancement is a final result of blood–brain barrier (BBB) leakage. The integrity of BBB can be assessed by MRI with injection of gadolinium contrast and measurement of contrast spillage using dynamic imaging. Various kinetic modeling of contrast movement through BBB have been proposed.[37,38] DCE PWI provides transfer constants such as K_{trans} (volume transfer constant between blood plasma and extravascular extracellular space [EES]), K_{ep} (rate constant between plasma and EES), and V_e (volume of the EES per unit volume of tissue). High-grade gliomas are known to have higher K_{trans} than low-grade

lesions. However, the superiority of K_{trans} against rCBV in glioma grading is still in controversy.[39,40]

In addition to permeability maps, T1 steady-state signal intensity curves help in the differential diagnosis of radiation necrosis and recurred tumor. Viable tumors have early and rapid increase of time-signal intensity curve, which correlates with the vascular phase of the lesion, whereas radiation necrosis has slow increase of time-signal intensity curve, suggesting leaky BBB (Fig. 7).[41]

The combination of conventional imaging, DSC, and DCE PWI can raise the accuracy of diagnosis in brain tumors.

SUMMARY

DTI and PWI are essential clinical tools in the primary diagnosis of brain tumors. The authors recommend a one-stop intra-axial brain tumor MRI protocol at 3 T (Table 1). DWI, DTI, and DSC PWI are integrated along with the conventional anatomic imaging. fMRI and MR spectroscopy are used as additional procedures in specific cases. In some institutes, fMRI is also implemented as a basic MRI protocol, but because the location of the tumor and the surgical plan might differ among patients, it is better performed as an additional examination.

In conclusion, high-field MRI is an essential clinical tool in the diagnosis and therapeutic plan for brain tumors. Multiparametric imaging with high-field MRI can raise the accuracy of lesion detection, differentiation, and prediction of prognosis of brain tumors. Ultra–high-field MRI and hybrid systems with positron emission tomography will be the next step in high-field imaging in neuro-oncology.

REFERENCES

1. Schmitz BL, Aschoff AJ, Hoffmann MH, et al. Advantages and pitfalls in 3T MR brain imaging: a pictorial review. AJNR Am J Neuroradiol 2005; 26(9):2229–37.
2. Pichler BJ, Kolb A, Nagele T, et al. PET/MRI: paving the way for the next generation of clinical multimodality imaging applications. J Nucl Med 2010;51(3): 333–6.
3. Nagae-Poetscher LM, Jiang H, Wakana S, et al. High-resolution diffusion tensor imaging of the brain stem at 3 T. AJNR Am J Neuroradiol 2004;25(8): 1325–30.
4. Guilfoyle DN, Helpern JA, Lim KO. Diffusion tensor imaging in fixed brain tissue at 7.0 T. NMR Biomed 2003;16(2):77–81.
5. Gillard JH, Papadakis NG, Martin K, et al. MR diffusion tensor imaging of white matter tract disruption in stroke at 3 T. Br J Radiol 2001;74(883):642–7.
6. Rocca MA, Ceccarelli A, Falini A, et al. Diffusion tensor magnetic resonance imaging at 3.0 tesla shows subtle cerebral grey matter abnormalities in patients with migraine. J Neurol Neurosurg Psychiatry 2006;77(5):686–9.
7. Ardekani S, Sinha U. Geometric distortion correction of high-resolution 3 T diffusion tensor brain images. Magn Reson Med 2005;54(5):1163–71.
8. Mori S, Crain BJ, Chacko VP, et al. Three-dimensional tracking of axonal projections in the brain by magnetic resonance imaging. Ann Neurol 1999;45(2):265–9.
9. Parker GJ, Wheeler-Kingshott CA, Barker GJ. Estimating distributed anatomical connectivity using fast marching methods and diffusion tensor imaging. IEEE Trans Med Imaging 2002;21(5):505–12.
10. Smirniotopoulos JG, Murphy FM, Rushing EJ, et al. Patterns of contrast enhancement in the brain and meninges. Radiographics 2007;27(2):525–51.
11. Giussani C, Poliakov A, Ferri RT, et al. DTI fiber tracking to differentiate demyelinating diseases from diffuse brain stem glioma. Neuroimage 2010; 52(1):217–23.
12. Price SJ, Burnet NG, Donovan T, et al. Diffusion tensor imaging of brain tumours at 3T: a potential tool for assessing white matter tract invasion? Clin Radiol 2003;58(6):455–62.
13. Byrnes TJ, Barrick TR, Bell BA, et al. Diffusion tensor imaging discriminates between glioblastoma and cerebral metastases in vivo. NMR Biomed 2011; 24(1):54–60.
14. Wang S, Kim S, Chawla S, et al. Differentiation between glioblastomas, solitary brain metastases, and primary cerebral lymphomas using diffusion tensor and dynamic susceptibility contrast-enhanced MR imaging. AJNR Am J Neuroradiol 2011;32(3): 507–14.
15. White ML, Zhang Y, Yu F, et al. Diffusion tensor MR imaging of cerebral gliomas: evaluating fractional anisotropy characteristics. AJNR Am J Neuroradiol 2011;32(2):374–81.
16. Saksena S, Jain R, Narang J, et al. Predicting survival in glioblastomas using diffusion tensor imaging metrics. J Magn Reson Imaging 2010;32(4): 788–95.
17. Hlatky R, Jackson EF, Weinberg JS, et al. intraoperative neuronavigation using diffusion tensor MR tractography for the resection of a deep tumor adjacent to the corticospinal tract. Stereotact Funct Neurosurg 2005;83(5–6):228–32.
18. Kamada K, Todo T, Masutani Y, et al. Combined use of tractography-integrated functional neuronavigation and direct fiber stimulation. J Neurosurg 2005; 102(4):664–72.
19. Laundre BJ, Jellison BJ, Badie B, et al. Diffusion tensor imaging of the corticospinal tract before and after mass resection as correlated with clinical motor findings: preliminary data. AJNR Am J Neuroradiol 2005;26(4):791–6.
20. Nimsky C, Ganslandt O, Merhof D, et al. Intraoperative visualization of the pyramidal tract by diffusion-tensor-imaging-based fiber tracking. Neuroimage 2006;30(4):1219–29.
21. Law N, Bouffet E, Laughlin S, et al. Cerebello-thalamo-cerebral connections in pediatric brain tumor patients: impact on working memory. Neuroimage 2011;56(4):2238–48.
22. Khong PL, Leung LH, Chan GC, et al. White matter anisotropy in childhood medulloblastoma survivors: association with neurotoxicity risk factors. Radiology 2005;236(2):647–52.
23. Shiroishi MS, Habibi M, Rajderkar D, et al. Perfusion and permeability MR imaging of gliomas. Technol Cancer Res Treat 2011;10(1):59–71.
24. Hakyemez B, Erdogan C, Bolca N, et al. Evaluation of different cerebral mass lesions by perfusion-weighted MR imaging. J Magn Reson Imaging 2006;24(4):817–24.
25. Law M, Cha S, Knopp EA, et al. High-grade gliomas and solitary metastases: differentiation by using perfusion and proton spectroscopic MR imaging. Radiology 2002;222(3):715–21.
26. Cha S. Perfusion MR imaging of brain tumors. Top Magn Reson Imaging 2004;15(5):279–89.
27. Kim HS, Kim JH, Kim SH, et al. Posttreatment high-grade glioma: usefulness of peak height position with semiquantitative MR perfusion histogram analysis in an entire contrast-enhanced lesion for predicting volume fraction of recurrence. Radiology 2010;256(3):906–15.
28. Sawlani RN, Raizer J, Horowitz SW, et al. Glioblastoma: a method for predicting response to antiangiogenic

chemotherapy by using MR perfusion imaging–pilot study. Radiology 2010;255(2):622–8.

29. Kong DS, Kim ST, Kim EH, et al. Diagnostic dilemma of pseudoprogression in the treatment of newly diagnosed glioblastomas: the role of assessing relative cerebral blood flow volume and oxygen-6-methylguanine-DNA methyltransferase promoter methylation status. AJNR Am J Neuroradiol 2011; 32(2):382–7.

30. Detre JA, Leigh JS, Williams DS, et al. Perfusion imaging. Magn Reson Med 1992;23(1):37–45.

31. Edelman RR, Siewert B, Darby DG, et al. Qualitative mapping of cerebral blood flow and functional localization with echo-planar MR imaging and signal targeting with alternating radio frequency. Radiology 1994;192(2):513–20.

32. Wu WC, Fernandez-Seara M, Detre JA, et al. A theoretical and experimental investigation of the tagging efficiency of pseudocontinuous arterial spin labeling. Magn Reson Med 2007;58(5):1020–7.

33. Lehmann P, Monet P, de Marco G, et al. A comparative study of perfusion measurement in brain tumours at 3 Tesla MR: Arterial spin labeling versus dynamic susceptibility contrast-enhanced MRI. Eur Neurol 2010;64(1):21–6.

34. Lupo JM, Lee MC, Han ET, et al. Feasibility of dynamic susceptibility contrast perfusion MR imaging at 3T using a standard quadrature head coil and eight-channel phased-array coil with and without SENSE reconstruction. J Magn Reson Imaging 2006;24(3): 520–9.

35. Hendrikse J, Petersen ET, Chng SM, et al. Distribution of cerebral blood flow in the nucleus caudatus, nucleus lentiformis, and thalamus: a study of territorial arterial spin-labeling MR imaging. Radiology 2010;254(3):867–75.

36. Chng SM, Petersen ET, Zimine I, et al. Territorial arterial spin labeling in the assessment of collateral circulation: comparison with digital subtraction angiography. Stroke 2008;39(12):3248–54.

37. Tofts PS, Kermode AG. Measurement of the blood-brain barrier permeability and leakage space using dynamic MR imaging. 1. Fundamental concepts. Magn Reson Med 1991;17(2):357–67.

38. Johnson G, Wetzel SG, Cha S, et al. Measuring blood volume and vascular transfer constant from dynamic, T(2)*-weighted contrast-enhanced MRI. Magn Reson Med 2004;51(5):961–8.

39. Cha S, Yang L, Johnson G, et al. Comparison of microvascular permeability measurements, K(trans), determined with conventional steady-state T1-weighted and first-pass T2*-weighted MR imaging methods in gliomas and meningiomas. AJNR Am J Neuroradiol 2006;27(2):409–17.

40. Law M, Yang S, Babb JS, et al. Comparison of cerebral blood volume and vascular permeability from dynamic susceptibility contrast-enhanced perfusion MR imaging with glioma grade. AJNR Am J Neuroradiol 2004;25(5):746–55.

41. Lacerda S, Law M. Magnetic resonance perfusion and permeability imaging in brain tumors. Neuroimaging Clin N Am 2009;19(4):527–57.

Inflammation High-Field Magnetic Resonance Imaging

Iris D. Kilsdonk, MD, Wolter L. de Graaf, MSc,
Frederik Barkhof, MD, PhD, Mike P. Wattjes, MD*

KEYWORDS

- High-field magnetic resonance imaging
- Neuroinflammation • Multiple sclerosis
- Clinically isolated syndrome

Key Points

- Multiple sclerosis (MS) is the most common chronic inflammatory demyelinating disorder of the central nervous system (CNS).
- MS has been subject to high-field magnetic resonance (MR) imaging research to a great extent.
- Using conventional sequences at higher magnetic field leads to an increased detection of focal inflammatory MS lesions in both white and gray matter.
- High-field MR imaging detects MS lesions particularly in anatomic regions that are important for the diagnosis, prognosis, and differential diagnosis of MS.
- Using quantitative sequences at high-field provided more insight in pathologic processes that cause (subtle) diffuse inflammatory changes and showed improved correlation with measures of clinical outcome.
- The use of high-field 3 T MR imaging does not lead to a significant earlier diagnosis of MS using the current McDonald criteria, which are based on 1.5 T.
- Future research on clinical relevance of high-field MR imaging in MS patients is warranted.
- Possibly this will lead to the development of more specific, high-field 3 T/7 T diagnostic criteria for MS.

Inflammatory diseases in the central nervous system (CNS) include a wide and heterogenic spectrum of diseases entities. In general, studies investigating the diagnostic value of higher magnetic field strengths in inflammatory CNS disease are limited. However, the most common inflammatory demyelinating disorder of the CNS, multiple sclerosis (MS), has been subject to high-field magnetic resonance (MR) imaging research to a great extent during the past years, and much data has been collected that might prove helpful in investigating other inflammatory CNS disorders. This article gives an overview of this data, focusing only on MS. The authors review the value of high-field MR in imaging inflammatory MS abnormalities by describing different imaging techniques. Furthermore, possibilities and challenges for the future of high-field MR imaging in MS are discussed.

MS is the most common inflammatory CNS disease in young adults that leads to relevant chronic disability,[1] and is typified by both pathologic and

---

Iris Kilsdonk is supported by a grant provided by the Noaber Foundation (Lunteren, The Netherlands). The authors have nothing to disclose.
Department of Radiology, VU University Medical Center, PO Box 7057, 1007 MB Amsterdam, The Netherlands
* Corresponding author.
E-mail address: m.wattjes@vumc.nl

Neuroimag Clin N Am 22 (2012) 135–157
doi:10.1016/j.nic.2012.02.010

Diagnostic Checklist

- The standard MR imaging protocol for the diagnosis of inflammatory central nervous system (CNS) diseases recommends brain and spinal cord imaging.
- It includes 3 sequences: fluid-attenuated inversion recovery (FLAIR) (brain), proton-density (PD)/T2-weighted fast spin echo (FSE) or turbo spin echo (TSE) (brain + spinal cord), and postcontrast T1-weighted (brain + spinal cord) images.
- High-field 3 T MR imaging detects more MS lesions in both gray and white matter of the brain, in anatomic regions that are important for the diagnosis of MS.
- The use of high-field 3 T MR imaging does not lead to a significant earlier diagnosis of MS using the current McDonald criteria, which are based on 1.5 T.
- High-field 3 T MR imaging therefore is safe and does not lead to field strength–induced overdiagnosis of MS because of false-positive detection of white matter lesions.
- The use of quantitative sequences at high-field MR imaging provides insight into pathologic processes and improves correlation with measures of clinical outcome, but is not included in clinical protocols.
- Future research should focus on the clinical relevance of (ultra) high-field MR imaging in terms of diagnostic criteria and individual patient care.

---

clinical heterogeneity. Pathologically, MS is described as multifocal areas of demyelination with loss of oligodendrocytes, astroglial scarring, and axonal injury. Damage can be focal (plaques) or diffuse (in diffusely abnormal and normal-appearing brain tissue [NABT]), occurs in both white matter (WM) and gray matter (GM), and is characterized by a combination of inflammation, demyelination, and neurodegeneration. Clinically, the disease displays heterogeneity in neurologic disability between and within patients.

MR imaging has been used increasingly over the past decades to depict inflammatory and neurodegenerative abnormalities, and has been established as the most important paraclinical tool in diagnosing MS.[2,3] This increasing use has led to the incorporation of MR imaging criteria for the demonstration of dissemination in space (DIS) and dissemination in time (DIT) into the International Panel (IP) diagnostic criteria for MS.[4–6] Besides ascertaining the diagnosis, MR imaging is used to exclude other conditions with similar clinical profiles,[7] and to monitor disease progression and treatment effects. Furthermore, MR imaging can be used to obtain prognostic information in the early course of the disease, being able to predict conversion to clinically definite MS (CDMS) and to predict long-term disability in patients with a clinically isolated syndrome (CIS) suggestive of MS.[8,9]

Much progress has been made in improving the dissociation between imaging and clinical disability in MS patients, the so-called clinico-radiological paradox, particularly with the application of advanced MR imaging techniques.[10] The assessment of brain atrophy can classify (GM

vs WM) and quantify tissue loss,[11] whereas relaxation-time mapping,[12] magnetization transfer ratio (MTR),[13] and diffusion tensor imaging (DTI)[14] are able to quantify the extent of structural changes within lesions and show occult damage to MS brain tissue, that is, outside focal lesions in NABT. Proton MR spectroscopy (^{1}H-MRS) provides information on the biochemical and metabolic nature of these changes, and functional MR imaging (fMRI) shows that the brain is capable of limiting clinical consequences of irreversible damage by a process called neuronal adaptation.[15,16]

In addition to developing advanced sequences and techniques to improve software of MR imaging, great strides have been made in improving hardware. Besides improvement in gradient and receiver coils, an important development is the introduction of high-field 3 T MR imaging scanners. At present these are widely available and increasingly used in many hospitals, particularly in MS centers.

Although high-field MR imaging seems a promising modality to depict and classify the heterogeneity of MS pathology, this article does not tackle the ongoing debate on the interrelation between inflammation, demyelination, and neurodegeneration of the disease.

HIGH-FIELD MR IMAGING IN MS: CONVENTIONAL IMAGING

The search for the impact of increasing magnetic field strengths on the visibility of MS lesions has existed since the introduction of MR imaging, as shown in studies comparing 0.5 T with

1.0 and 1.5 T.[17–19] At present, 3 T MR imaging is considered as high-field for clinical purposes, and field strengths of 4 T and above are considered ultrahigh-field.

One of the major advantages of moving to high-field MR imaging is the increase in signal-to-noise ratio (SNR) that follows an almost linear relation with magnetic field strength.[20] This gain in SNR can be used either to improve spatial resolution or to reduce scan time (or a combination of both), leading to higher image quality and faster image acquisition.

Detection of Inflammatory White Matter Pathology

Imaging guidelines for conventional brain MR imaging in the diagnosis of inflammatory CNS disease recommend a multisequence protocol consisting of 3 sequences (**Table 1**).[21,22] The first is a sagittal (preferably 3-dimensional [3D]) fluid-attenuated inversion recovery (FLAIR) sequence to depict the supratentorial brain, providing the highest sensitivity in detection of lesions close to the cerebrospinal fluid (juxtacortical and periventricular lesions). Second is proton-density (PD)/T2-weighted fast spin echo (FSE) or turbo spin echo (TSE) imaging, being highly sensitive for detection of WM lesions, particularly in the infratentorial WM. Final recommendations in the protocol are precontrast (optional) and postcontrast-enhanced T1-weighted images, which allow visualization of active lesions, that is, those associated with inflammatory activity and blood-brain barrier breakdown. For patients who present with symptoms at spinal cord level, or when brain MR imaging analysis is equivocal, the protocol recommends MR imaging of the spinal cord (post-contrast T1-weighted and FSE/TSE PD/T2-weighted sequences).

Images are evaluated for radiologic findings as seen in inflammatory diseases, concentrating on focal and diffuse WM and GM abnormalities. MR images obtained from patients with suspected MS are analyzed according to MR imaging criteria for DIS (Barkhof, Swanton),[23,24] and the recently revised IP diagnostic criteria for MS, which are based on magnetic field strengths of 0.5 to 1.5 T.[6,25] With 3 T MR imaging scanners being used more routinely in the clinical setting, one should question the accuracy of these criteria in determining lesion load in (suspected) MS. When comparing high (3 T/4 T) with lower (1.5 T) field-strength MR imaging in MS patients, a conclusive finding is an improved detection of WM lesions and contrast-enhanced lesions (**Table 2**).[26–31] Another important finding is that at high-field, more lesions are detected in anatomic regions important for establishing the diagnosis MS according to diagnostic criteria, such as periventricular, juxtacortical, and infratentorial WM lesions (**Fig. 1**).[31,32] The improvement in infratentorial lesion detection is also important in gaining information on prognosis of the disease, because these lesions have important prognostic value in the prediction of long-term disability in patients with CIS suggestive of MS.[8]

Detection of Gray Matter Pathology

GM pathology (cerebral cortex and deep GM structures) is a key feature of MS. It is already present in the earliest stages of the disease, and

---

Table 1
Standard imaging protocol for brain and spinal cord MR imaging in MS patients

Sequence	Orientation	Objective
Brain		
FLAIR	Sagittal + axial	Supratentorial brain, especially juxtacortical and periventricular lesions
PD/T2	Axial	Infratentorial lesions
T1 pregadolinium	Axial	Optional
T1 postgadolinium	Axial	Inflammatory lesions
Spinal Cord		
PD/T2	Sagittal	Focal demyelinating lesions
T1 postgadolinium	Sagittal	Inflammatory lesions

Abbreviations: FLAIR, fluid-attenuated inversion recovery; FSE, fast spin echo; MS, multiple sclerosis; MR, magnetic resonance; PD, proton-density weighted; SE, spin echo; TSE, turbo spin echo; T1w, T1-weighted; T2w, T2-weighted.

Table 2
MS lesion detection in white matter and gray matter using high-field MR imaging

Study, Year	Patients (N)	Field Strength Used (Sequence)	Most Important Results
White Matter			
Keiper et al,[26] 1998	CDMS (15)	1.5 T vs 4 T (T2w FSE)	WM lesion detection increase of 45%
Erskine et al,[27] 2005	SP (8)	1.5 T vs 4 T (T1w, PD/T2w)	WM lesion detection increase 46% Total WM lesion volume increase 60%
Sicotte et al,[28] 2003	RR, SP (25)	1.5 T vs 3 T (T1w ± Gd)	Increase in detection of CE WM lesions of 21% Lesion volume CE WM lesion increase 30% Total WM lesion volume increase 10%
Bachmann et al,[29] 2006	RR, PP, SP (22)	1.5 T vs 3 T (FLAIR)	3 T imaging superior in lesion conspicuity and quality Significantly more artifacts at 3 T Total WM lesion detection increase 42%
Nielsen et al,[30] 2006	Acute ON (28)	1.5 T vs 3 T (T1w SE ± Gd, PD/T2w TSE, FLAIR)	24% increase in detection of CE WM lesions, 26.5% increase in FLAIR lesions
Wattjes et al,[31] 2006	CIS (40)	1.5 T vs 3 T (T1w SE ± Gd, T2w TSE, FLAIR)	13% increase in WM lesion detection 7.5% increase in CE WM lesion detection Especially in the infratentorial, juxtacortical and periventricular anatomic region important for diagnosis
Gray Matter			
Wattjes et al,[32] 2007	CIS, CDMS (26)	3 T (2D-DIR, T2w TSE, FLAIR)	DIR detected a 7% and 15% increase in lesions compared with FLAIR and T2w imaging, respectively Especially in infratentorial region
Simon et al,[43] 2010	CIS, CDMS (34)	1.5 T vs 3 T (2D-DIR, T1w SE ± Gd, T2w TSE, FLAIR)	3 T DIR detected 192% more intracortical lesions and 30% more mixed WM/WM lesions than 1.5 T

Abbreviations: CDMS, clinically definite multiple sclerosis; CE, contrast-enhancing; CIS, clinically isolated syndrome; DIR, double inversion recovery; FLAIR, fluid-attenuated inversion recovery; FSE, fast spin echo; Gd, gadolinium; MR, magnetic resonance; MS, multiple sclerosis; ON, optic neuritis; PD, proton-density weighted; PP, primary progressive; RR, relapsing remitting; SE, spin echo; SP, secondary progressive; T1w, T1-weighted; T2w, T2-weighted; TSE, turbo spin echo; WM, white matter.

accumulates and accelerates more in the later and progressive phases.[33] GM damage can manifest as a mixture of focal demyelinating lesions and diffuse abnormalities. Early pathology studies already acknowledged the extensive involvement of GM in MS.[34,35]

Notwithstanding the recent focus of MR imaging research on GM abnormalities, thus far GM (especially subpial intracortical) lesions are still vastly underdetected by conventional in vivo MR imaging studies when compared with pathology studies. The sensitivity of conventional imaging techniques (T1, PD/T2, FLAIR) in detecting GM damage is poor, because these techniques lack the necessary contrast and resolution to visualize cortical demyelination.[36] The pathophysiology and histopathology of cortical lesions (less inflammatory cell infiltration, no complement activation or blood-brain-barrier damage) and low myelin content of GM, plus partial volume effects from cerebrospinal fluid (CSF) on MR imaging, all contribute to this lack of sensitivity.[37,38]

Improvement in the sensitivity of GM lesion detection was established with the introduction of the GM-specific double inversion recovery (DIR) sequence, higher resolution imaging of GM by the use of high-field MR imaging and, of course, the combination of these 2 methods. The development of DIR, which is not included in the conventional MR imaging protocol on a regular basis, leads to an improved (gray-white) contrast by depicting only GM. This is managed by using 2 inversion pulses leading to an attenuation of both CSF and WM.[39] Disadvantages are its rather low SNR resulting from the double signal-inversion pulses, and the propensity to (flow and pulsation) artifacts, particularly in the posterior fossa. The development of multislab and, later, single-slab 3D-DIR applications led to a great improvement[40]: a 5-fold increase in cortical lesions in MS patients was detected in comparison with conventional T2-weighted sequences.[41] In addition, an improved distinction was made between mixed GM-WM lesions and purely intracortical lesions.

The introduction of high-field imaging did not immediately lead to an increase in detection of cortical lesions, when applied in postmortem research using conventional PD sequences on a 4.7 T MR imaging system. Most GM lesions were still missed; contrast between GM and GM lesions was found to be very low, independent of sequence or field strength.[42] The combination of higher magnetic field strengths with DIR sequences in vivo seemed to be more successful in visualizing GM pathology. At 3 T, DIR was superior to the standard sequences in the detection of WM, mixed WM/GM, and intracortical GM lesions (see **Table 2**).[32,43] One of these studies also demonstrated superiority of DIR at 3 T over other sequences for infratentorial WM lesions, which is clinically highly important as stated earlier. Both studies made use of a 2-dimensional (2D)-DIR sequence; implementing 3D-DIR at higher magnetic field (3 T) might result in further improvement of lesion detection by reducing artifacts, but will be accompanied by an increase in acquisition time.

Improved depiction of GM damage was achieved in studies using ultrahigh-field strengths (7 T and higher),[44–48] the results of which are described in more detail later in this article.

The focus on how to depict GM damage has high clinical relevance, because cortical damage differs between MS disease types and stages,[49–52] and shows a relationship with physical as well as cognitive disability.[53,54] Furthermore, when including the presence of intracortical GM lesions in MR imaging diagnostic criteria, an increase in accuracy of these criteria has been reported.[55] However, an official introduction of GM lesions into the diagnostic criteria has not yet been made and needs further multicenter validation. A step in the right direction was recently made by developing consensus recommendations for MS cortical lesion scoring using DIR.[56]

Detection of Active Inflammatory Pathology

Magnetic field strength influences tissue relaxation times. With 3 T MR imaging, T1 (spin lattice/longitudinal) relaxation time increases by 20% to 40%, whereas T2 (spin spin/transverse) relaxation time decreases by about 5% to 10%.[57,58] When using T1-shortening contrast agents at higher field strengths, for example, paramagnetic gadolinium-based contrast agents, the overall longer high-field T1 relaxation times will create a relatively stronger effect of T1 reduction by the contrast agent. This effect causes a greater postcontrast signal intensity difference at 3 T in comparison with 1.5 T, which increases the detection of contrast-enhancing inflammatory lesions in MS (**Fig. 2**).[28,30,31,43] It may even allow dosage reduction at higher field strengths.[59] Nonetheless, because of decreased GM-WM contrast with increasing magnetic field, it remains a challenge to develop an SE T1 sequence for high-field MR imaging systems, which is the standard sequence used to detect inflammatory lesions at lower field strengths.

Paramagnetic contrast agents based on iron oxides such as (ultra) small particles of iron oxide ([U]SPIO), which have shown pluriformity of inflammatory MS pathology complementary to gadolinium-enhanced 1.5 T MR imaging, have not yet been applied at higher magnetic fields.[60]

Detection of Spinal Cord Pathology

MR imaging of the spinal cord has gained more importance in establishing the diagnosis of MS, particularly in the recent IP criteria.[6] As is known from standard field strength studies, conventional MR imaging shows asymptomatic spinal cord lesions in 30% to 40% of CIS patients and in up to 90% of CDMS patients.[61] Besides aiding in diagnosis and differential diagnosis,[62] imaging of spinal cord abnormalities is relevant because these are related to clinical outcome.[63,64] Advanced MR techniques are sensitive to tissue

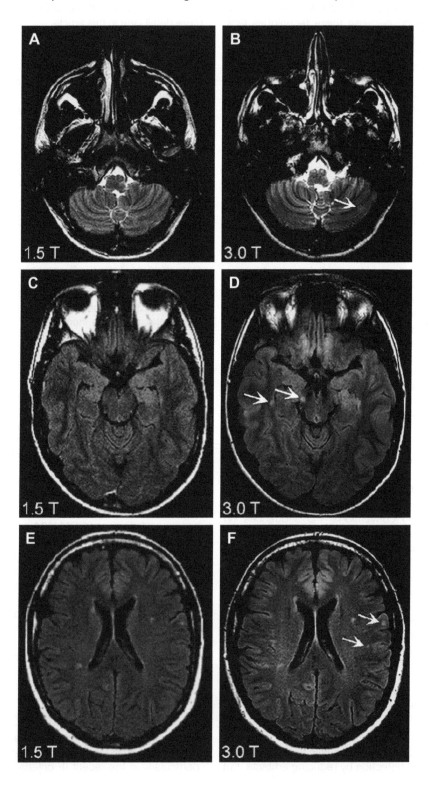

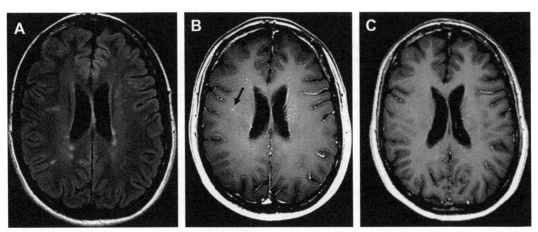

Fig. 2. Image examples of increased detection of contrast-enhanced inflammatory brain lesions at 3 T in comparison with 1.5 T. (*A*) Multiple lesions are seen in the 3 T FLAIR image of a relapsing remitting MS patient. (*B*) On 3 T postcontrast T1-weighted image, a contrast-enhancing lesion with a perivascular location can be visualized (*arrow*). (*C*) This lesion could not be identified on the corresponding 1.5 T postcontrast image.

damage in the spinal cord, and are related to measures of clinical outcome as well.[65–67]

Postmortem studies using high-field MR imaging showed a better visibility of MS spinal cord pathology including quantitative and GM abnormalities,[68–70] but the in vivo use of higher magnetic field strengths for imaging spinal cord remains problematic, mainly because of susceptibility, CSF, and pulsation artifacts. In contrast to brain MR imaging studies, in vivo comparison of 1.5 T and 3 T spinal cord MR imaging showed no significant differences in terms of lesion detection and correlations with clinical measures such as the Expanded Disability Status Scale (EDSS).[71] A recent MR imaging study investigating spinal cord volumes at 3 T described a decrease in cervical spinal cord volume in progressive forms of MS and a trend toward increased spinal cord volume in relapsing remitting (RR) MS/CIS patients, which the investigators refer to respectively as atrophy and inflammation/edema–related expansion.[72]

Clinical Value of Conventional High-Field MR imaging in Terms of Diagnostic Criteria

As described, studies investigating the influence of higher magnetic field strengths on lesion load measurement showed an evident improvement in lesion detection. However, the crucial question remains as to whether 3 T MR imaging scanners are of added clinical value in terms of an earlier diagnosis of MS. High-field 3 T MR imaging proved to be able to substantially influence classification of CIS patients according to Barkhof MR imaging criteria: 27.5% of the 40 patients studied fulfilled 1 additional criterion. Diagnostic classification in terms of DIS was mildly influenced: only 1 additional patient had DIS at 3 T on comparison with 1.5 T examinations.[73] During follow-up no additional patients showed DIT at 3 T compared with 1.5 T examination, neither to the revised IP criteria nor to the Swanton criteria.[74] Hence, when using the 2005 IP criteria, 3 T MR imaging does not lead to an earlier diagnosis of MS.[5] When

Fig. 1. Image examples of the higher sensitivity in the detection of inflammatory brain lesions at 3 T in comparison with 1.5 T. (*A, B*) A 23-year-old man presenting with unilateral optic neuritis. An inflammatory lesion in the left hemisphere of the cerebellum (*arrow*) was clearly identified on the T2-weighted turbo spin echo images at 3 T but not on the corresponding 1.5 T examination. (*C, D*) Axial fluid-attenuated inversion recovery (FLAIR) sections of the same patient. A small lesion in the brainstem and a lesion in the right temporal lobe (*arrows*) could be visualized on the 3 T image but not on the corresponding 1.5 T image. (*E, F*) Axial FLAIR sections of the supratentorial brain of a 45-year-old woman presenting with optic neuritis of her left eye. A small juxtacortical lesion (*arrow*) was prospectively identified on the 3 T image but was missed on the 1.5 T examination. Another lesion, which is probably a mixed white matter–gray matter lesion (*arrow*), is sharply delineated on the 3 T image but is more fuzzy and smaller on the 1.5 T image. (*Reproduced from* Wattjes MP, Lutterbey GG. Higher sensitivity in the detection of inflammatory brain lesions in patients with clinically isolated syndromes suggestive of multiple sclerosis using high-field MR imaging: an intraindividual comparison of 1.5 T with 3.0 T. Eur Radiol 2006;16:2070; with permission.)

retrospectively applying the data of this cohort to the more liberal 2010 revised IP criteria[6] that are based on MR imaging criteria developed by the MAGNIMS group,[25] again no earlier diagnosis of MS could be established at 3 T when compared with 1.5 T.[75] From these studies it can also be concluded that when using the revised IP criteria, 3 T MR imaging is safe and does not lead to field strength–influenced overdiagnosis of MS resulting from false-positive detection of WM lesions. However, this conclusion, together with the statement that in CIS patients there is no added clinical value of high-field 3 T MR imaging above standard 1.5 T MR imaging, might be too premature, because it was only based on one rather small, single-center, single-vendor data set. Future studies might lead to new and improved criteria for the diagnosis of MS, based on (ultra) high-field MR imaging in combination with novel sequences such as DIR.

ULTRAHIGH-FIELD MR IMAGING IN MS

Although high-field 3 T MR imaging showed advantages over lower field strength imaging, the true future of MR imaging in MS might reside in ultrahigh-field MR imaging systems (>4 T). Since 2000, when the US Food and Drug Administration (FDA) gave approval for in vivo high-field imaging with magnetic field strengths up to 8 T,[76] researchers worldwide started moving up to ultrahigh-field MR imaging. In MS research the ultrahigh-field machine most commonly used for in vivo brain imaging is a 7 T whole-body MR imaging scanner.

Implementation of in vivo 7 T MR imaging is technically challenging, because disadvantages of scanning at high-field strengths are even more distinct when using an ultrahigh magnetic field. From their own experience the authors can state that sequences that are robust at 1.5 and 3 T do not result in high-quality images at 7 T. The main problems are practical issues related to heterogeneity of the magnetic field and maximum specific absorption rate (SAR) limitations, leading to artifacts that make full brain coverage seemingly difficult. At present, the major drawbacks of 7 T MR imaging have been solved, and the first interesting observations of its application in MS research are being published. There are 2 crucial findings of ultrahigh-field MR imaging in MS: first, an increased detection of lesions when compared with lower field strengths (Table 3), as would be expected from increased resolution and SNR; second, the depiction of additional features of MS pathology, revealing a heterogeneity that is not visible at lower field strength.

Increased MS Lesion Detection Using Ultrahigh-Field MR imaging

Postmortem studies using ultrahigh magnetic field strengths discovered cortical lesions at 8 T that remained invisible at 1.5 T.[44] At histopathologic verification, often these cortical lesions could only be found after observing the 8 T MR images. A recent postmortem study showed that 3D-T2* gradient echo sequences and WM-attenuated turbo field echo sequences at 7 T were able to detect most cortical lesions verified by pathological examination.[47] Unfortunately, both postmortem studies used a limited number of patients, and further validation with a larger number of samples is warranted.

In vivo studies using ultrahigh magnetic field strength show increased detection of MS lesions in WM as well as in cortical GM.[45,46] The improvement in detection of cortical GM lesions is important, because the depiction of this type of lesions has been difficult at lower field strengths. Mainero and colleagues[46] found that 7 T MR images were able to differentiate cortical lesions in accordance with histopathologic lesion types (type 1: leukocortical; type 2: intracortical; type 3/4: subpial extending partly/completely through cortical layers). Type 3/4 was found to be the most frequent type of cortical plaques (50.2%), and this type was also related to higher EDSS scores. In vivo studies comparing advanced sequences between 7 T MR imaging and lower field strength do not exist, but the authors' own data show that 3D-FLAIR and 3D-DIR using magnetization preparation (MP) allows high-quality T2-weighted MR imaging in MS at 7 T,[77] and that 7 T 3D-FLAIR improves cortical lesion detection in comparison with 3 T (Fig. 3).

Visualizing Heterogeneity of MS Lesions at Ultrahigh-Field Strength

The main focus of ultrahigh-field imaging in MS patients thus far has been on heterogeneity of lesions, which is studied by making use of the increased magnetic susceptibility at higher field strength. Susceptibility-weighted imaging (SWI) identified the relationship between MS lesions and vasculature, and confirmed that MS lesions follow a strict perivascular distribution.[45,78–81] That perivenular inflammation plays a role in MS was already identified in histopathology studies, but the possibility to visualize it in vivo provides opportunities to further investigate what determines lesion location (in a longitudinal setting) and might help in differentiating MS from ischemic WM lesions.[82]

Table 3
MS lesion detection by MR imaging at ultrahigh magnetic field strength, postmortem and in vivo

Study, Year	Patients (N)	Field Strength (Sequence)	Most Important Results
Post Mortem			
Kangarlu et al,[44] 2007	SP (1)	1.5 T vs 8 T (GRE, T2w SE, FLAIR)	Detection of cortical lesions at 8 T that remained invisible at 1.5 T At histopathologic verification cortical lesions could only be found after observing 8 T images
Pitt et al,[47] 2010	SP (3)	7 T (3D T2* GRE, WM attenuated TFE)	Detection of 93% (3D T2* GRE) and 82% (WM attenuated TFE) of cortical lesions compared with pathological examination
In Vivo			
Kolia et al,[45] 2009	(12)	1.5 T vs 7 T (T1w, PD/T2w)	23% increased WM lesion detection at 7 T Better differentiation between juxtacortical and cortical lesions at 7 T
Mainero et al,[46] 2009	RR, SP (16)	7 T (3D-T1w MPRAGE, FLASH T2* GRE, T2w TSE)	7 T is able to classify cortical lesion according to histopathologic lesion type: type 1 (36.2%), type 2 (13.6%), type 3–4 (50.2%) Cortical lesion type 3–4 was related to higher EDSS score

Abbreviations: EDSS, Expanded Disability Status Scale; FLAIR, fluid-attenuated inversion recovery; FLASH, fast low-angle shot; GRE, gradient echo sequence; MPRAGE, magnetization-prepared rapid gradient echo; MR, magnetic resonance; MS, multiple sclerosis; PD, proton-density weighted; RR, relapsing remitting; SE, spin echo; SP, secondary progressive; T1w, T1-weighted; T2w, T2-weighted; TFE, turbo field echo; TSE, turbo spin echo; WM, white matter.

Another specific feature discovered by ultra-high-field SWI in a subset of MS lesions are hypo-intense rims **(Fig. 4)**.[45,47,79] Hammond and colleagues[79] explained these rims to reflect iron-rich macrophages at the periphery of a lesion, which may indicate the site of active inflammation in tissue and might be of help in staging the disease. Postmortem pathology studies have identified this iron accumulation in MS plaques as well.[83] Pitt and colleagues[47] reported the hypo-intense rims to correspond to increased density of activated microglia. Hypointense rims have not been conclusively identified at 1.5 T.[45]

At even higher field strengths (9.4 T), T2-weighted scanning was able to discriminate areas of remyelination and demyelination in postmortem MS lesions.[84] More recently, the same investi-gators studied 21 tissue samples of MS motor cortex, and found 28 GM cortical lesions that were visible on T2-weighted MR imaging as well as on sections immunostained for myelin basic protein.[48] Furthermore, a correlation between quantitative MR and quantitative histology was made, which suggested that in cortical GM, T1 relaxation-time differences may be a predictor of neuronal density and T2 relaxation-time differ-ences may predict myelin content. When these results can be translated into in vivo studies, for instance at 3 T or 7 T, they might possibly have a great impact on clinical translation of demyelin-ation and neuronal loss.

HIGH-FIELD MR IMAGING IN MS: QUANTITATIVE IMAGING

Several quantitative MR imaging modalities have been developed to gain more information con-cerning heterogeneity of pathologic substrates of MS abnormalities, with respect to the extent of inflammation, demyelination, axonal injury, gliosis, and remyelination as reported in pathology stud-ies.[85] These advanced techniques are also used

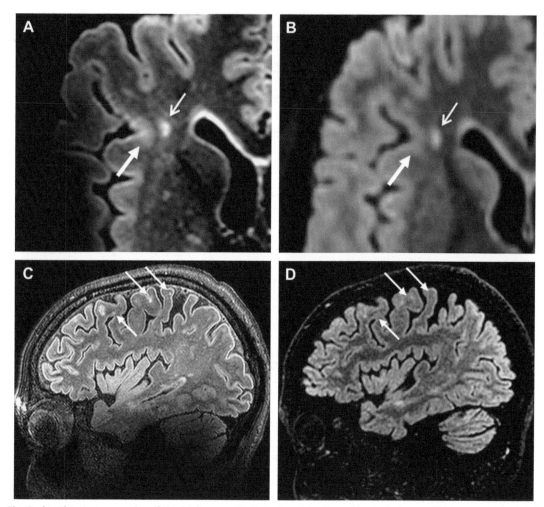

Fig. 3. (*A–D*) Image examples of the higher sensitivity in the detection of brain lesions at 7 T in comparison with 3 T. Axial reformatted (*A*) 7 T 3-dimensional magnetization-prepared (3D-MP)-FLAIR and (*B*) 3 T 3D-FLAIR images of a 37-year-old female secondary progressive MS patient. A cortical lesion (*closed arrowhead*) can be identified at 7 T, but not on the corresponding 3 T image. A deep white matter lesion (*open arrowhead*) is visible at both field strengths. Sagittal (*C*) 7 T 3D-MP-FLAIR and (*D*) 3 T 3D-FLAIR images of a 50-year-old male primary progressive MS patient. Arrows indicate examples of lesions visible at 7 T but not on the corresponding 3 T image; the images also show multiple lesions that are visible at both 7 T and 3 T.

to depict damage that is occult on conventional MR imaging, and to narrow the clinico-radiological dissociation between clinical disability and imaging findings. The availability of high-field MR imaging systems is beneficial to quantitative techniques such as proton magnetic resonance spectroscopy, diffusion-weighted imaging (DWI), and functional MR imaging in MS.

High-Field Proton Spectroscopy

Proton magnetic resonance spectroscopy (^{1}H-MRS) is a complementary modality to conventional MR imaging: it depicts and quantifies the biochemical and metabolic nature of tissue abnormalities.

Measuring metabolite changes in brains of MS patients has provided information on the pathogenesis and the natural history of the disease.[86] The most important metabolites that are quantified in MS spectroscopy are *N*-acetylaspartate (NAA), being a measure of axonal integrity, *myo*-inositol (mI), reflecting glial cell activity, and choline (Cho), an indicator of membrane turnover. In acute MS lesions mI and Cho are increased, indicating myelin breakdown, whereas NAA is reduced, reflecting axonal damage.[86,87] In chronic MS lesions Cho values return to normal, whereas the elevated mI and reduced NAA remain evident. Next to metabolic changes in focal lesions, ^{1}H-MRS also shows differences in metabolite concentrations in NABT

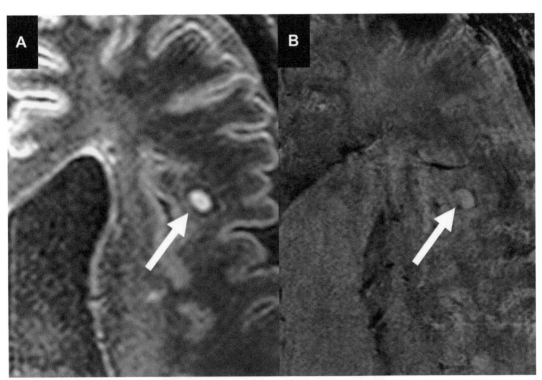

Fig. 4. Example of a deep white matter lesion in a 43-year-old male MS patient, which showed a hypointense ring at (*A*) 7 T 3D-MP-FLAIR (*arrow*) that can also be seen on (*B*) susceptibility-weighted imaging (SWI) (*arrow*), suggestive of iron deposition.

(normal-appearing WM [NAWM] and GM).[15,88,89] The NAA reduction in MS lesions on ^{1}H-MRS is related to greater clinical disability in MS patients.[90–92]

At higher magnetic field strengths there is an increase in the 2 main criteria on which spectrum quality depends, namely SNR and chemical shift. The increase in SNR results in more signal (higher metabolite peaks in relation to background noise), and the increase in chemical shift improves spectral resolution (metabolite separation). This process means that at high-field strength more precise metabolite quantification is possible. Increased spectral resolution at 3 T is capable of separating and individually quantifying glutamate, glutamine, and mI, the peaks of which are overlapping at 1.5 T (**Fig. 5**).[93–95] Furthermore, metabolite quantification has shown improved sensitivity and good reproducibility at 3 T.[93,94]

Moving to ultrahigh-field strength, these advantages become even more distinct: at 7 T ^{1}H-MRS a broad range of brain metabolites can be detected with increased sensitivity, total measurement time can be significantly reduced, or the spatial resolution significantly increased, relative to 4 T.[96] In addition, new metabolites can be investigated, such as γ-aminobutyric acid, as has been shown at 9.4 T in rats.[97]

The question remains: what is the added value of better metabolic quantification at higher magnetic field strengths for MS patients? Despite high-field ^{1}H-MRS studies of MS patients being limited, the published results are promising. As assessed by 3 T ^{1}H-MRS, significant axonal damage (decreased NAA) already becomes apparent during the first demyelinating episode in patients with CIS,[98,99] suggesting early neurodegeneration in MS. This finding contradicts that for glial cell activity (increased mI) at 3 T, which was not increased in CIS patients until later on in patients with a very early course of relapsing remitting MS (RRMS).[98] The decrease in NAA reflecting axonal injury in CIS patients also has a prognostic function in predicting the conversion to definite MS.[100]

3 T ^{1}H-MRS was used to study glutamate metabolism in MS patients, and showed a significant elevation in glutamate in acute, gadolinium-enhanced lesions as well as in NAWM, whereas no glutamate elevation was visible in chronic lesions. This finding might render quantification of glutamate suitable as a marker for active inflammation.[101]

Increasing magnetic field strength offers chances for new techniques, such as sodium 23 ([23]Na) imaging, which showed deviant sodium values in lesions, NAWM, and GM of RRMS

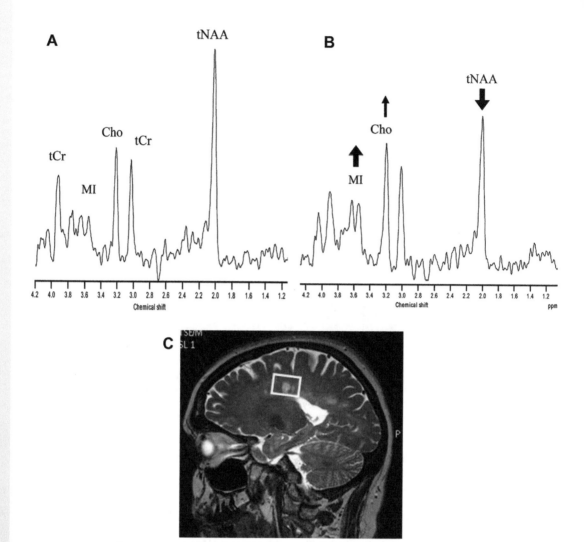

Fig. 5. Single-voxel ^{1}H-MR spectra (repetition time/echo time 2000/38 milliseconds) at 3 T from the centrum semi-ovale of a healthy control (*A*) and from an MS patient (*B*), where the MR spectroscopy volume includes a white matter lesion (*C*). The most prominent finding in the patient's spectrum is the strong decrease in the peak from *N*-acetyl components (tNAA). However, other metabolites such as *myo*-inositol (MI) and choline compounds (Cho) show characteristic alterations (increase) in their peak intensities. Note the multiplet of MI, which is not visible at lower field strengths because of overlap with glutamate and glutamine signals. tCr, total creatine. (*Courtesy of Dr Frank Träber, Radiologische Klinik der Universität Bonn.*)

patients. This finding might reflect changes in cellular and metabolic integrity, and has the potential to provide insight into pathophysiologic mechanisms of tissue injury.[102]

The only study using ^{1}H-MRS at 7 T in MS patients quantified glutathione (GSH), a marker of oxidative status.[103] Because of its low concentrations in the brain and its overlap with NAA, at lower field strengths this antioxidant is difficult to quantify. At 7 T, MS patients showed a significant reduction in GSH concentration in GM lesions when compared with healthy controls, implying a diminished protection against free radicals.

High-Field Diffusion Imaging

DWI measures Brownian motion of water molecules in tissues. Demyelination and remyelination in MS change the geometry of brain tissue orientation and thereby influence water diffusivity of tissues. Because of this, diffusion imaging has been widely used to study MS-related tissue damage. If not only total diffusivity but also the direction of the maximal diffusivity are measured, DWI is referred to as DTI. DTI quantifies diffusivity in MS patients, by measuring apparent diffusion coefficient (ADC), mean diffusivity (MD), and fractional anisotropy (FA), as well as radial and axial diffusivity.

In MS patients, DTI at 1.5 T provided information about tissue damage in focal lesions and in the NABT: compared with healthy controls, a decrease in anisotropy (FA) and an increase in diffusivity (ADC and MD) were reported.[104–106] DTI abnormalities are more pronounced in focal lesions than in NAWM and are most severe in T1 hypointense lesions, representing irreversible tissue damage.[14,107] The characteristics of enhancing MS lesions are not well defined: although FA values are consistently lower in enhancing than in nonenhancing lesions, MD values in enhancing lesions vary or do not seem to differ between enhancing and nonenhancing lesions.[107]

DTI alterations are more pronounced with increased disease duration and show a correlation with clinical disability.[104,108] The strongest correlation was found with the diffusion characteristics of T2 lesions and GM, with GM abnormalities being more severe in progressive disease.[109–111] Benedict and colleagues[112] reported a significant correlation between DTI values and cognitive dysfunction.

Despite the promising results of the application of 1.5 T DTI in MS research, the technique has shortcomings that can be amended by moving to a higher magnetic field. Diffusion imaging offers poor spatial resolution and marginal SNR because the use of diffusion gradients causes distortion and attenuation of signal. High-field DTI should be beneficial because of an increased SNR, although stronger susceptibility artifacts at higher field strengths decrease image quality. The implementation of high-field DTI faces several technical challenges. First, the mapping of many different diffusion directions is time consuming, a problem that is slightly more pronounced at higher magnetic field strength because increased T1 relaxation times need longer repetition times. Second, to limit bulk motion, DTI is in need of fast acquisition protocols. Rapid scanning is usually acquired by using spin echo single-shot echo-planar imaging (EPI) sequences which, unfortunately, at higher field have the disadvantage of image blurring and geometric distortions near air/tissue transitions. These difficulties have been largely overcome by combining high-field 3 T MR imaging scanners with parallel imaging techniques that reduce EPI artifacts and reduce acquisition times.[113–115] An example of DTI at high-field 3 T can be seen in **Fig. 6.**

The use of 3 T DTI in MS research has focused on anatomic regions that are difficult to study at lower field strength, such as GM. Ceccarelli and colleagues,[116] who reported that 3 T DTI is feasible

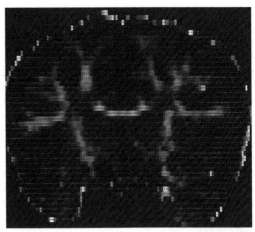

Fig. 6. Coronal 3 T DTI overlay of a male MS patient showing main fiber directions with reconstructed resolution of 1.0 × 1.0 × 2.4 mm. The application of a higher main magnetic field increases the accuracy of determination of fiber direction by higher SNR and decreases partial volume effects. (*Courtesy of Menno Schoonheim, VU University Medical Center, Amsterdam.*)

and shows decreased FA and increased MD in NAWM, made the first observations of DTI at high magnetic field, and confirmed abnormalities (increased water diffusivity and decreased GM volume) in the GM of MS patients. In a second study these investigators found that DTI at 3 T shows regional differences in WM damage between subtypes of MS, namely benign MS and RRMS.[117] In terms of global DTI metrics no differences were seen, which indicates that the topographic differences might be associated with clinical heterogeneity between different MS subtypes. Two other DTI studies at 3 T performed in MS patients related disability to corticospinal tract and optic tract abnormalities.[118,119]

High-Field Functional MR Imaging

When neurons are activated, blood flow to this specific brain region is increased. The oxygenated-deoxygenated hemoglobin ratio changes with it, causing small variations in the local magnetic field (T2*). fMRI measures these variations in blood oxygen level–dependent (BOLD) contrast and creates an indirect measure of brain activity. At standard field strength, fMRI has provided insight into different aspects of MS brain function, focusing on visual, cognitive, and motor networks. Compared with healthy controls, MS patients first show increased recruitment of brain regions for a specific task, followed by bilateral activation of these regions and at a later stage recruitment of additional brain regions.[120]

Comparing the results of brain function with those of structural damage using MR imaging in MS patients suggested the existence of brain plasticity: the capability of the MS brain to compensate for irreversible structural damage, so-called cortical reorganization/adaptation. That these cortical reorganization processes already occur in the earliest phases of the disease was shown in studies concerning CIS patients, in which functional changes were associated with the development to definite MS.[121,122] Functional changes in MS brains vary between disease types and different stages of the disease.[121–124] The interindividual efficacy of brain reorganization might play a major role in clarifying the clinical heterogeneity of MS.

Functional imaging benefits greatly from higher field strengths, firstly because of the increase in SNR and secondly because of the stronger magnetic susceptibility effects. The BOLD contrast increases with magnetic field strength (B0),[125,126] because the difference between deoxygenated blood (paramagnetic) and surrounding tissue (diamagnetic) increases with field strength, allocating a shorter echo time and, thus, higher SNR and shorter acquisition times. Higher signal and higher spatial resolution on high-field fMRI increase the reliability in localizing brain activity. More importantly, high-field fMRI enables the depiction of brain activity in additional (smaller) brain regions, which cannot be visualized at lower field strengths. While studying cognitive function at 3 T, Hoenig and colleagues[127] detected additional activation in cortical areas involved in higher executive motor functions when compared with functional 1.5 T MR imaging.

High-field fMRI in MS patients was used by Rocca and colleagues,[128] who focused on a part of the brain that could not be visualized with fMRI at standard field strength and reported increased activation of the mirror neuron system in patients with MS. These preliminary findings suggest a possibility that mirror neurons play a role in cortical reorganization. When the same study group focused only on primary progressive MS patients using fMRI, they saw an increased recruitment of cognition-related networks with the potential to limit the severity of cognitive impairment.[129]

In addition to focusing on changes in the extent of brain activation or on the additional recruited regions, high-field fMRI can be used in combination with other modalities to investigate functional and structural substrates of functional changes. During studies on motor and cognitive disability in MS patients,[130–132] DTI tractography integrated with fMRI at 3 T showed that functional connectivity is correlated with structural damage to some of the major brain WM bundles. This association between damage to specific WM tracts and changes on fMRI presents the opportunity for further investigation in a longitudinal setting to gain insight into functional reorganization of MS-related structural damage.

Further advantages of fMRI at higher field strength are the reduction of acquisition time and the possibility of following cortical stimulation in real time.[133]

High-Field Relaxation-Time Mapping

On standard 1.5 T MR imaging, T1 relaxation-time mapping in MS has shown abnormalities in NAWM and NAGM that are not visible on conventional images.[134,135] At (ultra) high-field strength, increased T1 relaxation times, together with increased SNR that enables the use of higher spatial resolution, are expected to enhance the sensitivity of detecting abnormal brain tissue. An example of a high-resolution T1 relaxation-time map of an MS brain at 7 T is shown in **Fig. 7**.

Although T2 relaxation times are less dependent on the main magnetic field, higher SNR and spatial resolution reduce partial volume effects and are

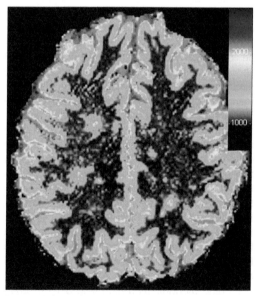

Fig. 7. High-resolution T1 relaxation-time map at 7 T of a female primary progressive MS patient. Whole-brain T1 maps with a spatial resolution of approximately 1 × 1 × 1.5 mm can be obtained in 5 minutes at 7 T. Compared with lower field strengths, accuracy is increased because of higher SNR and higher spatial resolution, reducing partial volume effects. This modality might help to detect damage to normal-appearing white and gray matter in MS.

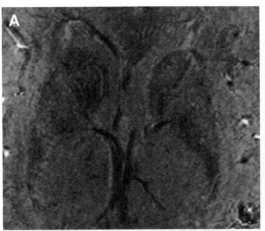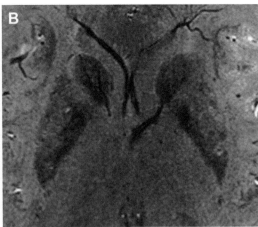

Fig. 8. 7 T SWI images from (*A*) a 42-year-old female healthy control and (*B*) a 48-year-old female MS patient. A lower signal intensity can be seen in the basal ganglia of the MS patient, which indicates more iron deposition, reflecting neurodegeneration.

therefore expected to improve T2 relaxation-time measurements at high-field strength.

NEURODEGENERATIVE ASPECTS OF NEUROINFLAMMATION

Besides neuroinflammation, MS also comprises neurodegenerative aspects, which can be visualized by (high-field) MR imaging. Atrophy can be quantified by using T1-weighted imaging, and shows a moderate correlation with the clinical status of MS patients.[11,136,137] Although atrophy measurements in MS patients have not yet been applied much at high-field strengths, they offer possibilities to look at specific regions such as the cortex or subcortical GM nuclei.

A second feature of neurodegeneration is pathologic iron deposition in the brain of MS patients, which is thought to be triggered by iron-mediated oxidative stress.[138] Iron deposition in MS can also be linked to inflammatory processes that cause local blood-brain barrier breakdown and promotion of macrophages to inflammation sites.[139,140]

Iron deposition in the brain, predominantly in the basal ganglia, is a function of increasing age,[141] but can also be a pathologic phenomenon of neurodegenerative disease.[142] High-field MR imaging is a valuable tool in imaging and quantifying iron deposition in MS brains, because high-field imaging is more sensitive to T2-shortening effects of iron-rich structures in the brain, causing hypointensities.[143,144] Magnetic susceptibility of protons influenced by local iron concentrations increase with magnetic field strength as well. Hence, (ultra) high-field studies using SWI lend themselves well to the imaging of pathologic iron deposition. Increased iron concentrations in deep GM nuclei of

MS patients have been depicted and quantified on high-field MR imaging (**Fig. 8**), with results related to clinical parameters such as cognitive performance and disease duration.[79,145,146]

For an overview of high-field MR imaging in neurodegenerative diseases, the reader is referred to the article by Luijten and colleagues elsewhere in this issue.

SUMMARY AND FUTURE PERSPECTIVES

Over the past years the impact of high-field MR imaging has been the subject of research in inflammatory CNS diseases such as MS. Both conventional and quantitative techniques take advantage of higher magnetic field strength. Using conventional high-field sequences leads to an increased detection of focal MS lesions, particularly WM lesions in anatomic regions that are important for the diagnosis, prognosis, and differential diagnosis of MS. Great strides have been made in the depiction of GM cortical lesions as well, by combining 3 T MR imaging with novel sequences such as DIR and by the introduction of ultrahigh-field systems. When adequate imaging of cortical abnormalities is feasible, this can be related to specific clinical symptoms. The use of high-field quantitative sequences provides more insight into the pathologic processes that cause (subtle) diffuse MS damage, and shows improved correlation with measures of clinical outcome.

One crucial question remains as to whether there is any added clinical value of high-field imaging in MS and whether 3 T MR imaging will therefore evolve to become the gold standard in imaging of MS patients in the future. 3 T MR imaging scanners are gradually being used more and more in the clinical setting while lacking explicit scientific foundation for their use, which gives rise to some debate.[147] Therefore, future research should focus on the clinical relevance of high-field MR imaging so as to justify the higher costs of high-field MR imaging scanners. As mentioned, the use of 3 T MR imaging does not lead to a significant earlier diagnosis of MS using the current IP diagnostic criteria based on the available data defined by imaging at 1.5 T. However, further studies are desired, including a larger study population or even the use of ultrahigh-field strength (7 T) MR imaging, which might lead to the development of more specific, high-field 3 T/7 T diagnostic criteria for MS.

In any case, high-field MR imaging will aid in understanding the pathogenesis and heterogeneity of MS, but more important is its role in individual patient care in diagnosing, monitoring disease progression, establishing prognosis, and monitoring treatment effects. The use of increasing field strengths will undoubtedly be part of this, and seems most promising if combined with other technical advancements such as refinements in quantitative techniques, development of new sequences, and improvement in hardware such as better coil technology.

ACKNOWLEDGMENTS

The authors would like to thank Professor Dr Peter R. Luijten and the 7 Tesla group from the University Medical Center Utrecht for creating the opportunity to use a 7 T MRI scanner and presenting **Figs. 2–4** and **7, 8**, Dr Frank Träber for providing **Fig. 5**, and Menno Schoonheim for providing **Fig. 6**.

REFERENCES

1. Compston A, Coles A. Multiple sclerosis. Lancet 2002;359:1221–31.
2. Young I, Hall A, Pallis C, et al. Nuclear magnetic resonance imaging of the brain in multiple sclerosis. Lancet 1981;14:1063–6.
3. Bakshi R, Thompson AJ, Rocca MA, et al. MRI in multiple sclerosis: current status and future prospects. Lancet Neurol 2008;7(7):615–25. Available at: http://linkinghub.elsevier.com/retrieve/pii/S1474442208701376. Accessed July 11, 2011.
4. McDonald WI, Compston A, Edan G, et al. Recommended diagnostic criteria for multiple sclerosis: guidelines from the International Panel on the diagnosis of multiple sclerosis. Ann Neurol 2001;50(1): 121–7. Available at: http://www.ncbi.nlm.nih.gov/pubmed/11456302. Accessed May 31, 2011.
5. Polman CH, Reingold SC, Edan G, et al. Diagnostic criteria for multiple sclerosis: 2005 revisions to the "McDonald Criteria." Ann Neurol 2005;58:840–6.
6. Polman CH, Reingold SC, Banwell B, et al. Diagnostic criteria for multiple sclerosis: 2010 revisions to the "McDonald criteria". Ann Neurol 2011;69: 292–302. Available at: http://doi.wiley.com/10.1002/ana.22366. Accessed March 9, 2011.
7. Charil A, Yousry TA, Rovaris M, et al. MRI and the diagnosis of multiple sclerosis: expanding the concept of "no better explanation". Lancet Neurol 2006;5(10):841–52. Available at: http://linkinghub.elsevier.com/retrieve/pii/S1474442206705725. Accessed January 6, 2011.
8. Minneboo A, Barkhof F, Polman CH, et al. Infratentorial lesions predict long-term disability in patients with initial findings suggestive of multiple sclerosis. Arch Neurol 2004;61(2):217–21. Available at: http://www.ncbi.nlm.nih.gov/pubmed/14967769. Accessed June 13, 2011.
9. Fisniku LK, Brex PA, Altmann DR, et al. Disability and T2 MRI lesions: a 20-year follow-up of patients with relapse onset of multiple sclerosis. Brain 2008;131(Pt 3):808–17. Available at: http://www.ncbi.nlm.nih.gov/pubmed/18234696. Accessed November 15, 2010.
10. Barkhof F. The clinico-radiological paradox in multiple sclerosis revisited. Curr Opin Neurol 2002;15(3):239–45. Available at: http://www.ncbi.nlm.nih.gov/pubmed/12045719. Accessed July 7, 2011.
11. Miller DH, Barkhof F, Frank JA, et al. Measurement of atrophy in multiple sclerosis: pathological basis, methodological aspects and clinical relevance. Brain 2002;125(Pt 8):1676–95. Available at: http://www.ncbi.nlm.nih.gov/pubmed/12135961. Accessed July 10, 2011.
12. MacKay AL, Vavasour IM, Rauscher A, et al. MR relaxation in multiple sclerosis. Neuroimaging Clin N Am 2009;19(1):1–26. Available at: http://www.ncbi.nlm.nih.gov/pubmed/19064196. Accessed June 20, 2011.
13. Ropele S, Fazekas F. Magnetization transfer MR imaging in multiple sclerosis. Neuroimaging Clin N Am 2009;19(1):27–36. Available at: http://www.ncbi.nlm.nih.gov/pubmed/19064197. Accessed August 19, 2010.
14. Rovaris M, Agosta F, Pagani E, et al. Diffusion tensor MR imaging. Neuroimaging Clin N Am 2009;19(1): 37–43. Available at: http://www.ncbi.nlm.nih.gov/pubmed/19064198. Accessed June 20, 2011.
15. Sajja BR, Wolinsky JS, Narayana PA. Proton magnetic resonance spectroscopy in multiple sclerosis. Neuroimaging Clin N Am 2009;19(1):45–58. Available at: http://www.pubmedcentral.nih.gov/articlerender.fcgi?artid=2615006&tool=pmcentrez&rendertype=abstract. Accessed August 19, 2010.

16. Filippi M, Rocca MA. Functional MR imaging in multiple sclerosis. Neuroimaging Clin N Am 2009; 19(1):59–70. Available at: http://www.ncbi.nlm.nih. gov/pubmed/19064200. Accessed June 20, 2011.

17. Schima W, Wimberger D, Schneider B, et al. Bedeu- tung der Magnetfeldstärke in der MR-Diagnostik der multiplen Sklerose: Ein Vergleich von 0,5 und 1,5 T. Rofo 1993;158:368–71. Available at: https:// www.thieme-connect.de/DOI/DOI?10.1055/s-2008- 1032665 [in German]. Accessed June 20, 2011.

18. Lee DH, Vellet AD, Eliasziw M, et al. MR imaging field strength: prospective evaluation of the diag- nostic accuracy of MR for diagnosis of multiple sclerosis at 0.5 and 1.5 T. Radiology 1995;194(1): 257–62. Available at: http://www.ncbi.nlm.nih.gov/ pubmed/7997564. Accessed June 20, 2011.

19. Filippi M, van Waesberghe JH, Horsfield MA, et al. Interscanner variation in brain MRI lesion load measurements in MS: implications for clinical trials. Neurology 1997;49(2):371–7. Available at: http:// www.ncbi.nlm.nih.gov/pubmed/9270564. Accessed June 6, 2011.

20. Willinek WA, Schild HH. Clinical advantages of 3.0 T MRI over 1.5 T. Eur J Radiol 2008;65(1):2–14. Available at: http://www.ncbi.nlm.nih.gov/pubmed/ 18162354. Accessed June 15, 2011.

21. Simon JH, Li D, Traboulsee A, et al. Standardized MR imaging protocol for multiple sclerosis: consor- tium of MS Centers consensus guidelines. AJNR Am J Neuroradiol 2006;27(2):455–61. Available at: http://www.ncbi.nlm.nih.gov/pubmed/16484429. Accessed November 18, 2010.

22. Wattjes MP, Lutterbey GG, Harzheim M, et al. Imaging of inflammatory lesions at 3.0 Tesla in patients with clinically isolated syndromes sug- gestive of multiple sclerosis: a comparison of fluid-attenuated inversion recovery with T2 turbo spin-echo. Eur Radiol 2006;16(7):1494–500. Avail- able at: http://www.ncbi.nlm.nih.gov/pubmed/16550354. Accessed May 30, 2011.

23. Barkhof F, Filippi M, Miller DH, et al. Comparison of MRI criteria at first presentation to predict conver- sion to clinically definite multiple sclerosis. Brain 1997;120(Pt 1):2059–69. Available at: http://www. ncbi.nlm.nih.gov/pubmed/9397021. Accessed January 6, 2011.

24. Swanton JK, Rovira A, Tintore M, et al. MRI criteria for multiple sclerosis in patients presenting with clinically isolated syndromes: a multicentre retro- spective study. Lancet Neurol 2007;6(8):677–86. Available at: http://www.ncbi.nlm.nih.gov/pubmed/ 17616439. Accessed August 19, 2010.

25. Montalban X, Tintoré M, Swanton J, et al. MRI criteria for MS in patients with clinically isolated syndromes. Neurology 2010;74(5):427–34. Available at: http:// www.ncbi.nlm.nih.gov/pubmed/20054006. Accessed April 30, 2011.

26. Keiper MD, Grossman RI, Hirsch JA, et al. MR identification of white matter abnormalities in multiple sclerosis: a comparison between 1.5 T and 4 T. AJNR Am J Neuroradiol 1998;19(8): 1489–93. Available at: http://www.ncbi.nlm.nih. gov/pubmed/9763383. Accessed June 20, 2011.

27. Erskine MK, Cook LL, Riddle KE, et al. Resolution- dependent estimates of multiple sclerosis lesion loads. Can J Neurol Sci 2005;32(2):205–12. Available at: http://www.ncbi.nlm.nih.gov/pubmed/ 16018156. Accessed June 20, 2011.

28. Sicotte NL, Voskuhl RR, Bouvier S, et al. Com- parison of multiple sclerosis lesions at 1.5 and 3.0 Tesla. Invest Radiol 2003;38(7):423–7. Available at: http://www.ncbi.nlm.nih.gov/pubmed/ 12821856. Accessed September 3, 2010.

29. Bachmann R, Reilmann R, Schwindt W, et al. FLAIR imaging for multiple sclerosis: a comparative MR study at 1.5 and 3.0 Tesla. Eur Radiol 2006;16(4): 915–21. Available at: http://www.ncbi.nlm.nih.gov/ pubmed/16365731. Accessed June 20, 2011.

30. Nielsen K, Rostrup E, Frederiksen JL, et al. Magnetic resonance imaging at 3.0 Tesla detects more lesions in acute optic neuritis than at 1.5 Tesla. Invest Radiol 2006;41(2):76–82. Available at: http://www.ncbi. nlm.nih.gov/pubmed/16428976. Accessed June 20, 2011.

31. Wattjes MP, Lutterbey GG, Harzheim M, et al. Higher sensitivity in the detection of inflammatory brain lesions in patients with clinically isolated syndromes suggestive of multiple sclerosis using high field MRI: an intraindividual comparison of 1.5 T with 3.0 T. Eur Radiol 2006;16(9):2067–73. Available at: http://www.ncbi.nlm.nih.gov/pubmed/16649033. Accessed May 30, 2011.

32. Wattjes MP, Lutterbey GG, Gieseke J, et al. Double inversion recovery brain imaging at 3T: diagnostic value in the detection of multiple sclerosis lesions. AJNR Am J Neuroradiol 2007;28(1):54–9. Available at: http://www.ncbi.nlm.nih.gov/pubmed/17213424. Accessed June 20, 2011.

33. Geurts JJ, Barkhof F. Grey matter pathology in multiple sclerosis. Lancet Neurol 2008;7(9): 841–51. Available at: http://www.ncbi.nlm.nih.gov/ pubmed/18703006. Accessed June 20, 2011.

34. Dawson J. The histology of disseminated sclerosis. Trans R Soc Edinburgh 1916;50:517–740.

35. Brownell B, Hughes JT. The distribution of plaques in the cerebrum in multiple sclerosis. J Neurol Neurosurg Psychiatr 1962;25:315–20. Available at: http://www.pubmedcentral.nih.gov/articlerender. fcgi?artid=495470&tool=pmcentrez&rendertype= abstract. Accessed June 20, 2011.

36. Kidd D, Barkhof F, McConnell R, et al. Cortical lesions in multiple sclerosis. Brain 1999;122(Pt 1): 17–26. Available at: http://www.ncbi.nlm.nih.gov/ pubmed/10050891. Accessed June 20, 2011.

37. Peterson JW, Bö L, Mörk S, et al. Transected neurites, apoptotic neurons, and reduced inflammation in cortical multiple sclerosis lesions. Ann Neurol 2001;50(3):389–400. Available at: http://www.ncbi.nlm.nih.gov/pubmed/11558796. Accessed June 20, 2011.

38. Bø L, Vedeler CA, Nyland HI, et al. Subpial demyelination in the cerebral cortex of multiple sclerosis patients. J Neuropathol Exp Neurol 2003; 62(7):723–32. Available at: http://www.ncbi.nlm.nih.gov/pubmed/12901699. Accessed January 31, 2011.

39. Redpath TW, Smith FW. Technical note: use of a double inversion recovery pulse sequence to image selectively grey or white brain matter. Br J Radiol 1994;67(804):1258–63. Available at: http://www.ncbi.nlm.nih.gov/pubmed/7874427. Accessed June 20, 2011.

40. Pouwels PJ, Kuijer JP, Mugler JP, et al. Human gray matter: feasibility of single-slab 3D double inversion-recovery high-spatial-resolution MR imaging. Radiology 2006;241(3):873–9. Available at: http://www.ncbi.nlm.nih.gov/pubmed/17053197. Accessed June 20, 2011.

41. Geurts JJ, Pouwels PJ, Uitdehaag BM, et al. Intracortical lesions in multiple sclerosis: improved detection with 3D double inversion-recovery MR imaging. Radiology 2005;236(1):254–60. Available at: http://www.ncbi.nlm.nih.gov/pubmed/15987979. Accessed June 20, 2011.

42. Geurts JJ, Blezer EL, Vrenken H, et al. Does high-field MR imaging improve cortical lesion detection in multiple sclerosis? J Neurol 2008;255(2): 183–91. Available at: http://www.ncbi.nlm.nih.gov/pubmed/18231704. Accessed June 20, 2011.

43. Simon B, Schmidt S, Lukas C, et al. Improved in vivo detection of cortical lesions in multiple sclerosis using double inversion recovery MR imaging at 3 Tesla. Eur Radiol 2010;20(7):1675–83. Available at: http://www.pubmedcentral.nih.gov/articlerender.fcgi?artid=2882050&tool=pmcentrez&rendertype=abstract. Accessed June 20, 2011.

44. Kangarlu A, Bourekas EC, Ray-Chaudhury A, et al. Cerebral cortical lesions in multiple sclerosis detected by MR imaging at 8 Tesla. AJNR Am J Neuroradiol 2007;28(2):262–6. Available at: http://www.ncbi.nlm.nih.gov/pubmed/17296991. Accessed June 20, 2011.

45. Kollia K, Maderwald S, Putzki N, et al. First clinical study on ultra-high-field MR imaging in patients with multiple sclerosis: comparison of 1.5T and 7T. AJNR Am J Neuroradiol 2009;30(4):699–702. Available at: http://www.ncbi.nlm.nih.gov/pubmed/19147714. Accessed October 1, 2010.

46. Mainero C, Benner T, Radding A, et al. In vivo imaging of cortical pathology in multiple sclerosis using ultra-high field MRI. Neurology 2009;73(12):941–8.

Available at: http://www.pubmedcentral.nih.gov/articlerender.fcgi?artid=2754332&tool=pmcentrez&rendertype=abstract. Accessed November 2, 2010.

47. Pitt D, Boster A, Pei W, et al. Imaging cortical lesions in multiple sclerosis with ultra-high-field magnetic resonance imaging. Arch Neurol 2010; 67(7):812–8. Available at: http://www.ncbi.nlm.nih.gov/pubmed/20625086. Accessed June 20, 2011.

48. Schmierer K, Parkes HG, So PW, et al. High field (9.4 Tesla) magnetic resonance imaging of cortical grey matter lesions in multiple sclerosis. Brain 2010;133(Pt 3):858–67. Available at: http://www.ncbi.nlm.nih.gov/pubmed/20123726. Accessed August 20, 2010.

49. Calabrese M, De Stefano N, Atzori M, et al. Detection of cortical inflammatory lesions by double inversion recovery magnetic resonance imaging in patients with multiple sclerosis. Arch Neurol 2007;64(10):1416–22. Available at: http://www.ncbi.nlm.nih.gov/pubmed/17923625. Accessed June 20, 2011.

50. Calabrese M, Gallo P. Magnetic resonance evidence of cortical onset of multiple sclerosis. Mult Scler 2009;15(8):933–41. Available at: http://www.ncbi.nlm.nih.gov/pubmed/19667021. Accessed June 20, 2011.

51. Calabrese M, Rocca MA, Atzori M, et al. Cortical lesions in primary progressive multiple sclerosis: a 2-year longitudinal MR study. Neurology 2009; 72(15):1330–6. Available at: http://www.ncbi.nlm.nih.gov/pubmed/19365054. Accessed December 20, 2010.

52. Calabrese M, Rocca MA, Atzori M, et al. A 3-year magnetic resonance imaging study of cortical lesions in relapse-onset multiple sclerosis. Ann Neurol 2010;67(3):376–83. Available at: http://www.ncbi.nlm.nih.gov/pubmed/20373349. Accessed June 20, 2011.

53. Calabrese M, Agosta F, Rinaldi F, et al. Cortical lesions and atrophy associated with cognitive impairment in relapsing-remitting multiple sclerosis. Arch Neurol 2009;66(9):1144–50. Available at: http://www.ncbi.nlm.nih.gov/pubmed/19752305. Accessed January 30, 2011.

54. Roosendaal SD, Moraal B, Pouwels PJ, et al. Accumulation of cortical lesions in MS: relation with cognitive impairment. Mult Scler 2009;15(6): 708–14. Available at: http://www.ncbi.nlm.nih.gov/pubmed/19435749. Accessed September 8, 2010.

55. Filippi M, Rocca MA, Calabrese M, et al. Intracortical lesions: relevance for new MRI diagnostic criteria for multiple sclerosis. Neurology 2010; 75(22):1988–94. Available at: http://www.ncbi.nlm.nih.gov/pubmed/21115953. Accessed July 11, 2011.

56. Geurts JJ, Roosendaal SD, Calabrese M, et al. Consensus recommendations for MS cortical

lesion scoring using double inversion recovery MRI. Neurology 2011;76(5):418–24. Available at: http://www.ncbi.nlm.nih.gov/pubmed/21209373. Accessed March 14, 2011.

57. Wansapura JP, Holland SK, Dunn RS, et al. NMR relaxation times in the human brain at 3.0 tesla. J Magn Reson Imaging 1999;9(4):531–8. Available at: http://www.ncbi.nlm.nih.gov/pubmed/10232510. Accessed June 23, 2011.

58. Willinek WA, Kuhl CK. 3.0 T neuroimaging: technical considerations and clinical applications. Neuroimaging Clin N Am 2006;16(2):217–28, ix. Available at: http://www.ncbi.nlm.nih.gov/pubmed/16731361. Accessed June 23, 2011.

59. Krautmacher C, Willinek WA, Tschampa HJ, et al. Brain tumors: full- and half-dose contrast-enhanced MR imaging at 3.0 T compared with 1.5 T—initial experience. Radiology 2005;237(3):1014–9. Available at: http://www.ncbi.nlm.nih.gov/pubmed/16237142. Accessed June 23, 2011.

60. Vellinga MM, Oude Engberink RD, Seewann A, et al. Pluriformity of inflammation in multiple sclerosis shown by ultra-small iron oxide particle enhancement. Brain 2008;131(Pt 3):800–7. Available at: http://www.ncbi.nlm.nih.gov/pubmed/18245785. Accessed November 3, 2010.

61. Lycklama G, Thompson A, Filippi M, et al. Spinal-cord MRI in multiple sclerosis. Lancet Neurol 2003;2(9):555–62. Available at: http://www.ncbi.nlm.nih.gov/pubmed/12941578. Accessed June 25, 2011.

62. Bot JC, Barkhof F, Lycklama à Nijeholt G, et al. Differentiation of multiple sclerosis from other inflammatory disorders and cerebrovascular disease: value of spinal MR imaging. Radiology 2002;223(1):46–56. Available at: http://www.ncbi.nlm.nih.gov/pubmed/11930047. Accessed July 11, 2011.

63. Losseff NA, Webb SL, O'Riordan JI, et al. Spinal cord atrophy and disability in multiple sclerosis. A new reproducible and sensitive MRI method with potential to monitor disease progression. Brain 1996;119(Pt 3):701–8. Available at: http://www.ncbi.nlm.nih.gov/pubmed/8673483. Accessed July 11, 2011.

64. Nijeholt GJ, van Walderveen MA, Castelijns JA, et al. Brain and spinal cord abnormalities in multiple sclerosis. Correlation between MRI parameters, clinical subtypes and symptoms. Brain 1998;121(Pt 4):687–97. Available at: http://www.ncbi.nlm.nih.gov/pubmed/9577394. Accessed July 11, 2011.

65. Kendi AT, Tan FU, Kendi M, et al. MR spectroscopy of cervical spinal cord in patients with multiple sclerosis. Neuroradiology 2004;46(9):764–9. Available at: http://www.ncbi.nlm.nih.gov/pubmed/15258708. Accessed June 25, 2011.

66. Agosta F, Absinta M, Sormani MP, et al. In vivo assessment of cervical cord damage in MS patients: a longitudinal diffusion tensor MRI study. Brain 2007;130(Pt 8):2211–9. Available at: http://www.ncbi.nlm.nih.gov/pubmed/17535835. Accessed August 20, 2010.

67. Ciccarelli O, Wheeler-Kingshott CA, McLean MA, et al. Spinal cord spectroscopy and diffusion-based tractography to assess acute disability in multiple sclerosis. Brain 2007;130(Pt 8):2220–31. Available at: http://www.ncbi.nlm.nih.gov/pubmed/17664178. Accessed April 21, 2011.

68. Nijeholt GJ, Bergers E, Kamphorst W, et al. Post-mortem high-resolution MRI of the spinal cord in multiple sclerosis: a correlative study with conventional MRI, histopathology and clinical phenotype. Brain 2001;124(Pt 1):154–66. Available at: http://www.ncbi.nlm.nih.gov/pubmed/11133795. Accessed June 25, 2011.

69. Bot JC, Blezer EL, Kamphorst W, et al. The spinal cord in multiple sclerosis: relationship of high-spatial-resolution quantitative MR imaging findings to histopathologic results. Radiology 2004;233(2):531–40. Available at: http://www.ncbi.nlm.nih.gov/pubmed/15385682. Accessed June 212011.

70. Gilmore CP, Geurts JJ, Evangelou N, et al. Spinal cord grey matter lesions in multiple sclerosis detected by post-mortem high field MR imaging. Mult Scler 2009;15(2):180–8. Available at: http://www.ncbi.nlm.nih.gov/pubmed/18845658. Accessed June 25, 2011.

71. Stankiewicz JM, Neema M, Alsop DC, et al. Spinal cord lesions and clinical status in multiple sclerosis: A 1.5 T and 3 T MRI study. J Neurol Sci 2009;279(1–2):99–105. Available at: http://www.pubmedcentral.nih.gov/articlerender.fcgi?artid=2679653&tool=pmcentrez&rendertype=abstract. Accessed September 8, 2010.

72. Klein JP, Arora A, Neema M, et al. A 3T MR imaging investigation of the topography of whole spinal cord atrophy in multiple sclerosis. AJNR Am J Neuroradiol 2011;32(6):1138–42. Available at: http://www.ncbi.nlm.nih.gov/pubmed/21527570. Accessed June 20, 2011.

73. Wattjes MP, Harzheim M, Kuhl CK, et al. Does high-field MR imaging have an influence on the classification of patients with clinically isolated syndromes according to current diagnostic MR imaging criteria for multiple sclerosis? AJNR Am J Neuroradiol 2006;27(8):1794–8. Available at: http://www.ncbi.nlm.nih.gov/pubmed/16971638. Accessed May 30, 2011.

74. Wattjes MP, Harzheim M, Lutterbey GG, et al. Does high field MRI allow an earlier diagnosis of multiple sclerosis? J Neurol 2008;255(8):1159–63. Available at: http://www.ncbi.nlm.nih.gov/pubmed/18446305. Accessed May 30, 2011.

75. Kilsdonk ID, Barkhof F, Wattjes MP. 2010 Revisions to McDonald criteria for diagnosis of MS: impact of 3 Tesla MRI. Ann Neurol 2011;70(1):182–3.

76. Available at: http://www.fda.gov/downloads/MedicalDevices/DeviceRegulationandGuidance/GuidanceDocuments/ucm072688.pdf. Accessed July 11, 2011.

77. de Graaf WL, Zwanenburg JJ, Visser F, et al. Lesion detection at 7 Tesla in multiple sclerosis using 3D magnetisation prepared 3D-FLAIR and 3D-DIR. Eur Radiol 2012;22(1):221–31.

78. Ge Y, Zohrabian VM, Grossman RI. Seven-Tesla magnetic resonance imaging: new vision of microvascular abnormalities in multiple sclerosis. Arch Neurol 2008;65(6):812–6. Available at: http://www.pubmedcentral.nih.gov/articlerender.fcgi?artid=2579786&tool=pmcentrez&rendertype=abstract. Accessed September 24, 2010.

79. Hammond KE, Metcalf M, Carvajal L, et al. Quantitative in vivo magnetic resonance imaging of multiple sclerosis at 7 Tesla with sensitivity to iron. Ann Neurol 2008;64(6):707–13. Available at: http://www.ncbi.nlm.nih.gov/pubmed/19107998. Accessed June 21, 2011.

80. Tallantyre EC, Brookes MJ, Dixon JE, et al. Demonstrating the perivascular distribution of MS lesions in vivo with 7-Tesla MRI. Neurology 2008;70(22):2076–8. Available at: http://www.ncbi.nlm.nih.gov/pubmed/18505982. Accessed June 28, 2011.

81. Tallantyre EC, Morgan PS, Dixon JE, et al. A comparison of 3T and 7T in the detection of small parenchymal veins within MS lesions. Invest Radiol 2009;44(9):491–4. Available at: http://www.ncbi.nlm.nih.gov/pubmed/19652606. Accessed September 8, 2010.

82. Tallantyre EC, Dixon JE, Donaldson I, et al. Ultra-high-field imaging distinguishes MS lesions from asymptomatic white matter lesions. Neurology 2011;76(6):534–9. Available at: http://www.pubmedcentral.nih.gov/articlerender.fcgi?artid=3053180&tool=pmcentrez&rendertype=abstract. Accessed June 21, 2011.

83. LeVine SM. Iron deposits in multiple sclerosis and Alzheimer's disease brains. Brain Res 1997;760(1–2):298–303. Available at: http://www.ncbi.nlm.nih.gov/pubmed/9237552. Accessed June 21, 2011.

84. Schmierer K, Parkes HG, So PW. Direct visualization of remyelination in multiple sclerosis using T2-weighted high-field MRI. Neurology 2009;72(5):472. Available at: http://www.pubmedcentral.nih.gov/articlerender.fcgi?artid=2635938&tool=pmcentrez&rendertype=abstract. Accessed June 21, 2011.

85. Lassmann H, Brück W, Lucchinetti C. Heterogeneity of multiple sclerosis pathogenesis: implications for diagnosis and therapy. Trends Mol Med 2001;7(3):115–21. Available at: http://www.ncbi.nlm.nih.gov/pubmed/11286782. Accessed September 26, 2010.

86. De Stefano N, Filippi M. MR spectroscopy in multiple sclerosis. J Neuroimaging 2007;17(Suppl 1):31S–5S. Available at: http://www.ncbi.nlm.nih.gov/pubmed/17425732. Accessed July 8, 2011.

87. Matthews PM, De Stefano N, Narayanan S, et al. Putting magnetic resonance spectroscopy studies in context: axonal damage and disability in multiple sclerosis. Semin Neurol 1998;18(3):327–36. Available at: http://www.ncbi.nlm.nih.gov/pubmed/9817537. Accessed July 8, 2011.

88. Miller DH, Thompson AJ, Filippi M. Magnetic resonance studies of abnormalities in the normal appearing white matter and grey matter in multiple sclerosis. J Neurol 2003;250(12):1407–19. Available at: http://www.ncbi.nlm.nih.gov/pubmed/14673572. Accessed July 9, 2011.

89. Wattjes MP, Barkhof F. High field MRI in the diagnosis of multiple sclerosis: high field-high yield? Neuroradiology 2009;51(5):279–92. Available at: http://www.ncbi.nlm.nih.gov/pubmed/19277621. Accessed May 30, 2011.

90. Davie CA, Barker GJ, Thompson AJ, et al. ^{1}H magnetic resonance spectroscopy of chronic cerebral white matter lesions and normal appearing white matter in multiple sclerosis. J Neurol Neurosurg Psychiatr 1997;63(6):736–42. Available at: http://www.pubmedcentral.nih.gov/articlerender.fcgi?artid=2169838&tool=pmcentrez&rendertype=abstract. Accessed June 21, 2011.

91. De Stefano N, Matthews PM, Antel JP, et al. Chemical pathology of acute demyelinating lesions and its correlation with disability. Ann Neurol 1995;38(6):901–9. Available at: http://www.ncbi.nlm.nih.gov/pubmed/8526462. Accessed July 9, 2011.

92. De Stefano N, Matthews PM, Fu L, et al. Axonal damage correlates with disability in patients with relapsing-remitting multiple sclerosis. Results of a longitudinal magnetic resonance spectroscopy study. Brain 1998;121:1469–77. Available at: http://www.ncbi.nlm.nih.gov/pubmed/9712009. Accessed July 9, 2011.

93. Srinivasan R, Vigneron D, Sailasuta N, et al. A comparative study of myo-inositol quantification using LCmodel at 1.5 T and 3.0 T with 3 D ^{1}H proton spectroscopic imaging of the human brain. Magn Reson Imaging 2004;22(4):523–8. Available at: http://www.ncbi.nlm.nih.gov/pubmed/15120172. Accessed September 8, 2010.

94. Schubert F, Gallinat J, Seifert F, et al. Glutamate concentrations in human brain using single voxel proton magnetic resonance spectroscopy at 3 Tesla. Neuroimage 2004;21(4):1762–71. Available at: http://www.ncbi.nlm.nih.gov/pubmed/15050596. Accessed June 21, 2011.

95. Hurd R, Sailasuta N, Srinivasan R, et al. Measurement of brain glutamate using TE-averaged PRESS at 3T. Magn Reson Med 2004;51(3):435–40. Available at: http://www.ncbi.nlm.nih.gov/pubmed/15004781. Accessed August 3, 2010.

96. Tkác I, Oz G, Adriany G, et al. In vivo ^{1}H NMR spectroscopy of the human brain at high magnetic fields: metabolite quantification at 4T vs. 7T. Magn Reson Med 2009;62(4):868–79. Available at: http://www.pubmedcentral.nih.gov/articlerender.fcgi?artid=2843548&tool=pmcentrez&rendertype=abstract. Accessed June 21, 2011.

97. Bielicki G, Chassain C, Renou JP, et al. Brain GABA editing by localized in vivo (1)H magnetic resonance spectroscopy. NMR Biomed 2004;17(2):60–8. Available at: http://www.ncbi.nlm.nih.gov/pubmed/15052553. Accessed August 26, 2010.

98. Wattjes MP, Harzheim M, Lutterbey GG, et al. Axonal damage but no increased glial cell activity in the normal-appearing white matter of patients with clinically isolated syndromes suggestive of multiple sclerosis using high-field magnetic resonance spectroscopy. AJNR Am J Neuroradiol 2007;28(8):1517–22. Available at: http://www.ncbi.nlm.nih.gov/pubmed/17846203. Accessed July 9, 2011.

99. Wattjes MP, Harzheim M, Lutterbey GG, et al. High field MR imaging and [1]H-MR spectroscopy in clinically isolated syndromes suggestive of multiple sclerosis: correlation between metabolic alterations and diagnostic MR imaging criteria. J Neurol 2008;255(1):56–63. Available at: http://www.ncbi.nlm.nih.gov/pubmed/18080854. Accessed June 21, 2011.

100. Wattjes MP, Harzheim M, Lutterbey GG, et al. Prognostic value of high-field proton magnetic resonance spectroscopy in patients presenting with clinically isolated syndromes suggestive of multiple sclerosis. Neuroradiology 2008;50(2):123–9. Available at: http://www.ncbi.nlm.nih.gov/pubmed/17982745. Accessed November 9, 2010.

101. Srinivasan R, Sailasuta N, Hurd R, et al. Evidence of elevated glutamate in multiple sclerosis using magnetic resonance spectroscopy at 3 T. Brain 2005;128(Pt 5):1016–25. Available at: http://www.ncbi.nlm.nih.gov/pubmed/15758036. Accessed June 21, 2011.

102. Inglese M, Madelin G, Oesingmann N, et al. Brain tissue sodium concentration in multiple sclerosis: a sodium imaging study at 3 tesla. Brain 2010;133(Pt 3):847–57. Available at: http://www.pubmedcentral.nih.gov/articlerender.fcgi?artid=2842511&tool=pmcentrez&rendertype=abstract. Accessed November 23, 2010.

103. Srinivasan R, Ratiney H, Hammond-Rosenbluth KE, et al. MR spectroscopic imaging of glutathione in the white and gray matter at 7 T with an application

104. Rovaris M, Gass A, Bammer R, et al. Diffusion MRI in multiple sclerosis. Neurology 2005;65(10):1526–32. Available at: http://www.ncbi.nlm.nih.gov/pubmed/16301477. Accessed June 21, 2011.

105. Goldberg-Zimring D, Mewes AU, Maddah M, et al. Diffusion tensor magnetic resonance imaging in multiple sclerosis. J Neuroimaging 2005;15(4 Suppl):68S–81S. Available at: http://www.ncbi.nlm.nih.gov/pubmed/16385020. Accessed June 21, 2011.

106. Pagani E, Bammer R, Horsfield MA, et al. Diffusion MR imaging in multiple sclerosis: technical aspects and challenges. AJNR Am J Neuroradiol 2007;28(3):411–20. Available at: http://www.ncbi.nlm.nih.gov/pubmed/17353305. Accessed October 26, 2010.

107. Filippi M, Iannucci G, Cercignani M, et al. A quantitative study of water diffusion in multiple sclerosis lesions and normal-appearing white matter using echo-planar imaging. Arch Neurol 2000;57(7):1017–21. Available at: http://www.ncbi.nlm.nih.gov/pubmed/10891984. Accessed June 21, 2011.

108. Cercignani M, Inglese M, Pagani E, et al. Mean diffusivity and fractional anisotropy histograms of patients with multiple sclerosis. AJNR Am J Neuroradiol 2001;22(5):952–8. Available at: http://www.ncbi.nlm.nih.gov/pubmed/11337342. Accessed November 2, 2010.

109. Rocca MA, Cercignani M, Iannucci G, et al. Weekly diffusion-weighted imaging of normal-appearing white matter in MS. Neurology 2000;55(6):882–4. Available at: http://www.ncbi.nlm.nih.gov/pubmed/10994017. Accessed June 7, 2011.

110. Bozzali M, Cercignani M, Sormani MP, et al. Quantification of brain gray matter damage in different MS phenotypes by use of diffusion tensor MR imaging. AJNR Am J Neuroradiol 2002;23(6):985–8. Available at: http://www.ncbi.nlm.nih.gov/pubmed/12063230. Accessed June 22, 2011.

111. Vrenken H, Pouwels PJ, Geurts JJ, et al. Altered diffusion tensor in multiple sclerosis normal-appearing brain tissue: cortical diffusion changes seem related to clinical deterioration. J Magn Reson Imaging 2006;23(5):628–36. Available at: http://www.ncbi.nlm.nih.gov/pubmed/16565955. Accessed June 7, 2011.

112. Benedict RH, Bruce J, Dwyer MG, et al. Diffusion-weighted imaging predicts cognitive impairment in multiple sclerosis. Mult Scler 2007;13(6):722–30. Available at: http://www.ncbi.nlm.nih.gov/pubmed/17613599. Accessed June 23, 2011.

113. Pruessmann KP, Weiger M, Scheidegger MB, et al. SENSE: sensitivity encoding for fast MRI. Magn Reson Med 1999;42(5):952–62. Available at: http://www.ncbi.nlm.nih.gov/pubmed/10542355. Accessed June 23, 2011.

114. Okada T, Miki Y, Fushimi Y, et al. Diffusion-tensor fiber tractography: intraindividual comparison of 3.0-T and

1.5-T MR imaging. Radiology 2006;238(2):668–78. Available at: http://www.ncbi.nlm.nih.gov/pubmed/16396839. Accessed June 23, 2011.

115. Jaermann T, Crelier G, Pruessmann KP, et al. SENSE-DTI at 3 T. Magn Reson Med 2004;51(2): 230–6. Available at: http://www.ncbi.nlm.nih.gov/pubmed/14755645. Accessed June 23, 2011.

116. Ceccarelli A, Rocca MA, Falini A, et al. Normal-appearing white and grey matter damage in MS. A volumetric and diffusion tensor MRI study at 3.0 Tesla. J Neurol 2007;254(4):513–8. Available at: http://www.ncbi.nlm.nih.gov/pubmed/17401516. Accessed June 23, 2011.

117. Ceccarelli A, Rocca MA, Pagani E, et al. The topographical distribution of tissue injury in benign MS: a 3T multiparametric MRI study. Neuroimage 2008; 39(4):1499–509. Available at: http://www.ncbi.nlm.nih.gov/pubmed/18155611. Accessed December 29, 2010.

118. Reich DS, Zackowski KM, Gordon-Lipkin EM, et al. Corticospinal tract abnormalities are associated with weakness in multiple sclerosis. AJNR Am J Neuroradiol 2008;29(2):333–9. Available at: http://www.pubmedcentral.nih.gov/articlerender.fcgi?artid=2802714&tool=pmcentrez&rendertype=abstract. Accessed June 7, 2011.

119. Naismith RT, Xu J, Tutlam NT, et al. Disability in optic neuritis correlates with diffusion tensor-derived directional diffusivities. Neurology 2009;72(7):589–94. Available at: http://www.pubmedcentral.nih.gov/articlerender.fcgi?artid=2672917&tool=pmcentrez&rendertype=abstract. Accessed November 9, 2010.

120. Rocca MA, Filippi M. Functional MRI in multiple sclerosis. J Neuroimaging 2007;17(Suppl 1): 36S–41S. Available at: http://www.ncbi.nlm.nih.gov/pubmed/17425733. Accessed July 11, 2011.

121. Rocca MA, Mezzapesa DM, Falini A, et al. Evidence for axonal pathology and adaptive cortical reorganization in patients at presentation with clinically isolated syndromes suggestive of multiple sclerosis. Neuroimage 2003;18(4):847–55. Available at: http://www.ncbi.nlm.nih.gov/pubmed/12725761. Accessed June 23, 2011.

122. Filippi M, Rocca MA, Mezzapesa DM, et al. Simple and complex movement-associated functional MRI changes in patients at presentation with clinically isolated syndromes suggestive of multiple sclerosis. Hum Brain Mapp 2004;21(2):108–17. Available at: http://www.ncbi.nlm.nih.gov/pubmed/14755598. Accessed June 23, 2011.

123. Rocca MA, Colombo B, Falini A, et al. Cortical adaptation in patients with MS: a cross-sectional functional MRI study of disease phenotypes. Lancet Neurol 2005; 4(10):618–26. Available at: http://www.ncbi.nlm.nih.gov/pubmed/16168930. Accessed May 25, 2011.

124. Rocca MA, Absinta M, Ghezzi A, et al. Is a preserved functional reserve a mechanism limiting clinical impairment in pediatric MS patients? Hum Brain Mapp 2009;30(9):2844–51. Available at: http://www.ncbi.nlm.nih.gov/pubmed/19107755. Accessed June 23, 2011.

125. Ogawa S, Lee T, Kay A, et al. Brain magnetic resonance imaging with contrast dependent on blood oxygenation. Proc Natl Acad Sci U S A 1990; 87(24):9868. Available at: http://www.pnas.org/content/87/24/9868.short. Accessed June 23, 2011.

126. Gati JS, Menon RS, Ugurbil K, et al. Experimental determination of the BOLD field strength dependence in vessels and tissue. Magn Reson Med 1997;38(2): 296–302. Available at: http://www.ncbi.nlm.nih.gov/pubmed/9256111. Accessed June 23, 2011.

127. Hoenig K, Kuhl CK, Scheef L. Functional 3.0-T MR assessment of higher cognitive function: are there advantages over 1.5-T imaging? Radiology 2005; 234(3):860–8. Available at: http://www.ncbi.nlm.nih.gov/pubmed/15650039. Accessed June 23, 2011.

128. Rocca MA, Tortorella P, Ceccarelli A, et al. The "mirror-neuron system" in MS: a 3 tesla fMRI study. Neurology 2008;70(4):255–62. Available at: http://www.ncbi.nlm.nih.gov/pubmed/18077798.

129. Rocca MA, Riccitelli G, Rodegher M, et al. Functional MR imaging correlates of neuropsychological impairment in primary-progressive multiple sclerosis. AJNR Am J Neuroradiol 2010;31(7):1240–6. Available at: http://www.ncbi.nlm.nih.gov/pubmed/20299439. Accessed June 23, 2011.

130. Rocca MA, Pagani E, Absinta M, et al. Altered functional and structural connectivities in patients with MS: a 3-T study. Neurology 2007;69(23):2136–45. Available at: http://www.ncbi.nlm.nih.gov/pubmed/18056577. Accessed June 24, 2011.

131. Rocca MA, Absinta M, Valsasina P, et al. Abnormal connectivity of the sensorimotor network in patients with MS: a multicenter fMRI study. Hum Brain Mapp 2009;30(8):2412–25. Available at: http://www.ncbi.nlm.nih.gov/pubmed/19034902. Accessed June 24, 2011.

132. Ceccarelli A, Rocca MA, Valsasina P, et al. Structural and functional magnetic resonance imaging correlates of motor network dysfunction in primary progressive multiple sclerosis. Eur J Neurosci 2010;31(7): 1273–80. Available at: http://www.ncbi.nlm.nih.gov/pubmed/20345920. Accessed June 23, 2011.

133. Scarabino T, Giannatempo GM, Popolizio T, et al. 3.0-T functional brain imaging: a 5-year experience. Radiol Med 2007;112(1):97–112. Available at: http://www.ncbi.nlm.nih.gov/pubmed/17310287. Accessed June 23, 2011.

134. Vrenken H, Rombouts SA, Pouwels PJ, et al. Voxel-based analysis of quantitative T1 maps demonstrates that multiple sclerosis acts throughout the normal-appearing white matter. AJNR Am J Neuroradiol 2006;27:868–74.

135. Vrenken H, Geurts J, Knol D, et al. Whole-brain T1 mapping in multiple sclerosis: global changes of normal-appearing gray and white matter1. Radiology 2006;240(3):811–20. Available at: http://radiology.rsna.org/content/240/3/811.short. Accessed July 27, 2011.

136. Bermel RA, Bakshi R. The measurement and clinical relevance of brain atrophy in multiple sclerosis. Lancet Neurol 2006;5(2):158–70. Available at: http://www.ncbi.nlm.nih.gov/pubmed/16426992. Accessed July 10, 2011.

137. Giorgio A, Battaglini M, Smith SM, et al. Brain atrophy assessment in multiple sclerosis: importance and limitations. Neuroimaging Clin N Am 2008;18(4): 675–86. Available at: http://www.ncbi.nlm.nih.gov/pubmed/19068408. Accessed July 10, 2011, xi.

138. Stankiewicz J, Panter SS, Neema M, et al. Iron in chronic brain disorders: imaging and neurotherapeutic implications. Neurotherapeutics 2007;4(3): 371–86. Available at: http://www.pubmedcentral.nih.gov/articlerender.fcgi?artid=1963417&tool=pmcentrez&rendertype=abstract. Accessed July 10, 2011.

139. Craelius W, Migdal M, Luessenhoop C, et al. Iron deposits surrounding multiple sclerosis plaques. Arch Pathol Lab Med 1982;106(3):397–9.

140. Lassmann H, Brück W, Lucchinetti CF. The immunopathology of multiple sclerosis: an overview. Brain Pathol 2007;17(2):210–8. Available at: http://www.ncbi.nlm.nih.gov/pubmed/17388952. Accessed June 30, 2011.

141. Hallgren B, Sourander P. The effect of age on the non-haemin iron in the human brain. J Neurochem 1958;3(1):41–51. Available at: http://www.ncbi.nlm.nih.gov/pubmed/13611557. Accessed July 10, 2011.

142. Ropele S, de Graaf W, Khalil M, et al. MRI assessment of iron deposition in multiple sclerosis. J Magn Reson Imaging 2011;34(1):13–21. Available at: http://www.ncbi.nlm.nih.gov/pubmed/21698703. Accessed July 11, 2011.

143. Drayer B, Burger P, Hurwitz B, et al. Reduced signal intensity on MR images of thalamus and putamen in multiple sclerosis: increased iron content? AJR Am J Roentgenol 1987;149(2):357–63. Available at: http://www.ncbi.nlm.nih.gov/pubmed/3496764. Accessed July 10, 2011.

144. Bakshi R, Shaikh ZA, Janardhan V. MRI T2 shortening ('black T2') in multiple sclerosis: frequency, location, and clinical correlation. Neuroreport 2000; 11(1):15–21. Available at: http://www.ncbi.nlm.nih.gov/pubmed/10683822. Accessed February 28, 2011.

145. Ge Y, Jensen JH, Lu H, et al. Quantitative assessment of iron accumulation in the deep gray matter of multiple sclerosis by magnetic field correlation imaging. AJNR Am J Neuroradiol 2007;28(9): 1639–44. Available at: http://www.ncbi.nlm.nih.gov/pubmed/17893225. Accessed July 11, 2011.

146. Khalil M, Enzinger C, Langkammer C, et al. Quantitative assessment of brain iron by R(2)* relaxometry in patients with clinically isolated syndrome and relapsing-remitting multiple sclerosis. Mult Scler 2009;15(9):1048–54. Available at: http://www.ncbi.nlm.nih.gov/pubmed/19556316. Accessed July 11, 2011.

147. Barkhof F, Pouwels PJ, Wattjes MP. The Holy Grail in diagnostic neuroradiology: 3T or 3D? Eur Radiol 2011;21(3):449–56. Available at: http://www.pubmedcentral.nih.gov/articlerender.fcgi?artid=3032195&tool=pmcentrez&rendertype=abstract. Accessed July 4, 2011.

High-Field Imaging of Neurodegenerative Diseases

M.J. Versluis, MSc[a],*, J. van der Grond, PhD[a],
M.A. van Buchem, MD, PhD[a], P. van Zijl, PhD[b,c],
A.G. Webb, PhD[a]

KEYWORDS

- Neurodegenerative disease • 7 Tesla • Spectroscopy
- High-resolution imaging • MR angiography
- Susceptibility-weighted imaging

Key Points

- Preliminary studies have shown that high-field MR imaging is possible in patients with neurodegenerative diseases.
- High-field MR imaging is sensitive to detect the perivenous location of MS lesions and the frequent cortical involvement, difficult to visualize at lower field strengths.
- Visualization of the lenticulostriate arteries is possible in patients with CADASIL.
- Localized spectroscopy in patients can be performed in small anatomic structures allowing for improved metabolite quantification, including glutamate.
- High-resolution structural imaging revealed local changes in the hippocampus in patients with AD or HS.
- A new type of image contrast based on signal phase has been developed called quantitative magnetic susceptibility imaging.

POTENTIAL OF HIGH-FIELD MAGNETIC RESONANCE IMAGING FOR NEURODEGENERATIVE DISEASES

The increase in static magnetic field strength for clinical magnetic resonance (MR) imaging scanners has resulted in significant improvements in image quality. There is almost universal improvement in the diagnostic value of 3 T versus 1.5 T clinical neurologic MR imaging scans, and 3 T scanners are routinely used for a broad range of applications. The need for increased sensitivity to

early indicators of neurodegeneration with the goal of identifying potential biomarkers for diagnosis and the monitoring of treatment is one of the driving forces behind the interest in further increasing the magnetic field strength. The well-characterized signal-to-noise ratio (SNR) increase with field strength can be used for reduced acquisition times or higher spatial resolution. The increased sensitivity of image contrast (particularly in T_2^*-weighted sequences) to tissue iron levels has great potential for the detection of early diffuse depositions that may lead to neurotoxic effects.

The authors have nothing to disclose.
[a] Department of Radiology, C.J. Gorter Center for High Field MR, Leiden University Medical Center, Albinusdreef 2, 2333 ZA Leiden, The Netherlands
[b] Department of Radiology and Radiological Sciences, Johns Hopkins University School of Medicine, Traylor Building, Room 217, 720 Rutland Avenue, Baltimore, MD 21205, USA
[c] F.M. Kirby Research Center for Functional Brain Imaging, Kennedy Krieger Institute, 707 North Broadway Street, Baltimore, MD 21205, USA
* Corresponding author.
E-mail address: m.j.versluis@lumc.nl

<table>
<tr><td>

Diagnostic Checklist

Despite the limited number of clinical studies that have been performed, 7 T MR imaging has been shown to provide high sensitivity for:

- High-resolution MR angiography using a TOF technique to visualize small arteries, such as the lenticulostriate arteries in patients with CADASIL
- Detection of iron depositions in basal ganglia, a common finding in many patients with neurodegenerative diseases
- Detection of lesions in patients with MS, specifically the sensitivity to detect the presence of a central vein within the lesions is increased compared to lower field strengths
- Detection of cerebral microbleeds, a common finding in many patients with neurodegenerative diseases
- Imaging with high detail of the hippocampal substructures, a region of interest for patients with HS, or AD
- Detection of brain metabolites using MR spectroscopy in small anatomical structures, such as the putamen and the caudate nucleus, that could provide further insight in neurodegenerative disease processes

</td></tr>
</table>

There is a new type of image contrast based on signal phase, but this contrast depends on the brain orientation[1] and its interpretation needs to be further developed, which is the topic of a relatively new approach called quantitative magnetic susceptibility imaging.[2–5] In addition, the orientation of WM bundles also affects this contrast, which has to be described using a susceptibility tensor.[1,2] The longer T_1 value of both blood and tissue results in higher-quality MR angiography with improved background suppression. Furthermore, the increased difference in chemical shift between the proton signals of different metabolites has an advantage for MR spectroscopy in quantifying more metabolites than previously possible.[6,7]

Initial imaging studies of multiple sclerosis (MS) patients at 7 T seem promising in detecting more lesions with higher structural detail,[8–10] especially in gray matter (GM). In addition to the improved spatial resolution and SNR, the increased contrast in MR angiography[11] and cortical layer contrast in $T_2{}^*$-weighted imaging[12] have already demonstrated the potential of 7 T MR imaging. However, many intrinsic challenges remain in obtaining high-quality MR data at field strengths of 7 T and higher.

CHALLENGES

The main challenges are related to creating a homogeneous magnetic field (B_0) and radiofrequency (RF) field B_1 over the whole brain. A higher magnetic field strength results in increased sensitivity to magnetic susceptibility–induced field variations. On a microscopic scale this effect enhances the contrast within cortical layers,[12,13] basal ganglia,[14] and small venous structures,[15–17] and results in greater white matter (WM) heterogeneity.[18] However, large-scale magnetic field variations induced by, for example, air-tissue interfaces (static) or respiration (dynamic), can lead to undesired signal loss and image deformations. Most modern high-field MR imaging scanners are equipped with higher-order shim gradients to improve the static field homogeneity. Careful optimization of sequence parameters and image-correction algorithms has shown that it is possible to acquire high-quality images even from sequences such as echo-planar imaging, which are particularly susceptible to static magnetic field inhomogeneities. Equally problematic, the amplitude of dynamically fluctuating magnetic fields caused by respiration or body movements also increases with field strength. It has been shown that corrections for these dynamic effects are possible both prospectively and retrospectively. Using dedicated hardware or sequences,[19–21] image quality can be restored reasonably well.

Another fundamental challenge at 7 T is producing a highly homogeneous RF field, B_1, with high efficiency, to minimize tissue heating. B_1 inhomogeneities are due primarily to the dielectric properties of tissue, which result in partial constructive and destructive interactions from RF wave behavior.[22] Tissue conductivity produces conduction currents in tissue, which dampens the electromagnetic (EM) field as it penetrates through tissue, producing a phase shift in the traveling RF. This process not only results in significant image inhomogeneity and areas of signal loss, but may also give rise to local heating, expressed as the specific absorption rate (SAR) from interaction with the electric field. The dielectric properties of tissue produce displacement currents in tissue and inductive losses caused by eddy currents, and also alter the RF wavelength in tissue. The effective wavelength of electromagnetic energy in tissue is approximately 13 cm at 7 T. The brain has dimensions on the same order as the wavelength. This situation limits the applicability of conventional volume coils, such as the birdcage[23] and transverse electromagnetic (TEM) resonator,[24] which produce homogeneous transmit fields at 1.5 T and 3 T, but cannot produce the same homogeneous fields at 7 T.[22] The inhomogeneous RF field in combination with increased tissue heating leads to important sequence considerations. SAR-intensive protocols involving sequences such as fast spin echo and fluid-attenuated inversion recovery (FLAIR) cannot simply be copied from lower field strengths. Solutions are discussed in the section on future prospects and challenges.

Despite these challenges, 7 T MR imaging is beginning to be used in a clinical setting and the theoretical benefits of 7 T, namely higher SNR, sensitivity to iron, improved MR angiography, and spectroscopy are being confirmed. Although thus far only a limited number of patient studies have been performed at 7 T and many of the proposed techniques still need further validation. Initial imaging studies of MS patients at 7 T seem promising in detecting more lesions with higher structural detail,[8–10] especially in GM. In addition to the improved spatial resolution and SNR, the increased contrast in MR angiography[11] and the detection of cortical layer contrast in T_2^*-weighted imaging[12] have already demonstrated the potential of 7 T MR imaging.

NEURODEGENERATIVE DISEASES

This section describes some of the clinical studies with 7 T MR imaging that have been performed to date in patients suffering from neurodegenerative diseases. A selection of the used sequences is given in **Table 1**.

CADASIL

Cerebral autosomal dominant arteriopathy with subcortical infarcts and leukoencephalopathy (CADASIL) is a hereditary form of small-vessel disease that is caused by a mutation in the Notch3 gene. Pathologically, degeneration of the small smooth vessels is observed together with fibrous thickening of the small vessels. Clinical characteristics of the disease are cognitive loss, migrainous headaches, strokelike episodes, and dementia. In addition, cerebral blood flow is known to be reduced in CADASIL patients. However, the exact mechanism remains unclear, and most findings regarding vessel wall pathology come from ex vivo studies. In vivo MR angiography can potentially provide valuable information on the hemodynamic changes in CADASIL patients. The most affected vessels are the leptomeningeal arteries supplying the WM and the lenticulostriate perforating arteries supplying the deep gray nuclei. At lower field strengths, MR angiography has been unable to visualize these arteries because of their small diameter. However, recent studies performed at

7 T show sufficient enhancements in resolution and contrast, enabling visualization of the lenticulostriate arteries.[11,25,26] The method that is most suited is time-of-flight (TOF) MR angiography, whereby the contrast is generated by the fresh inflow of blood with a gradient echo sequence that is relatively SAR friendly. The prolonged T_1 relaxation times at 7 T result in improved background saturation compared with lower field strengths, increasing the contrast between the vessel lumen and surrounding tissue. In addition, the increase in SNR can be traded for a very high spatial resolution. In a recent study this was confirmed by visualization of significant lengths of the lenticulostriate arteries[27] in patients with CADASIL and control subjects. **Fig. 1** shows an example of a coronal maximum-intensity projection of the lenticulostriate arteries in a healthy control subject and in a patient with CADASIL. A small field-of-view (FOV) 3-dimensional TOF MR angiography technique was used with an isotropic resolution of $0.23 \times 0.23 \times 0.23$ mm^3 and 161 slices, resulting in a scan duration of 11 minutes. From these data sets, the number of visible arteries at different locations with respect to the middle and anterior cerebral artery, the cross-sectional area, and length of the arteries were determined. No significant differences were found between patients and controls in any of the measures. In addition, no association was found between the luminal diameters and lacunar infarct load in the basal ganglia and basal ganglia hypointensities on separately acquired T_2-, T_2^*-, or T_1-weighted scans.[27] These results suggest that basal ganglia damage in CADASIL is likely not caused by vascular mechanisms. The lack of association between age and disease duration with these vascular measurements further supports the finding that generalized narrowing of luminal diameters of lenticulostriate arteries does not play a significant role in the pathophysiology of CADASIL.

Another common MR imaging finding in patients with CADASIL are hypointensities on T_2^*-weighted images[27,28] caused by iron-containing hemosiderin deposits in cerebral microbleeds (CMBs). **Fig. 2** shows CMBs observed bilaterally in the thalamus of a 35-year-old patient with CADASIL on T_2^*- and T_1-weighted images. Initial results have shown diffuse areas of T_2^* hypointensity in the basal ganglia, most commonly caused by diffuse iron deposition in CADASIL.[29] Such diffuse areas have also been described in other neurodegenerative diseases such as Alzheimer disease (AD). Nevertheless, whether iron deposition is exclusively a neurodegenerative process or whether it can also be caused by vascular mechanisms is unsure. High-field T_2^*-weighted MR imaging is

Table 1
Selection of recommended sequences applied in clinical studies of neurodegenerative diseases at 7 T

Sequence	Resolution (mm³)	TR (ms)/TE (ms)/FA	Slices/Orientation	Specific Parameters	Parallel Imaging	Scan Duration	Refs.
3D TOF	$0.23 \times 0.23 \times 0.23$	16/4.1/30°	161/Transverse		RL = 3	10 min 40 s	25,27
2D T_2^*	$0.24 \times 0.24 \times 1$	1770/25/60°	46/Transverse	Retrospective f_0 correction	RL = 2.2	10 min 00 s	18,20
2D T_2	$0.5 \times 0.5 \times 1$	3000/56/90°	35/Transverse	Turbo factor = 12, refocusing angle = 105°		9 min 09 s	27
3D T_1	$0.9 \times 0.9 \times 0.9$	4.2/1.87/7°	193/Sagittal	TI = 1300 ms, turbo factor = 350	AP × RL = 2 × 2.5	2 min 30 s	
3D FLAIR	$0.8 \times 0.8 \times 0.8$	8000/300/90°	225/Sagittal	TI = 2200 ms, T_{2prep} = 100 ms, refocusing angle = 70°	AP × RL = 2.5 × 2.5	12 min 30 s	39

More details can be found in the text and in the referenced studies.

Abbreviations: 2D, 2-dimensional; 3D, 3-dimensional; AP, anterior-posterior; FLAIR, fluid-attenuated inversion recovery; FA, flip angle; RL, right-left; TE, echo time; TI, inversion time; TOF, time-of-flight; TR, repetition time; T_{2prep}, T_2 preparation echo time.

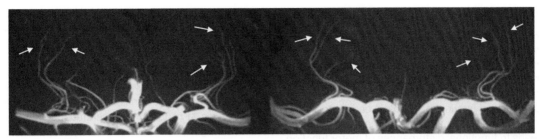

Fig. 1. Coronal maximum-intensity projections of a 32-year-old healthy control (*left*) and a 32-year-old patient with CADASIL (*right*). The arrows indicate the lenticulostriate arteries. Excellent visualization of large portions of the lenticulostriate arteries was possible, due to the high spatial resolution and contrast between the artery and surrounding tissue. No significant differences in length, diameter, and number of lenticulostriate arteries was found, suggesting that basal ganglia damage in patients with CADASIL is not caused by luminal narrowing of these vessels.

extremely sensitive to changes in the local magnetic field, such as those generated by iron-rich regions. These changes in local magnetic field lead to decreased signal intensity on magnitude images and an increased frequency shift (relative to non–iron-containing brain tissue) on phase images. Preliminary data of high-resolution T_2*-weighted images using a 2-dimensional gradient echo sequence obtained with a resolution of $0.24 \times 0.24 \times 1$ mm[329] demonstrated increased iron deposition in the globus pallidus and the caudate nucleus. These findings were based on both magnitude images and unwrapped phase images. Both approaches gave similar results, but the phase-shift measurements showed larger differences, emphasizing the sensitivity of phase to iron-induced changes in the brain.

In summary, high-field MR imaging can provide useful additional information in understanding CADASIL abnormalities, given the high-resolution TOF images, sensitivity to CMBs,[30] and diffuse iron deposition.

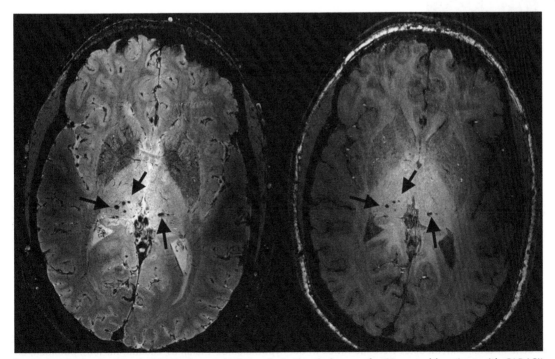

Fig. 2. Cerebral microbleeds (CMB) observed bilaterally in the thalamus of a 35-year-old patient with CADASIL, visualized on a T_2*-weighted (*left*) and T_1-weighted (*right*) scan. The arrows point to the CMB. Accurate visualization of CMB is possible at high magnetic field strengths because of the induced susceptibility effect of hemosiderin deposits in the microbleeds. The sensitivity to detect CMB is highest on T_2*-weighted scans.

Huntington Disease

Huntington disease (HD) is a neurodegenerative autosomal dominant disorder caused by a gene mutation on the short arm of chromosome 4. A repeat expansion of the cytosine-adenine-guanine gene leads to an abnormally increased synthesis of huntingtin, a protein causing neuronal damage and brain atrophy. Ultimately the disease leads to functional disturbances of motor function, cognition, and behavior. Brain atrophy measurements, particularly of the striatum, are considered the MR imaging hallmark of the disease, showing changes up to a decade before clinical manifestations of the disease occur. The exact disease mechanism underlying these volume changes remains unclear. Several proposed theories include impaired energy metabolism and the degeneration of neurons caused by neuronal overstimulation (excitotoxicity). MR spectroscopy offers additional insight into which processes may play a role in these volume changes, by measuring, for example, N-acetylaspartate (NAA), creatine, and glutamate

concentrations. If the neuronal integrity were to be compromised, NAA would be expected to be reduced. Changes in energy deposition may be reflected in total creatine signals. By contrast, an increase in glutamate levels would reflect overstimulation of neurons. Lower-field MR spectroscopy studies have shown conflicting results, especially for findings in glutamate concentrations.[31] Higher field strength provides improved spectral resolution, allowing more metabolites to be quantified.[6,7] This quantification can be done with better spatial localization (smaller volumes) owing to increased SNR. In a study by Van den Bogaard and colleagues,[31] localized MR spectroscopy was performed using a stimulated echo acquisition mode (STEAM) sequence in the caudate nucleus, putamen, thalamus, hypothalamus, and frontal lobe in patients with manifest and premanifest HD. Using 7 T MR spectroscopy, 6 metabolites were identified in all of these nuclei: choline, creatine, glutamine + glutamate, total NAA, myo-inositol, and lactate; this despite the significant brain atrophy, which led to reduced SNR. **Fig. 3** shows MR spectra in the

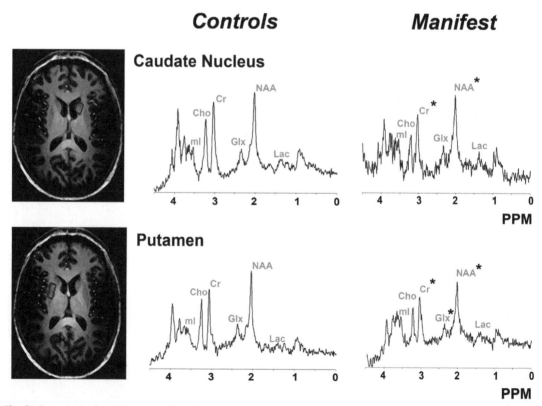

Fig. 3. Representative MR spectra from the caudate nucleus and putamen in a control subject and manifest HD patient. In total, 6 metabolites were identified in the hypothalamus, thalamus, caudate nucleus, putamen, and the prefrontal region. In the caudate nucleus and putamen, a significant decrease in NAA and creatine levels was found in manifest HD patients. Glutamate levels were found to decrease significantly in the putamen. Significance changes are depicted by asterisks, P<.05. Cho, choline; Cr, creatine; Glx, glutamate + glutamine; Lac, lactate; ml, myo-inositol; NAA, N-acetylaspartate; PPM, parts per million.

caudate nucleus and putamen of control subjects and manifest patients. Lower concentrations of creatine and NAA were found in the caudate nucleus and the putamen, and a reduction of glutamate in the putamen, of manifest HD patients. Moreover, an association between disease severity and metabolic levels of NAA, creatine, and glutamate was demonstrated. The results from this study indicate affected energy metabolism in HD patients reflected in lower creatine concentrations, and a decrease in neuronal integrity reflected in lower NAA concentrations. In contrast to other studies, a lower concentration of glutamate was found in the putamen of manifest patients. This study showed that 7 T allows measurement of reliable glutamate concentrations, thereby obtaining additional insight in the disease process.

In summary, the increased spectral and spatial resolution of 7 T MR spectroscopy offer capabilities that are not possible at lower field strengths. It allows for the examination of metabolites in small anatomic structures that are important in many neurodegenerative diseases, such as the caudate nucleus and putamen, in clinically acceptable scanning times.

Multiple Sclerosis

Research in MS has been most active since the introduction of 7 T MR imaging scanners. MS manifests itself through demyelinating lesions that can be detected by MR imaging. Conventional protocols use FLAIR and dual inversion recovery (DIR) sequences to suppress signal from cerebrospinal fluid (CSF) or from both CSF and WM, respectively, to highlight WM lesions. In addition, gadolinium contrast agents can be administered to distinguish active lesions from older lesions on T_1-weighted images. Histology has revealed that lesions not only occur in WM but also frequently affect GM, and that MS lesions have a preference for a perivenular location. The high spatial resolution and sensitivity of high-field MR imaging facilitates the detection of GM lesions and the perivenous location of lesions, which is more difficult at lower field strengths.

To make effective use of the high contrast generated by venous blood and to circumvent the difficulties implementing B_1-sensitive and SAR-intensive sequences such as FLAIR and DIR, many studies have focused on T_2*-weighted sequences. Using this type of contrast it was found that between 50% and 87% of lesions contain a central vein.[9,10,32–34] Compared with lower field strengths, a significantly lower number of lesions containing a central vein was found. At 1.5 T no central venous structure was observed in any of the detected lesions,[9] whereas twice as many lesions with a central vein were detected at 7 T than were detected at 3 T.[10] **Fig. 4** shows a large WM lesion visualized using T_2*-weighted MR imaging, comparing 7 T and 3 T.[10] It is immediately apparent that the contrast within the lesion is enhanced at 7 T and that the perivenous location of the lesion can be appreciated.

The presence of a central vein in WM lesions may be an imaging characteristic that helps differentiating MS-related lesions from other WM

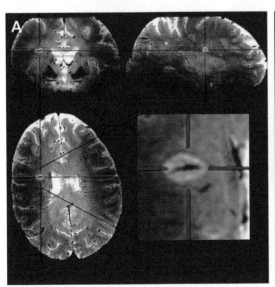
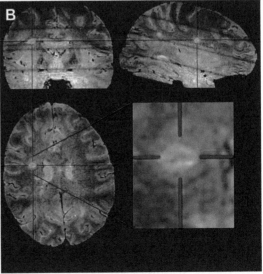

Fig. 4. T_2*-weighted MR imaging shows more detail of central veins in MS lesions at 7 T than at 3 T. T_2* images of a patient with MS showing a large lesion with a perivenous orientation. On the 7 T image (*A*), the vein can be seen in more detail than on the equivalent 3 T image (*B*). (*Courtesy of* Dr Emma Tallantyre.)

lesions. This aspect may be important in designing therapies targeted at MS lesions and monitoring disease progression, and also may help to provide insight into the mechanisms of lesion formation.[32] The presence of a central vessel has been found to be highly indicative of MS-specific lesions. In a comparison between MS patients and subjects with WM lesions that were nonspecific to MS, 80% of MS lesions had a perivenous location compared with only 19% in WM lesions not related to MS.[34] The high sensitivity of 7 T in detecting perivascular signal changes is due to the susceptibility effect of venous blood. The effect of induced changes in the local magnetic field scales linearly with the applied magnetic field strength. Therefore, the use of a sensitive method such as a T_2*-weighted sequence at high-field strength greatly improves the contrast generated by venous blood.

Besides WM lesions, GM lesions are a frequent finding in MS. GM MS lesions, however, can be very difficult to detect at lower field strengths. The increased spatial resolution at 7 T increases the number of visible GM lesions. **Fig. 5** shows an example of an MS patient with a cortical GM lesion.[35] In one study no GM lesions were detected in patients at 1.5 T, whereas 44% of the lesions detected at 7 T showed cortical involvement.[9] This finding was confirmed by other studies

at 7 T.[35,36] In line with other neurodegenerative diseases, higher iron deposition is expected in patients with MS. The high sensitivity to iron of 7 T has led to the investigation of MS lesions using phase images.[8,36,37] However, initial studies found that phase images have a lower sensitivity in detecting MS lesions[36] than do the magnitude images. Between 8% and 21% of WM lesions show a characteristic ring around the lesion that is not readily visible on magnitude images.[8,36] This ring is thought to occur via iron-rich macrophages and, as such, may provide information about the extent of inflammation around the MS lesion.[9,36]

T_2*-weighted sequences were identified as being the most sensitive in detecting lesions, in comparison with other sequences[36] and lower field strength.[9] Recently, progress has been made in reducing the SAR requirements of FLAIR and DIR sequences at 7 T while maintaining comparable or improved contrast and spatial resolution.[38,39] A recent study has shown the applicability of high-field FLAIR and DIR sequences in detecting MS lesions.[40]

In summary, MS research at 7 T is promising. The difficulty in designing FLAIR and DIR sequences at 7 T has to date resulted in the most frequent use of T_2*-weighted sequences to

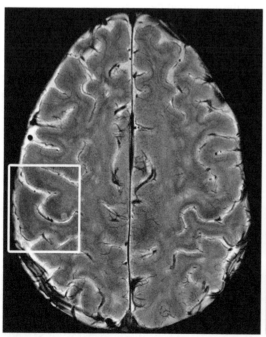 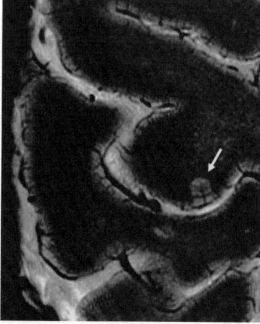

Fig. 5. Axial T_2*-weighted image (195 × 260 μm) of an MS patient with a cortical GM lesion at 7 T. Image on the right is an enlargement of the region around the GM lesion (*boxed area on the left*), demonstrating fine detail within the cortical lesion at this high magnetic field, and fine spatial resolution. Arrow indicates the GM lesion. (*Courtesy of* Drs Vigneron, Metcalf, and Pelletier.)

detect MS lesions. The high contrast and spatial resolution of this sequence provides an additional type of sequence to investigate MS lesions, especially suited for high magnetic field strengths.

Other Neurodegenerative Diseases

There have been several other clinical studies regarding neurodegenerative diseases at 7 T. Most studies use the same contrast mechanisms as mentioned in the previous sections. In amyotrophic lateral sclerosis (ALS) patients, 7 T MR imaging was used to investigate the presence of CMBs. In animal models of this disease, deposits of hemosiderin and CMBs were found; by contrast, no CMBs were found in sporadic ALS patients.[41] Regarding patients with AD, a limited number of studies has been published. One of the hallmarks of AD is the presence amyloid beta plaques, a protein thought to be associated with iron. The small size of these plaques (typically smaller than 150 μm)[42] makes direct in vivo visualization difficult although not impossible. Using localized coils and a limited FOV, a resolution of the same order of magnitude as individual plaques has been obtained in a reasonable scan time.[43] Susceptibility-weighted imaging (SWI) after processing was performed to enhance the sensitivity to susceptibility changes,[44] such as induced by iron. The results of this study suggest that plaques can be visualized using this technique. It remains unclear, however, whether the observed signal voids represent individual plaques or not. In addition to the presence of plaques, early in the process of the disease brain atrophy occurs. One of the first brain regions affected by AD is the hippocampus; however, not all subsections of the hippocampus are affected in a similar way. These different subregions can be distinguished using high-resolution T_2*-weighted imaging sequences. One study has shown that in the very early stage of AD, changes can be observed in the hippocampal subregion, CA1 apical neuropil.[45] From postmortem studies this region is known to be among the earliest affected in the brain, and this was confirmed in vivo at 7 T. Along the same lines are findings in patients with hippocampal sclerosis (HS), in whom accurate visualization of subregions within the hippocampus is important for diagnosis. HS leads to atrophy of the intrahippocampal cortical field CA1 to CA4 regions, and to disruption of the internal hippocampal structure. In a study of focal epilepsy patients with HS, the intrahippocampal cortical fields were well visualized on T_2- and T_2*-weighted sequences.[46] Regional differences in hippocampal atrophy were shown between patients. In a different study, similar findings were reported using T_1- and T_2-weighted imaging. Hippocampal abnormalities were observed in all patients. Using 7 T MR imaging, localized atrophy in the Ammon horn was observed in patients with temporal lobe epilepsy.[47]

A small number of patients with Parkinson disease (PD) has been studied at 7 T. The symptoms of PD can sometimes be reduced by deep brain stimulation, which is a neurosurgical technique that relies on the accurate placement of electrodes. Using high-resolution SWI, high contrast can be generated between the iron-rich basal ganglia. It has been shown that high-quality images can be obtained that help to guide the placement of these electrodes.[48,49]

FUTURE PROSPECTS AND CHALLENGES

In general, the theoretical gain in SNR and sensitivity of high-field MR imaging to, for example, diffuse iron accumulation have been shown to be achievable in practice. Transmit RF field inhomogeneity is still a major concern, but by using dedicated sequences that are less sensitive to these inhomogeneities some of these effects can be circumvented.[50,51] By placing high dielectric materials close to the brain, the transmit field becomes more homogeneous.[52,53] The coverage toward the cerebellum in particular is improved, and the effect of high signal centrally in the brain is reduced. The ultimate solution, although currently only in the technical development phase, is the use of multiple transmit channels to improve the transmit homogeneity. Preliminary results already show some added value, and one can anticipate that it will not take long before this technique is used in a clinical setting.

Sequence adaptations have not been trivial; the increased RF deposition and inhomogeneous transmit field preclude the simple translation from lower field strength protocols to 7 T. However, all conventional image contrasts (T_1-, T_2-, T_2*-weighted, and FLAIR) are currently available with high image quality. To limit the need for additional scans at lower field strength, it is important to have these image contrasts available.

Magnetic susceptibility–induced field changes scale linearly with the applied field strength, which leads to an increased sensitivity to iron accumulation in the brain[13,14] and WM heterogeneity[18] detected in T_2*-weighted sequences. An adverse effect is that the sensitivity to unwanted field changes is also increased. Air-tissue interfaces at the edge of the brain or near the sinuses generate a static inhomogeneous magnetic field. Shim gradients, up to third order, are used to compensate for these changes. However, the

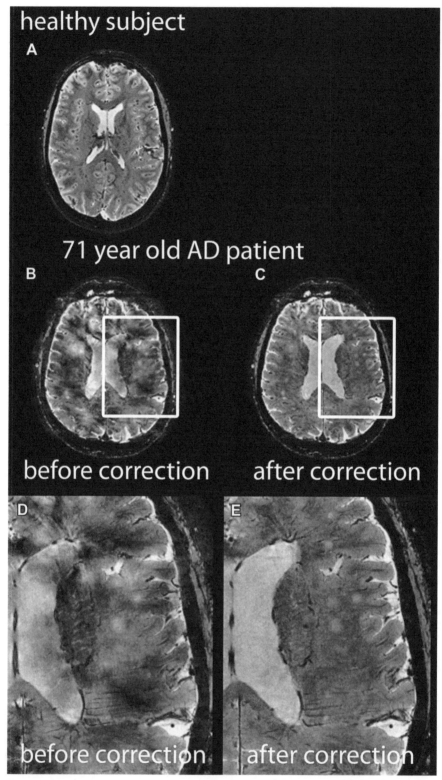

Fig. 6. T$_2$*-weighted images obtained in a healthy subject (*A*), showing the high image quality and contrast that can be obtained. Application of the same sequence in patients with AD leads to frequent image degradation (*B*, *D*) caused by fluctuating magnetic fields during image acquisition. Using a navigator echo correction technique, it is possible to measure and correct for these dynamic fluctuations and improve image quality significantly (*C*, *E*). Correction techniques like these improve image quality at high field strength.

effects of dynamic susceptibility changes are also enhanced, leading to ghosting and image blurring. It has been shown that breathing[19,54] and body movements[55] can lead to substantial magnetic field changes in the brain. In a study in AD patients, image artifacts were observed that were related to dynamic magnetic field changes.[20] **Fig. 6** shows a transverse slice from a T_2^*-weighted sequence in a healthy subject and an AD patient. The image quality is severely reduced in the AD patient. After navigator-based image correction for the effects of the magnetic field changes, most image artifacts are suppressed. Still more advanced is to measure the field changes in real time using separate field probes that are positioned around the brain,[21,56] but this may not be clinically practical.

There has been rapid development of sequences and hardware since the introduction of 7 T MR systems. As a result, most conventional sequences are available and high-quality images are obtained in the brain. Based on the results to date, 7 T MR imaging is showing potential to be valuable in investigating neurodegenerative diseases. In patients with MS an increased number of lesions can be detected and, more importantly, there is greater sensitivity in detecting GM lesions. In addition to the increased sensitivity, the pathophysiology of these lesions can be studied more extensively at high-field strength. It was shown that most MS lesions have a clear vascular component. However, some lesions also showed up on phase images surrounded by a hypointense rim, possibly reflecting the area of inflammation or potentially a susceptibility effect. In patients with HD it was possible to quantify metabolite levels, including glutamate, in very small regions of interest, providing valuable information about possible disease mechanisms. The sensitivity to iron and the high spatial resolution leads to a clearer depiction of the substantia nigra and other deep GM nuclei in PD.

Even though only a limited number of clinical studies has been performed thus far, it is expected that the contribution of 7 T MR imaging, especially in the field of neurodegenerative diseases, will increase over time. Many of the initial problems related to magnetic and RF field inhomogeneities and the lack of optimized sequences have been solved or improved.

REFERENCES

1. Lee J, Shmueli K, Fukunaga M, et al. Sensitivity of MRI resonance frequency to the orientation of brain tissue microstructure. Proc Natl Acad Sci U S A 2010;107:5130–5.

2. Liu C. Susceptibility tensor imaging. Magn Reson Med 2010;63(6):1471–7.

3. Wharton S, Bowtell R. Whole-brain susceptibility mapping at high field: a comparison of multiple- and single-orientation methods. Neuroimage 2010; 53(2):515–25.

4. Schweser F, Deistung A, Lehr BW, et al. Quantitative imaging of intrinsic magnetic tissue properties using MRI signal phase: an approach to in vivo brain iron metabolism? Neuroimage 2011;54(4): 2789–807.

5. de Rochefort L, Liu T, Kressler B, et al. Quantitative susceptibility map reconstruction from MR phase data using Bayesian regularization: validation and application to brain imaging. Magn Reson Med 2010; 63(1):194–206.

6. Tkác I, Oz G, Adriany G, et al. In vivo ^{1}H NMR spectroscopy of the human brain at high magnetic fields: metabolite quantification at 4T vs. 7T. Magn Reson Med 2009;62(4):868–79.

7. Mekle R, Mlynárik V, Gambarota G, et al. MR spectroscopy of the human brain with enhanced signal intensity at ultrashort echo times on a clinical platform at 3T and 7T. Magn Reson Med 2009;61(6): 1279–85.

8. Hammond KE, Metcalf M, Carvajal L, et al. Quantitative in vivo magnetic resonance imaging of multiple sclerosis at 7 Tesla with sensitivity to iron. Ann Neurol 2008;64(6):707–13.

9. Kollia K, Maderwald S, Putzki N, et al. First clinical study on ultra-high-field MR imaging in patients with multiple sclerosis: comparison of 1.5T and 7T. AJNR Am J Neuroradiol 2009;30(4):699–702.

10. Tallantyre EC, Morgan PS, Dixon JE, et al. A comparison of 3T and 7T in the detection of small parenchymal veins within MS lesions. Invest Radiol 2009; 44(9):491–4.

11. Kang CK, Park CW, Han JY, et al. Imaging and analysis of lenticulostriate arteries using 7.0-Tesla magnetic resonance angiography. Magn Reson Med 2009;61(1):136–44.

12. Duyn JH, van Gelderen P, Li TQ, et al. High-field MRI of brain cortical substructure based on signal phase. Proc Natl Acad Sci U S A 2007;104(28): 11796–801.

13. Fukunaga M, Li TQ, van Gelderen P, et al. Layer-specific variation of iron content in cerebral cortex as a source of MRI contrast. Proc Natl Acad Sci U S A 2010;107(8):3834–9.

14. Yao B, Li TQ, Gelderen P, et al. Susceptibility contrast in high field MRI of human brain as a function of tissue iron content. Neuroimage 2009;44(4): 1259–66.

15. Conijn MM, Geerlings MI, Luijten PR, et al. Visualization of cerebral microbleeds with dual-echo T2*-weighted magnetic resonance imaging at 7.0 T. J Magn Reson Imaging 2010;32(1):52–9.

16. Koopmans P, Manniesing R, Niessen W, et al. MR venography of the human brain using susceptibility

weighted imaging at very high field strength. MAGMA 2008;21(1):149–58.

17. Theysohn JM, Kraff O, Maderwald S, et al. 7 tesla MRI of microbleeds and white matter lesions as seen in vascular dementia. J Magn Reson Imaging 2011;33(4):782–91.

18. Li TQ, van Gelderen P, Merkle H, et al. Extensive heterogeneity in white matter intensity in high-resolution T2*-weighted MRI of the human brain at 7.0 T. Neuroimage 2006;32(3):1032–40.

19. Van Gelderen P, de Zwart JA, Starewicz P, et al. Real-time shimming to compensate for respiration-induced B0 fluctuations. Magn Reson Med 2007; 57(2):362–8.

20. Versluis MJ, Peeters JM, van Rooden S, et al. Origin and reduction of motion and f0 artifacts in high resolution T2*-weighted magnetic resonance imaging: application in Alzheimer's disease patients. Neuroimage 2010;51(3):1082–8.

21. Wilm BJ, Barmet C, Pavan M, et al. Higher order reconstruction for MRI in the presence of spatiotemporal field perturbations. Magn Reson Med 2011;65(6):1690–701.

22. Webb AG, Collins CM. Parallel transmit and receive technology in high-field magnetic resonance neuroimaging. Int J Imaging Syst Technol 2010;20(1):2–13.

23. Hayes CE, Edelstein WA, Schenck JF, et al. An efficient, highly homogeneous radiofrequency coil for whole-body NMR imaging at 1.5 T. J Magn Reson 1985;63:622–8.

24. Vaughan JT, Hetherington HP, Otu JO, et al. High frequency volume coils for clinical NMR imaging and spectroscopy. Magn Reson Med 1994;32(2): 206–18.

25. Kang CK, Park CA, Kim KN, et al. Non-invasive visualization of basilar artery perforators with 7T MR angiography. J Magn Reson Imaging 2010;32(3): 544–50.

26. Zwanenburg JJ, Hendrikse J, Takahara T, et al. MR angiography of the cerebral perforating arteries with magnetization prepared anatomical reference at 7T: Comparison with time-of-flight. J Magn Reson Imaging 2008;28(6):1519–26.

27. Liem MK, van der Grond J, Versluis MJ, et al. Lenticulostriate arterial lumina are normal in cerebral autosomal-dominant arteriopathy with subcortical infarcts and leukoencephalopathy. Stroke 2010; 41(12):2812–6.

28. Jouvent E, Poupon C, Gray F, et al. Intracortical infarcts in small vessel disease. Stroke 2011;42(3): e27–30.

29. Liem MK, Oberstein SA, Versluis MJ, et al. Diffuse iron deposition in the putamen and caudate nucleus in CADASIL: comparing phase and magnitude images at 7 Tesla. Proceedings of the International Society of Magnetic Resonance in Medicine. Montreal (Canada), 2011.

30. Conijn MM, Geerlings MI, Biessels G-J, et al. Cerebral microbleeds on MR imaging: comparison between 1.5 and 7T. AJNR Am J Neuroradiol 2011; 32(6):1043–9.

31. van den Bogaard SJA, Dumas EM, Teeuwisse WM, et al. Exploratory 7-Tesla magnetic resonance spectroscopy in Huntington's disease provides in vivo evidence for impaired energy metabolism. J Neurol 2011;258(12):2230–9.

32. Ge Y, Zohrabian VM, Grossman RI. Seven-Tesla magnetic resonance imaging: new vision of microvascular abnormalities in multiple sclerosis. Arch Neurol 2008;65(6):812–6.

33. Tallantyre EC, Brookes MJ, Dixon JE, et al. Demonstrating the perivascular distribution of MS lesions in vivo with 7-Tesla MRI. Neurology 2008;70(22): 2076–8.

34. Tallantyre EC, Dixon JE, Donaldson I, et al. Ultra-high-field imaging distinguishes MS lesions from asymptomatic white matter lesions. Neurology 2011;76(6): 534–9.

35. Metcalf M, Xu D, Okuda DT, et al. High-resolution phased-array MRI of the human brain at 7 Tesla: initial experience in multiple sclerosis patients. J Neuroimaging 2010;20(2):141–7.

36. Mainero C, Benner T, Radding A, et al. In vivo imaging of cortical pathology in multiple sclerosis using ultra-high field MRI. Neurology 2009;73(12): 941–8.

37. Hammond KE, Lupo JM, Xu D, et al. Development of a robust method for generating 7.0 T multichannel phase images of the brain with application to normal volunteers and patients with neurological diseases. Neuroimage 2008;39(4):1682–92.

38. Zwanenburg J, Hendrikse J, Visser F, et al. Fluid attenuated inversion recovery (FLAIR) MRI at 7.0 Tesla: comparison with 1.5 and 3.0 Tesla. Eur Radiol 2010;20(4):915–22.

39. Visser F, Zwanenburg JJ, Hoogduin JM, et al. High-resolution magnetization-prepared 3D-FLAIR imaging at 7.0 Tesla. Magn Reson Med 2010;64(1):194–202.

40. de Graaf WL, Zwanenburg JJM, Visser F, et al. Lesion detection at seven Tesla in multiple sclerosis using magnetisation prepared 3D-FLAIR and 3D-DIR. Eur Radiol 2012;22(1):221–31.

41. Verstraete E, Biessels GJ, van Den Heuvel MP, et al. No evidence of microbleeds in ALS patients at 7 Tesla MRI. Amyotroph Lateral Scler 2010;11(6): 555–7.

42. van Rooden S, Maat-Schieman ML, Nabuurs RJ, et al. Cerebral amyloidosis: postmortem detection with human 7.0-T MR imaging system. Radiology 2009;253(3):788–96.

43. Nakada T, Matsuzawa H, Igarashi H, et al. In vivo visualization of senile-plaque-like pathology in Alzheimer's disease patients by MR microscopy on a 7T system. J Neuroimaging 2008;18(2):125–9.

44. Haacke EM, Xu Y, Cheng YC, et al. Susceptibility weighted imaging (SWI). Magn Reson Med 2004; 52(3):612–8.

45. Kerchner GA, Hess CP, Hammond-Rosenbluth KE, et al. Hippocampal CA1 apical neuropil atrophy in mild Alzheimer disease visualized with 7-T MRI. Neurology 2010;75(15):1381–7.

46. Breyer T, Wanke I, Maderwald S, et al. Imaging of patients with hippocampal sclerosis at 7 Tesla: initial results. Acad Radiol 2010;17(4):421–6.

47. Henry TR, Chupin M, Lehéricy S, et al. Hippocampal sclerosis in temporal lobe epilepsy: findings at 7 T[1]. Radiology 2011;261(1):199–209.

48. Abosch A, Yacoub E, Ugurbil K, et al. An assessment of current brain targets for deep brain stimulation surgery with susceptibility-weighted imaging at 7 Tesla. Neurosurgery 2010;67(6):1745–56.

49. Cho ZH, Min HK, Oh SH, et al. Direct visualization of deep brain stimulation targets in Parkinson disease with the use of 7-tesla magnetic resonance imaging. J Neurosurg 2010;113(3):639–47.

50. Moore J, Jankiewicz M, Zeng H, et al. Composite RF pulses for -insensitive volume excitation at 7 Tesla. J Magn Reson 2010;205(1):50–62.

51. Henning A, Fuchs A, Murdoch JB, et al. Slice-selective FID acquisition, localized by outer volume suppression (FIDLOVS) for (1)H-MRSI of the human brain at 7 T with minimal signal loss. NMR Biomed 2009;22(7):683–96.

52. Haines K, Smith NB, Webb AG. New high dielectric constant materials for tailoring the distribution at high magnetic fields. J Magn Reson 2010;203(2):323–7.

53. Snaar JEM, Teeuwisse WM, Versluis MJ, et al. Improvements in high-field localized MRS of the medial temporal lobe in humans using new deformable high-dielectric materials. NMR Biomed 2011; 24(7):873–9.

54. Van de Moortele PF, Pfeuffer J, Glover GH, et al. Respiration-induced B0 fluctuations and their spatial distribution in the human brain at 7 Tesla. Magn Reson Med 2002;47(5):888–95.

55. Barry RL, Williams JM, Klassen LM, et al. Evaluation of preprocessing steps to compensate for magnetic field distortions due to body movements in BOLD fMRI. Magn Reson Imaging 2010;28(2):235–44.

56. Barmet C, Zanche ND, Pruessmann KP. Spatiotemporal magnetic field monitoring for MR. Magn Reson Med 2008;60(1):187–97.

High-Field Magnetic Resonance Imaging for Epilepsy

Horst Urbach, MD, PhD

KEYWORDS

- MR imaging • High-field MR imaging • Epilepsy
- Drug-resistant epilepsy • Epilepsy surgery

Key Points

- High-field magnetic resonance (MR) imaging is currently the state-of-the-art technique for the detection and characterization of epileptogenic lesions.
- An increased signal-to-noise ratio helps to increase the spatial resolution while maintaining a high contrast between normal cortex and epileptogenic lesion.
- Subtle epileptogenic lesions are more frequently overlooked than invisible on high-quality MR imaging.

The primary goal of MR imaging in epilepsy patients is to detect an epileptogenic lesion, defined as a radiographic lesion that causes seizures.[1] These lesions are often subtle, do not change during the life span, and may even be missed by careful visual inspection.[2-5]

According to the recent International League Against Epilepsy (ILAE) classification, genetic (formerly idiopathic epilepsy syndromes with a proven or presumed genetic cause), structural, and/or metabolic and unknown epilepsy syndromes are distinguished.[6] Genetic epilepsy syndromes with a typical generalized electroencephalography (EEG) pattern involving bilaterally distributed networks are not caused by underlying structural lesions. However, whether an individual patient really suffers from a genetic epilepsy syndrome or has focal seizures with rapid secondary generalization is often unknown, not referred to the radiologist, or not adequately addressed by the radiologist.

If a patient has a first seizure, the goal of MR Imaging is rather to rule out an acute disease (eg, sinus thrombosis, encephalitis) than to visualize a subtle epileptogenic lesion. This approach justifies a lower temporal and logistic effort and involves acquisition of other sequences and contrast-medium injections, in comparison with MR imaging in patients with drug-resistant focal epilepsies. In these patients, especially if a focal epileptogenic lesion has not yet been detected with routine MR imaging, 3 T MR imaging has been proved to be superior to 1.5 T MR imaging.[7,8] Detectability of epileptogenic lesions at 3 T is improved by an increased contrast-to-noise ratio (CNR) and spatial, and thus anatomic, resolution. Because epilepsy patients are often uncooperative or mentally retarded, the length of an individual sequence should not be much longer than 5 minutes. In some instances, especially in children, MR imaging under general anesthesia or sedation is needed.

Many questions arise after an epileptogenic lesion has been detected and epilepsy surgery is considered. These questions involve the epileptogenicity of a lesion and the resectability with respect to its location in areas of eloquent cortex

The author has nothing to disclose.
Department of Radiology/Neuroradiology, University of Bonn Medical Center, Sigmund Freud Str. 25, D-53105 Bonn, Germany
E-mail address: urbach@uni-bonn.de

Neuroimag Clin N Am 22 (2012) 173–189
doi:10.1016/j.nic.2012.02.008
1052-5149/12/$ – see front matter © 2012 Elsevier Inc. All rights reserved.

Diagnostic Checklist

Do not start MR imaging without information about:

- Seizure type
- Seizure frequency (single vs multiple seizures, seizures in context of an acute disease)
- Semiology of the seizure
- Suspected etiology (genetic/idiopathic, structural/metabolic, unknown)

Check if MR images show:

- Sufficient gray/white matter contrast
- Appropriate spatial resolution
- Symmetric visualization of unaffected anatomic structures for allowing side comparisons

Interpret MR imaging

- In a clinical context as described above
- Incorporating electroencephalography findings if possible

---

or white matter tracts. Such questions may be addressed using DTI, MR spectroscopy, and/or functional MR imaging, which also benefit from high-field MR imaging, however, the present article focuses on structural MR imaging and the detection of characteristic epileptogenic lesions.

THEORETICAL CONSIDERATIONS
Signal-to-Noise Ratio

According to the increasing number of parallel spins at higher field strengths (as derived from the Boltzmann equation), the signal increases in proportion to the field strength B_0 (signal to noise $\sim B_0$). The signal theoretically doubles from 1.5 to 3 T, and in practice it increases by a factor of around 1.8. However, this higher signal-to-noise ratio (SNR) can be used to increase the CNR and the spatial resolution, or to decrease the acquisition time (**Fig. 1**).[9]

Relaxation Times

Relaxation times are a function of the applied magnetic field strength.[10] With increasing field strength, spin-lattice or longitudinal relaxation time T1 increases by 20% to 40% for most tissue.[11] At the same time, spin-spin or transversal relaxation time T2 decreases. T1 and T2 relaxation times of biological fluids such as water (ie, cerebrospinal fluid) and blood are constant between 1.5 T and 3 T; the strong prolongation of T1 of solid tissue (ie, brain) at 3 T leads to an overall lower tissue contrast on T1-weighted images.

Larmor Frequency

According to the relationship between the Larmor precession frequency and the magnetic field strength ($\omega = \gamma B_0$), the Larmor frequency increases from 63.9 MHz at 1.5 T to 127.8 MHz at 3 T.

Chemical Shift, Susceptibility, and B_1 Homogeneity

Chemical shift increases proportionally with the field strength, that is, from 220 Hz at 1.5 T to 440 Hz at 3 T. The shorter echo time (TE) at 3 T potentially decreases the sensitivity to pulsation and motion artifacts. Susceptibility, defined as the extent to which a material becomes magnetized when placed within a magnetic field, scales in proportion to the field strength, which can be both an advantage (**Fig. 2**) and disadvantage. Susceptibility can affect local tissue resonance frequencies (spin-spin relaxation) and lead to dephasing and signal loss typically in gradient echo pulse sequences. The relaxation time T2* that describes the susceptibility-induced signal loss is shortened at 3 T compared with 1.5 T.

Radiofrequency Power Deposition

Radiofrequency (RF) energy deposition is monitored by measuring the specific absorption rate (SAR), which must not exceed 4 W/kg over a 15-minute period. For comparison, RF energy deposition of most mobile phones is in the range of 0.5 to 0.75 W/kg. Because RF energy deposition scales with the square of B_0 in the range from 1.5 T to 3 T, SAR limits will be reached much earlier, limiting especially fast pulse sequences with high RF energy deposition, such as fast spin-echo sequences.

Adaption of Imaging Protocols

SAR limitations, different relaxation times, and increased susceptibility are the most important

Recommended basic MR protocol acquired at 3 T (based on Philips Intera)

	\multicolumn{6}{c}{Sequence Type}					
	3D T1 FFE	FLAIR TSE	T2 TSE	FLAIR TSE	T2 TSE	FLAIR TSE
Orientation	Sagittal	Sagittal	Axial	Coronal	Coronal	Axial
FOV	256	240	230	230	240	256
RFOV	0.95	0.9	0.8	0.8	0.9	1
Matrix	256	256	512	256	512	256
Scan%	100	72.6	80	70.6	80	100
TI	833	2850		2850		2850
TR/TE	8.2	12000	3272	12000	5765	12000
TE	3.7	120	80	140	120	140
Flip angle	8	140	90	90	90	90
R-factor		No	No	No	3	No
Slice thickness	1	3.5	5	3	2	2
Interslice gap	0	0	1	0	0	0
No. of slices	140	40	24	40	40	60
No. of excitations	1	1	1	1	6	1
Acquired voxel size (mm)	1 × 1 × 1	0.98 × 1.26 × 3.5	0.57 × 0.72 × 5	0.9 × 1.27 × 3	0.47 × 0.64 × 2	1 × 1 × 2
Reconstructed voxel size (mm)	1 × 1 × 1	0.49 × 0.49 × 3.5	0.45 × 0.45 × 5	0.45 × 0.45 × 3	0.23 × 0.23 × 2	1 × 1 × 2
Acquisition time	3 min 11 s	4 min 48 s	1 min 58 s	4 min 00 s	4 min 53 s	5 min 24 s

Abbreviations: 3D, 3-dimensional; FFE, fast field echo; FLAIR, fluid-attenuated inversion recovery; FOV, field of view; R-factor, reduction factor; RFOV, rectangular field of view; T1, T1-weighted; T2, T2-weighted; TE, echo time; TI, inversion time; TR, repetition time; TSE, turbo spin echo.

Special sequences are added to the protocol based on imaging findings or clinical hints: if there is an epileptogenic lesion other than hippocampal sclerosis, nonenhanced and contrast-enhanced spin-echo sequences are added. Contrast-medium injections are needed to characterize a lesion but not to find it.[12]

If lesions contain areas with signal loss on T2-weighted images suggesting hemosiderin deposits or calcifications or if patients present with a trauma anamnesis, T2-weighted gradient echo sequences or, as of more recently, susceptibility-weighted sequences (SWI) are added.

3 T scanners allowing the generation of 3-dimensional (3D) fluid-attenuated inversion recovery (FLAIR) sequences with isotropic voxels depict the whole brain with high spatial resolution and are, in addition, usable for multiplanar reformations and voxel-based analyses.[2,3,13] An elegant reformation is the planar surface (pancake) view, which facilitates anatomic orientation and is helpful in determining the boundaries of epileptogenic lesions. This view is generated by defining a path along the brain surface on coronal reformations, and constructing a planar curved surface view enabled by parallel shifting in an anterior and posterior direction (see **Figs. 7** and **8** later in this article).[14]

Diffusion-weighted imaging (DWI) and diffusion tensor imaging (DTI) reversible splenium lesions are helpful in characterizing so-called reversible splenium lesions, which occur more often if antiepileptic drugs are reduced or withdrawn in order to provoke epileptic seizures during presurgical workup.[15]

parameters to be adapted at 3 T.[9] Parallel imaging reduces RF energy deposition by reducing the number of phase-encoding readouts (determined by the reduction factor R) at a given TE, or it allows for the reduction of echo-train length in, for example, echo planar imaging (EPI), yielding a shorter effective TE.[16,17] This approach allows a substantial reduction in image distortion and improves image quality. In addition, the shorter TE is more motion resistant and reduces blurring in the image. Moreover, as the application of high R-factors are limited by the parallel imaging inherent signal loss (S ~ $1/\sqrt{R}$), the abundant

SNR at 3 T can be used to implement R-factors of greater than 2.[18]

Another way to reduce SAR is to acquire 3D sequences and sequences with variable refocusing flip angle. However, 2-dimensional (2D) FLAIR sequences with in-plane resolutions of less than 1 mm and slice thicknesses between 2 and 5 mm still have a higher CNR than 3D FLAIR sequences with isotropic, typically 1-mm^3 voxels, which are useful for the generation of multiplanar reformations and voxel-based analyses.

With respect to T1-weighted spin echo images, gray matter/white matter contrast is reduced at 3 T

Additional MR sequences for 3 T (based on Philips Achieva)						
	Sequence					
	T1 TSE	T2 FFE	DWI	DTI	SWI	3D FLAIR
Orientation	Coronal	Axial	Axial	Axial	Axial	Sagittal
FOV	230	230	256	256	220	250
RFOV	0.8	0.8	1	1	0.8	100
Matrix	256	256	128	128	256	228
Scan%	79.9	79.9	97.8	98.4	100	100
TI						1600
TR	550	601	3151	11374	16	4800
TE	13	18	69	63	23	309
Flip angle	90	18	90	90	10	90
R-factor	No	No	3 AP	2.2 AP	1.5 RL	2.5 AP, 2 RL
Slice thickness	5	5	5	2	1	1.1
Interslice gap	1	1	1	0	0	0
No. of slices	24	24	24	60	200	327
No. of excitations	1	1	2	1	1	2
Acquired voxel size (mm)	0.9 × 1.12 × 5	0.9 × 1.12 × 5	2 × 2.4 × 5	2 × 2.03 × 2	1 × 1 × 1	1.1 × 1.1 × 1.1
Reconstructed voxel size (mm)	0.45 × 0.45 × 5	0.45 × 0.45 × 5	1 × 1 × 5	2 × 2 × 2	0.43 × 0.43 × 0.5	0.43 × 0.43 × 0.55
Acquisition time	4 min 33 s	1 min 41 s	1 min 09 s	6 min 26 s	3 min 17 s	4 min 43 s

Abbreviations: AP, anterior-posterior; RL, right-left.

for several reasons. T1 relaxation times of gray and white matter lengthen and converge. Shielding effects induced by eddy currents prevent central parts of the image from being properly excited,[19] which results in reduced signal intensity of the basal ganglia region. Stronger magnetization transfer effects reduce signal intensity and contrast. T1-weighted gradient echo images provide a good contrast between gray and white matter; however, contrast enhancement is different and may remain undetected on gradient echo images.

A recent survey about the distribution of epileptogenic lesions operated on in a large epilepsy surgery center shows hippocampal sclerosis (HS) as the most common and also almost constant lesion over time. The number of long-term epilepsy-associated tumors (LEATs) and of patients negative on MR imaging has decreased, whereas the number of focal cortical dysplasias (FCDs) has steadily increased.[5] These main groups of epileptogenic lesions are now described in detail:

HIPPOCAMPAL SCLEROSIS
Background

HS is by far the most common cause of temporal lobe epilepsy and is found in approximately half of patients undergoing resective surgery.[20] Resective surgery, either by anterior two-thirds temporal lobe resection or selective amgydalohippocampectomy, results in complete seizure relief in at least 58% of patients. Conversely, with medical therapy only 8% of patients achieve freedom from seizures.[21]

Imaging

On MR imaging, the sclerotic hippocampus is atrophic and has an increased signal intensity on FLAIR and T2-weighted fast spin-echo images. This pattern is best visualized on thin (2–3 mm thick) coronal images perpendicular to the longitudinal axis of the hippocampus. CNR is higher on FLAIR than on T2-weighted images (**Figs. 3 and 4**); however, already normal limbic structures have an increased FLAIR signal intensity compared with the remaining cortex.[22] High-resolution T2-weighted fast spin-echo images at 3 T visualize hippocampal substructures precisely (see **Figs. 3 and 4**) and are therefore suited to detect mild forms of HS, which, however, account for only around 5% of epilepsy surgery series.[23,24] Associated lesions such as amygdala atrophy, entorhinal cortex atrophy, atrophy of ipsilateral corpus mamillare, atrophy of ipsilateral fornix,

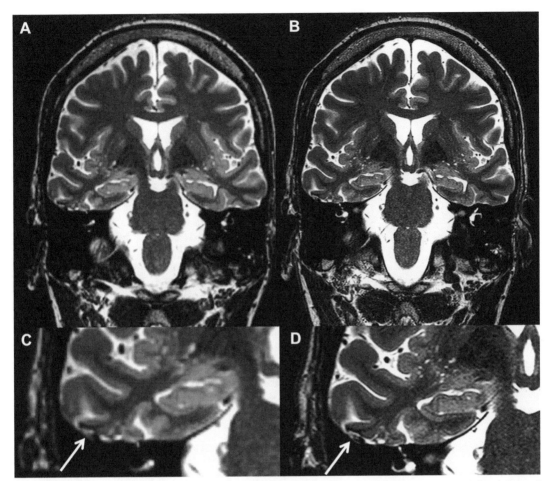

Fig. 1. A circumscribed temporobasal cortical contusion (*arrow*) is better visible on a T2-weighted fast spin sequence with higher spatial resolution (*B, D*: 0.47 × 0.64 × 2 mm vs *A, C*: 0.93 × 0.93 × 2 mm).

and gray/white matter demarcation loss of the anterior temporal lobe are also better visualized on 3 T than on 1.5 T MR imaging.

EPILEPSY-ASSOCIATED TUMORS
Background

Neuroepithelial tumors are found in 20% to 30% of patients with long-term drug-resistant epilepsy.[25] Clinically, 2 different groups exist in this cohort. The first group contains typical epilepsy-associated tumors such as gangliogliomas, dysembryoplastic neuroepithelial tumors (DNTs), pleomorphic xanthoastrocytomas (pXAs), supratentorial pilocytic astrocytomas, World Health Organization (WHO) grade I, and, recently added to the WHO classification, angiocentric gliomas with an usually benign behavior.[26] The second group consists of diffuse astrocytomas (WHO grade II) and oligodendrogliomas (WHO grade II), with a 5-year-survival rate of 50% to 65%, and

a few anaplastic cases, classified as WHO grade III, with a median survival time of 2 to 3 years.

Imaging

Gangliogliomas are consistently located in the cortex or in the cortex and subcortical white matter, and have a spatial preponderance for the parahippocampal and lateral temporo-occipital gyri (**Fig. 5**). The classic imaging features are the combination of intracortical cyst(s), a circumscribed area of cortical (and subcortical) signal increase on FLAIR and T2-weighted images, and a contrast-enhancing nodule. Calcifications are present in one-third of cases. If contrast enhancement is absent (in approximately 50% of cases), gangliogliomas may be difficult to distinguish from cortical dysplasias. The benefit of 3 T MR imaging is the visualization of highly diagnostic intracortical cysts and of different (cystic and solid) tumor components (see **Fig. 5**).

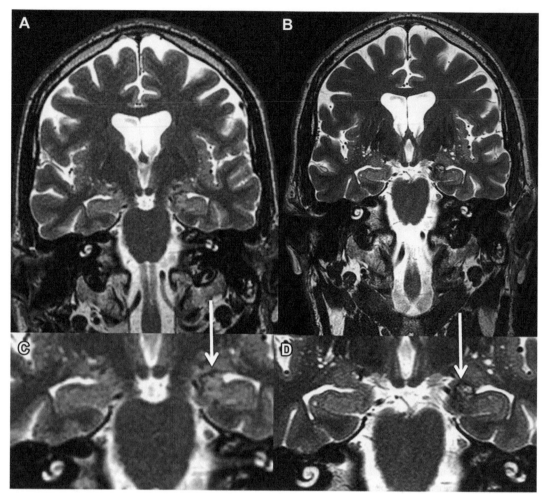

Fig. 2. A cavernoma in the left hippocampal head was overlooked on a T2-weighted fast spin echo sequence at 1.5 T (*A, C: arrow*). Because of higher susceptibility, it is clearly visible on the same sequence at 3 T (*B, D: arrow*).

DNTs are characterized by the so-called glioneuronal element, containing oligodendrocyte-like cells attached to bundles of axons and neurons floating in a myxoid interstitial fluid.[27] The oligodendrocyte-like cells cause misclassifications as WHO grade II oligodendrogliomas or astrocytomas in around 15% of cases (**Fig. 6G–I**).[28] On MR imaging, the glioneuronal element appears as usually multilobulated cysts in the cortex or in the cortex and subcortical white matter, which are either oriented in a ball-like fashion or are perpendicular to the cortical surface (see **Fig. 6**). Smaller cysts in the vicinity of the tumor are highlighted by 3 T MR imaging, and are highly diagnostic. Parts of the glioneuronal element may show contrast enhancement, which may vary on follow-up examinations in such a way that sharply marginated contrast-enhancing nodules occur while others have disappeared.[28]

pXAs are rare (2% in the Bonn epilepsy surgery series),[25] epilepsy-associated astrocytic tumors with superficial location in the cerebral hemispheres and involvement of the meninges. Two-thirds of patients are younger than 20 years. pXAs are in most cases WHO grade II tumors; for tumors with significant mitotic activity (5 or more mitoses per 10 high-power fields) the term pXA with anaplastic features is used, and a significant portion of pXAs dedifferentiates to glioblastomas. On MR imaging, so-called meningeocerebral contrast enhancement on T1-weighted spin-echo images reflects the extensive involvement of the subarachnoid space; however, it is not present in all cases. Some tumors have white matter edema on T2-weighted and FLAIR images, and calcifications and a space-occupying effect are possible.

Angiocentric gliomas are variably infiltrative tumors with histopathological features of both astrocytomas and ependymomas.[29,30] On MR imaging, they are located in the cortex and subcortical white matter with a stalklike extension to the lateral

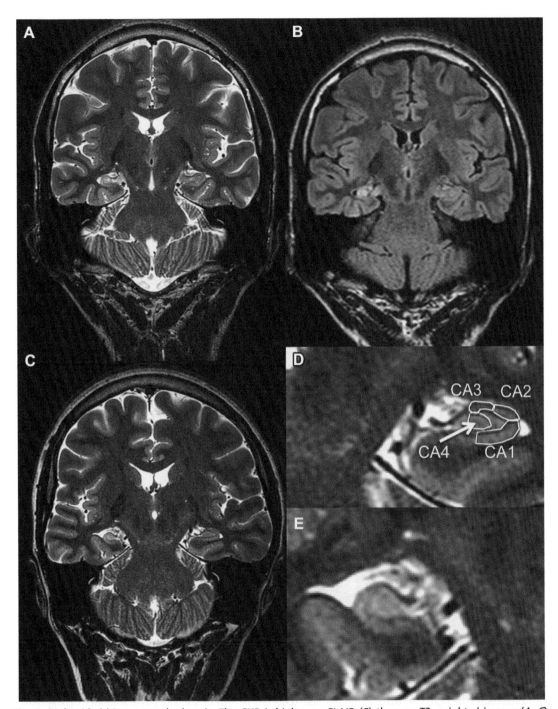

Fig. 3. Right-sided hippocampal sclerosis. The CNR is higher on FLAIR (*B*) than on T2-weighted images (*A, C*); however, T2-weighted images show anatomic details more clearly. On high-resolution T2-weighted images it is possible to visualize hippocampal substructures. (*D*) The sectors of the left hippocampus with the arrow pointing to the CA4 sector. (*E*) A grade IV hippocampal sclerosis according to Wyler, with atrophy and increased signal of all Sommer sectors.

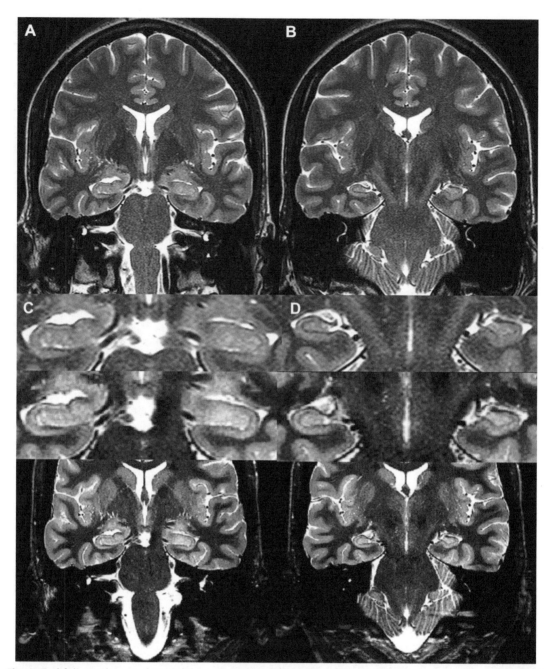

Fig. 4. End folium sclerosis of the left hippocampus. High-resolution T2-weighted fast spin-echo images from 2 different vendors (*A*, *B*: Philips Intera 3 T; *C*, *D*: Siemens Trio 3 T) reveal a better delineation of hippocampal substructures on the right side than on the left side. (*Courtesy of* Prof Dr C.E. Elger, Department of Epileptology, University of Bonn.)

ventricle. On T1-weighted SE sequences, the involved cortical gyri are isointense with an intrinsic rim of hyperintense appearance. On T2-weighted and FLAIR sequences the tumors are hyperintense. There is typically no calcification or contrast enhancement.

MALFORMATIONS OF CORTICAL DEVELOPMENT
Background

Malformations of cortical development (MCDs) and FCD, an MCD subtype in which the abnormality is strictly or largely intracortical,[31] are increasingly

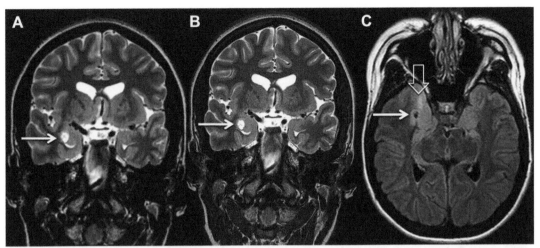

Fig. 5. Small ganglioglioma, WHO grade I, of the right amygdala and anterior uncus. The different tumor components with a cystic portion (*A–C: arrow*) and a solid portion (*C: hollow arrow*) are highlighted on high-resolution MR imaging (*A*: 0.93 × 0.93 × 2 mm; *B*: 0.47 × 0.64 × 2 mm).

recognized in patients with drug-refractory epilepsies. MCDs are radiologically and conceptually classified according to the stage in which normal cortical development was first disturbed.[32] Histopathological classification considers arrangement of cortical neurons, immature, giant, and dysplastic neurons, and so-called balloon cells.[31,33] Two types are distinguished. Type I FCDs are cytoarchitectural abnormalities without (type IA) or with giant or immature neurons (type IB), but without dysmorphic neurons or balloon cells. Type II FCDs contain dysmorphic neurons (type IIA) or dysmorphic neurons and balloon cells (type IIB). In addition to FCDs, Palmini and colleagues[31] describe the category of mild malformations of cortical development (mMCD) with ectopic neurons placed either in or adjacent to layer 1 or outside layer 1.

A significant number of patients with epilepsies and/or physical and intellectual disabilities are, for several reasons, never operated on. These lesions are classified according to Barkovich and colleagues,[32] taking genetic and pathophysiological considerations into account. Lesions resulting from disturbed neuronal migration (lissencephaly/subcortical band heterotopia, cobblestone complex/congenital muscular dystrophy syndromes, heterotopias) or from disturbed cortical organization (polymicrogyria/schizencephaly) are typically bilateral; in many diseases involved genes and pathomechanisms have been clarified in the meantime.[34,35] For example, a specific type I lissencephaly in males and subcortical band heterotopia in females are caused by the same gene defect and are therefore classified as one disease.[34]

Lesions, however, are sometimes very subtle, and either appear to be or are truly unilateral.

High-field MR imaging including voxel-based analyses and careful inspection of typically affected brain regions may facilitate detection of these lesions.[13]

Imaging

From an imaging point of view, 4 patterns in patients with FCDs can be distinguished:

1. Increased white matter signal approaching the signal of gray matter on FLAIR and T2-weighted sequences (gray–white matter demarcation loss)
2. Altered cortical thickness
3. Altered cortical signal and relief
4. Altered cortical thickness/signal and distinct funnel-shaped subcortical hyperintensity.

Type IIB FCDs, also referred to as FCD with Taylor balloon cell type or transmantle dysplasia, are characterized on MR imaging by their funnel-shaped FLAIR hyperintensity tapering toward the lateral ventricle (see **Figs. 6** and **7**).[36–38] Lesions are on surgical specimens identical or similar to cortical tubers of tuberous sclerosis, and may indeed represent a forme fruste or phenotypic variation of tuberous sclerosis. Type IIB FCDs also show histologic similarities to extensive malformation hemimegalencephaly. However, many lesions are very subtle and are typically located at the bottom of a somewhat deeper sulcus.[32,39] These bottom-of-sulcus dysplasias are easily overlooked but may be highlighted with voxel-based analyses.[2,3]

Type IIA FCDs are generally more difficult to detect because the only abnormality may be an

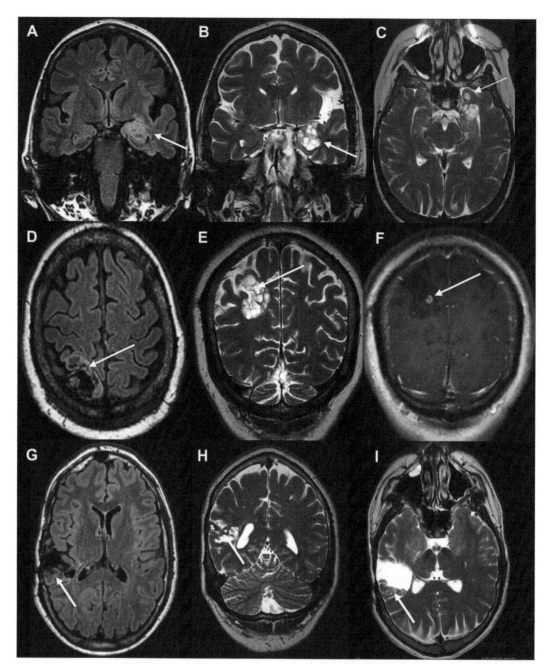

Fig. 6. Three examples of a dysembryoplastic neuroepithelial tumor (DNT) in the left amygdala (*A–C*), the right superior parietal lobule (*D–F*), and the dorsal superior temporal gyrus (*G–I*). Note the multicystic appearance, the MR imaging hallmark of this tumor (*A, B, D, E, G, H: arrow*). Smaller cysts in the vicinity of the tumor (*C: arrow*) are highly diagnostic. Smaller cysts are difficult to delineate on 3-mm FLAIR sequences (*A*); larger cysts are hypointense (*D*). Contrast enhancement occurs in 25% of cases, is typically ringlike (*F: arrow*), and may vary on follow-up MR imaging. Fifteen percent of DNTs are, as in the case displayed in *G–I*, mistaken for oligodendrogliomas: Note the anterior resection cavity and multiple tiny cysts at its posterior border (*G–I: arrow*).

altered cortical thickness or relief. mMCD and FCDs type 1 either appear normal on MR imaging or may show the pattern described as gray–white matter demarcation loss. It is difficult to assess the diagnostic yield of MR imaging for these lesions because interobserver agreement among neuropathologists is low,[40] and what is described as gray–white matter demarcation loss by some investigators is denominated FCD type I by others.[41–43] Moreover, another rare, recently

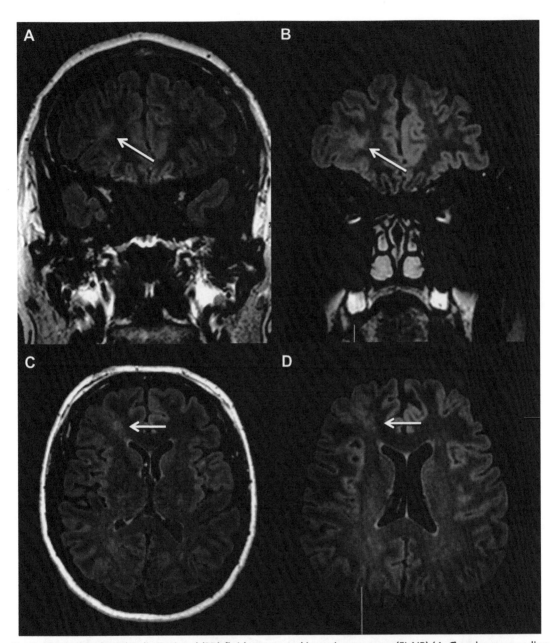

Fig. 7. Coronal and axial 2-dimensional (2D) fluid-attenuated inversion recovery (FLAIR) (*A, C*) and corresponding reformatted 3-dimensional (3D) FLAIR slices (*B, D*). Although the contrast-to-noise ratio (CNR) is higher on 2D FLAIR sequences, image quality is comparable. If there is a difference at all, is the subcortical hyperintensity of an focal cortical dysplasia (FCD) IIB (*arrow*), best visible on the axial 2D FLAIR slice (*arrow* in *C*) and the cortical involvement on the coronal 3D FLAIR image (*B*).

described and not yet classified mild dysplasia, so-called oligodendroglial hyperplasia, shows the pattern of gray–white matter demarcation loss.[44] From a prognostic point of view, it is worth mentioning that the proportion of patients with seizures and of seizure-free patients after surgery is significantly higher in FCD type II patients than in FCD type I and mMCD patients.[42,45] Complete resection of the cortical lesion, not the subcortical

funnel-shaped hyperintensity, is crucial to achieve freedom from seizures.[2,3,46]

Lissencephalic brains have a smooth surface on MR imaging with an abnormally thick cortex, including areas of absent gyration (agyria) and abnormally wide gyri (pachygyria). Type I lissencephalies are morphologically and pathogenetically distinguished from cobblestone (type II) lissencephalies associated with congenital muscular dystrophies.

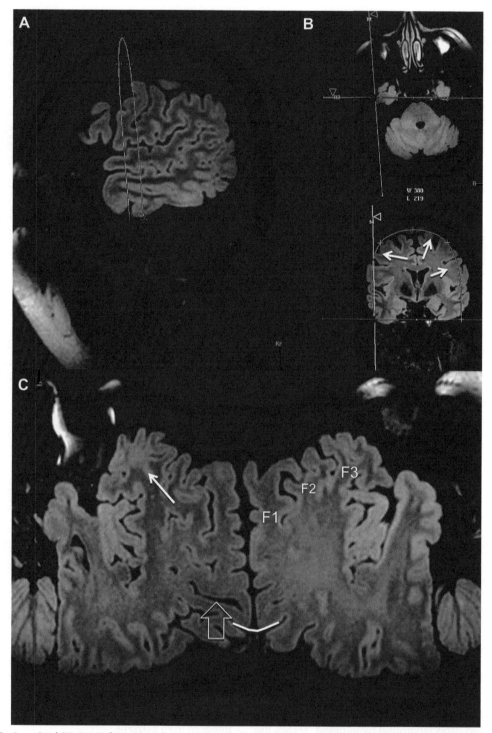

Fig. 8. A sagittal 3D FLAIR fast spin-echo sequence with isotropic voxel (*A*) is reformatted in axial and coronal orientations (*B*). A path is created along the brain surface on the coronal image (*B, arrows*). The curved planar surface view (*C*) displays both hemispheres in a mirrorlike fashion. The FCD type IIB is located in the right inferior frontal gyrus with its tail extending into the subcortical white matter (*C, arrow*). F1, superior frontal gyrus; F2, middle frontal gyrus; F3, inferior frontal gyrus; hollow arrow, central sulcus; curved line, pars marginalis cinguli.

Common associated malformations of type I lissencephalies include rounded hippocampi, enlarged posterior portions of the lateral ventricles, flat anterior portion of the corpus callosum, and very variable hypoplasia of the cerebellum, especially the midline vermis.[34] What appears to be pachygyria on low-resolution MR imaging is often polymicrogyria displayed with high-resolution MR imaging (Figs. 9 and 10).

In subcortical band heterotopia, a smooth band of neurons that never reached the true cortex lies beneath a normal-appearing cortex. This band has a variable thickness, and thin bands are easily overlooked but are highlighted by voxel-based morphometric analysis.[13]

Heterotopias are gray matter structures, which are either bandlike and subcortically located (subcortical band heterotopia), nodular or linearly ordered along the ventricular margins, or circumscribed in the white matter (subcortical heterotopia).

Polymicrogyria can be focal, multifocal, or diffuse, and unilateral, bilateral-asymmetric, and bilateral

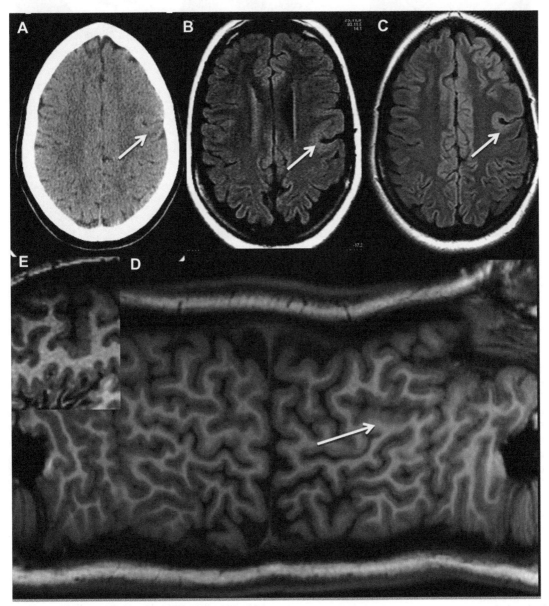

Fig. 9. An 18-year-old girl presented with a first secondary generalized tonic-clonic seizure. Her father had observed that it started with clonic jerking in the right mouth angle. Axial computed tomography (A), 1.5 T FLAIR (B), and 3 T FLAIR (C) images revealed an abnormal gyrus (A–C: arrow). Only the planar surface reformation (D) displays the lesion as focal polymicrogyria (arrow). For comparison, see the sagittal T1-weighted 3D image (E).

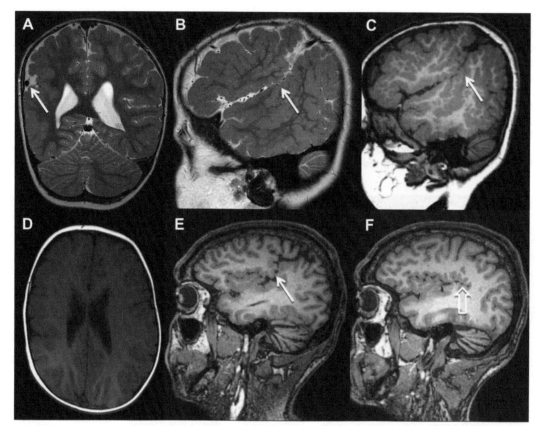

Fig. 10. Unilateral, right-sided polymicrogyria in a 16-year-old boy with secondarily generalized seizures (A–D) and a 39-year-old man with generalized seizures (E, F). Polymicrogyria is best visible on 3D T1-weighted gradient echo images with isotropic images (C) in comparison with lower resolved images (A: 0.47 × 0.64 × 2 mm; D: 5 × 0.9 × 1.12 mm). A steeper course of the Sylvian fissure (B, C, E: arrow) and enlarged draining veins (A: arrow) may indicate polymicrogyria. Preferential location of polymicrogyria is the posterior end of the Sylvian fissure. As perisylvian polymicrogyria is a common, genetically determined disease, one must carefully examine the opposite side, which may show subtle findings (F: arrow).

symmetric. The most common location is around the posterior portions of the Sylvian fissure (60%–70% of cases), which typically takes a steeper course (see Fig. 10). This region should be carefully inspected on sagittal 3D T1-weighted gradient echo images. Note that the cortical surface shows multiple small gyri, or it appears thick and bumpy or, paradoxically, smooth because the outer cortical layer (molecular layer) fuses over the microsulci. The overlying subarachnoid space is focally widened and may contain enlarged flow void structures representing anomalous venous drainage (in approximately 50% of cases) (see Fig. 10).[47]

VASCULAR MALFORMATIONS
Background

Vascular malformations include arteriovenous malformations (AVMs), cavernous hemangiomas (cavernomas), dural arteriovenous fistulas, developmental venous anomalies (venous angiomas), and capillary telangiectasias. Only the first 2 lesion types are typically associated with chronic epileptic seizures; they represent fewer than 10% of patients in epilepsy surgery series.[20] Cavernomas are much more common than AVMs and dural arteriovenous fistulas, which may explain why epilepsy is the presenting clinical feature in 79% of cavernomas, compared with 17% of AVMs.[48,49]

Imaging

Detection and delineation of AVMs and cavernomas clearly benefit from high-field MR imaging, because of the higher susceptibility (for cavernomas) at higher field strength (see Fig. 2). A higher SNR allows assessment of the spatial relationship between the vascular malformations and its vicinity, especially on high-resolution T2-weighted fast spin-echo images. Another clear advantage is the higher spatial resolution of 3 T time-of-flight angiography and higher quality of time-resolved contrast-enhanced MR angiography.[50,51]

TRAUMA AND OTHER CORTICAL SCARS
Background

Trauma is the cause of epilepsy in around 4% of cases. It is also worth mentioning that posttraumatic lesions may be result but not the cause of epileptic seizures. In addition, a significant number of scars results from encephalitis and other infections.

Imaging

Primary brain parenchymal injuries comprise cortical contusions and diffuse axonal injuries. Cortical contusions occur in locations where the brain is adjacent to bony protuberances or dural folds: basal frontal lobe, temporal pole and inferior surface, and parasagittal (gliding contusions). These locations should be carefully looked for, especially on high-resolution T2-weighted fast spin-echo images, because lesions may be invisible on T2-weighted gradient echo images because of susceptibility artifacts (see **Fig. 1**). Diffuse axonal injury is characterized by multiple punctate hypointense lesions on T2-weighted gradient echo sequences. Specific locations are the gray/white matter interfaces, the corpus callosum, and the dorsolateral upper brainstem. Cortical scars in convexity locations are best displayed on FLAIR sequences. Such scars are characterized by cortex atrophy and hyperintensity, and associated sulcus widening. The outcome of postsurgical seizure is poor for posttraumatic lesions and gyral scars, most likely because visible lesions on MR imaging represent just the tip of the iceberg.[20]

SUMMARY

Epileptogenic lesions are often small and do not change throughout life. Moreover, several genetically determined epilepsy syndromes exist, which by definition are not caused by structural lesions. Both cause a certain degree of uncertainty, whether an epileptogenic lesion is overlooked or is just not present. High-field MR imaging at 3 T is currently the state of the art for patients with suspected structural epilepsies in whom an epileptogenic lesion has not yet been found. A higher SNR is used to increase the spatial resolution while maintaining a high contrast between normal cortex and the epileptogenic lesion.

REFERENCES

1. Rosenow F, Lüders H. Presurgical evaluation of epilepsy. Brain 2001;124(Pt 9):1683–700.

2. Wagner J, Weber B, Urbach H, et al. Morphometric MRI analysis improves detection of focal cortical dysplasia type II. Brain 2011;134(Pt 10):2844–54.

3. Wagner J, Wellmer J, Urbach H, et al. Focal cortical dysplasia type IIb: completeness of cortical, not subcortical resection is necessary for seizure freedom. Epilepsia 2011;52(8):1418–24.

4. Bien CG, Szinai M, Wagner J, et al. Characteristics and surgical outcome of patients with refractory MRI-negative epilepsies. Arch Neurol 2009;66(12):1491–9.

5. Bien CG, Raabe AL, Schramm J, et al. Long-term developments in presurgical evaluation and surgical treatment of epilepsy at one tertiary center: Part II: surgical outcome. Epilepsia 2010;51(Suppl 4):6.

6. Berg AT, Berkovic SF, Brodie M, et al. Revised terminology and concepts for organization of seizures and epilepsies: report of the ILAE commission on classification and terminology, 2005-2009. Epilepsia 2010;51(4):676–85.

7. Phal PM, Usmanov A, Nesbit GM, et al. Qualitative comparison of 3-T and 1.5-T MRI in the evaluation of epilepsy. AJR Am J Roentgenol 2008;191(3):890–5.

8. Knake S, Triantafyllou C, Wald LL, et al. 3T phased array MRI improves the presurgical evaluation in focal epilepsies: a prospective study. Neurology 2005;65(7):1026–31.

9. Willinek WA, Kuhl CK. 3.0 T neuroimaging: technical considerations and clinical applications. Neuroimaging Clin N Am 2006;16(2):217–8.

10. Wansapura JP, Holland SK, Dunn RS, et al. NMR relaxation times in the human brain at 3.0 T. J Magn Reson Imaging 1999;9(4):531–8.

11. Lin C, Bernstein MA, Huston J, et al. In-vivo and in-vitro measurements of T1 relaxation at 3.0T. In: Proceedings of the 9th Meeting ISMRM. Glasgow, 2001. p. 1685.

12. Elster AD, Mirza W. MR imaging in chronic partial epilepsy: role of contrast enhancement. AJNR Am J Neuroradiol 1991;12(1):165–70.

13. Huppertz HJ, Wellmer J, Staack AM, et al. Voxel-based 3-D MRI analysis helps to detect subtle forms of subcortical band heterotopia. Epilepsia 2008; 49(5):772–85.

14. Hattingen E, Hattingen J, Clusmann H, et al. Planar brain surface reformations for localization of cortical brain lesions. Zentralbl Neurochir 2004;65(2):75–80.

15. Nelles M, Bien CG, Kurthen M, et al. Transient splenium lesions in presurgical epilepsy patients: incidence and pathogenesis. Neuroradiology 2006; 48(7):443–8.

16. Pruessmann KP, Weiger M, Scheidegger MB, et al. SENSE: sensitivity encoding for fast MRI. Magn Reson Med 1999;42(5):952–62.

17. Bammer R, Keeling SL, Augustin M, et al. Improved diffusion-weighted single-shot-echo-planar imaging in stroke using sensitivity encoding (SENSE). Magn Reson Med 2001;46(3):548–54.

18. Willinek WA, Schild HH. Clinical advantages of 3.0T MRI over 1.5T. Eur J Radiol 2008;65(1):2–14.

19. Hoult DI, Phil D. Sensitivity and power deposition in a high-field imaging experiment. J Magn Reson Imaging 2000;12(1):46–67.

20. Urbach H, Hattingen J, von Oertzen J, et al. MRI in the presurgical evaluation of patients with drug-resistant epilepsy. AJNR Am J Neuroradiol 2004; 25(6):919–26.

21. Wiebe S, Blume WT, Girvin JP, et al. A randomized, controlled trial of surgery for temporal lobe epilepsy. N Engl J Med 2001;38:154–63.

22. Hirai T, Korogi Y, Yoshizumi Y, et al. Limbic lobe of the human brain: evaluation with turbo fluid-attenuated inversion recovery MR imaging. Radiology 2000; 215(2):470–5.

23. Blümcke I, Pauli E, Clusmann H, et al. A new clinico-pathological classification system for mesial temporal sclerosis. Acta Neuropathol 2007;113(3): 235–44.

24. Thom M, Liagkouras I, Elliot KJ, et al. Reliability of patterns of hippocampal sclerosis as predictors of postsurgical outcome. Epilepsia 2010;51(9):1801–8.

25. Luyken C, Blümcke I, Fimmers R, et al. The spectrum of long-term epilepsy associated tumors: long-term seizure and tumor outcome and neurosurgical aspects. Epilepsia 2003;44(6):822–30.

26. Louis DN, Ohgaki H, Wiestler OD, et al. The 2007 WHO classification of tumours of the central nervous system. Acta Neuropathol 2007;114(2):97–109.

27. Daumas-Duport C, Pietsch T, Lantos PL. Dysembryoplastic neuroepithelial tumour. In: Kleihues P, Cavenee K, editors. Pathology and genetic of tumours of the nervous system. Lyon (France): IARC press; 2000. p. 103–6.

28. Campos AR, Clusmann H, von Lehe M, et al. Simple and complex dysembryoplastic neuroepithelial tumors (DNT): clinical profile, MRI and histopathology. Neuroradiology 2009;51(7):433–43.

29. Lellouch-Tubiana A, Boddaert N, Bourgeois M, et al. Angiocentric neuroepithelial tumor (ANET): a new Epilepsy-related clinicopathological entity with distinctive MRI. Brain Pathol 2005;15(4):281–6.

30. Wang M, Tihan T, Rojiani AM, et al. Monomorphous angiocentric glioma: a distinctive epileptogenic neoplasm with features of infiltrating astrocytoma and ependymoma. J Neuropathol Exp Neurol 2005;64(10):875–81.

31. Palmini A, Najm I, Avanzini G, et al. Terminology and classification of the cortical dysplasias. Neurology 2004;62(6 Suppl 3):S2–8.

32. Barkovich AJ, Kuzniecky RI, Jackson GD, et al. A developmental and genetic classification for malformations of cortical development. Neurology 2005;65(12):1873–87.

33. Blümcke I, Thom M, Aronica E, et al. The clinico-pathologic spectrum of focal cortical dysplasias: a consensus classification proposed by an ad hoc Task Force of the ILAE Diagnostic Methods Commission. Epilepsia 2011;52(1):158–74.

34. Dobyns WB. The clinical patterns and molecular genetics of lissencephaly and subcortical band heterotopia. Epilepsia 2010;51(Suppl 1):5–9.

35. Leventer RJ, Jansen A, Pilz DT, et al. Clinical and imaging heterogeneity of polymicrogyria: a study of 328 patients. Brain 2010;133(Pt 5):1415–27.

36. Taylor DC, Falconer MA, Bruton CJ, et al. Focal dysplasia of the cerebral cortex in epilepsy. J Neurol Neurosurg Psychiatry 1971;34(4):369–87.

37. Barkovich AJ, Kuzniecky RI, Bollen AW, et al. Focal transmantle dysplasia: a specific malformation of cortical development. Neurology 1997;49(4):1148–52.

38. Urbach H, Scheffler B, Heinrichsmeier T, et al. Focal cortical dysplasia of Taylor's balloon cell type: a clinicopathological entity with characteristic neuroimaging and histopathological features, and favorable postsurgical outcome. Epilepsia 2002;43(1):33–40.

39. Besson P, Andermann F, Dubeau F, et al. Small focal cortical dysplasia lesions are located at the bottom of a deep sulcus. Brain 2008;131(Pt 12): 3246–55.

40. Chamberlain WA, Cohen ML, Gyure KA, et al. Interobserver and intraobserver reproducibility in focal cortical dysplasia (malformations of cortical development). Epilepsia 2009;50(12):2593–8.

41. Hildebrandt M, Pieper T, Winkler P, et al. Neuropathological spectrum of cortical dysplasia in children with severe focal epilepsies. Acta Neuropathol 2005;110(1):1–11.

42. Krsek P, Maton B, Korman B, et al. Different features of histopathological subtypes of pediatric focal cortical dysplasia. Ann Neurol 2008;63(6): 758–69.

43. Fauser S, Huppertz HJ, Bast T, et al. Clinical characteristics in focal cortical dysplasia: a retrospective evaluation in a series of 120 patients. Brain 2006; 129(Pt 7):1907–16.

44. Hamilton BE, Nesbit GM. MR imaging identification of oligodendroglial hyperplasia. AJNR Am J Neuroradiol 2009;30(7):1412–3.

45. Lerner JT, Salaman N, Hauptman JS, et al. Assessment of surgical outcomes for mild type I and severe type II cortical dysplasia: a critical review and the UCLA experience. Epilepsia 2009;50(6): 1310–35.

46. Krsek P, Maton B, Jayakar P, et al. Incomplete resection of focal cortical dysplasia is the main predictor of poor postsurgical outcome. Neurology 2009; 72(3):217–23.

47. Hayashi N, Tsutsumi Y, Barkovich AJ. Polymicrogyria without porencephaly/schizencephaly. MRI analysis of the spectrum and the prevalence of macroscopic findings in the clinical population. Neuroradiology 2002;44(8):647–55.

48. Moran NF, Fish DR, Kitchen N, et al. Supratentorial cavernous haemangiomas and epilepsy: a review of the literature and case series. J Neurol Neurosurg Psychiatry 1999;66(5):561–8.

49. Zhao J, Wang S, Li J, et al. Clinical characteristics and surgical results of patients with cerebral arteriovenous malformations. Surg Neurol 2005; 63(2):156–61.

50. Willinek WA, Born M, Simon B, et al. 3.0 T time of flight MR angiography: comparison with 1.5 T—initial experience. Radiology 2003;229(3):913–20.

51. Hadizadeh D, Gieseke J, von Falkenhausen M, et al. Subsecond temporal resolution 4D-MR angiography: Spetzler-Martin classification of cerebral arteriovenous malformations as compared to DSA. Radiology 2008;246(1):205–13.

Stroke: High-Field Magnetic Resonance Imaging

Karl-Olof Lövblad, MD*, Sven Haller, MSc, MD,
Vitor Mendes Pereira, MSc, MD

KEYWORDS

- Stroke • Magnetic resonance imaging • Perfusion
- Diffusion • High-field imaging

Key Points

- Imaging must be fast and comprehensive (20 mins).
- Exclude hemorrhage with T2*/susceptibility-weighted imaging.
- Demonstrate/exclude ischemia with diffusion-weighted imaging/diffusion tensor imaging.
- Demonstrate tissue at risk with perfusion.
- Demonstrate occlusion with time of flight.
- Demonstrate/exclude proximal carotid disease with neck magnetic resonance angiography.

In industrialized countries, cerebrovascular disease is 1 of the top 3 causes of morbidity and mortality of the general population, making it a priority for any health care system. Since the arrival of thrombolysis for cerebral stroke, there has been a complete change in paradigm when it comes to approaching patients with acute stroke. Indeed, previously, the outcome was bleak for most patients with very little beyond reeducation available if they survived the initial event. Following the National Institute of Neurological Disorders and Stroke and the European Cooperative Acute Stroke trials,[1,2] intravenous thrombolysis established itself as the treatment modality for patients being recruited within 3 hours after the initial event; following recent studies in Europe, intravenous therapy can now be applied up to 4.5 hours[3] and there is an evolving understanding that using alternative therapies it may be possible to go beyond even this strict time window. Since then, there has been an unprecedented parallel evolution in advances in both imaging and treatment for stroke. During the 1990s there was an explosion of imaging modalities with the development at first of new magnetic resonance (MR) techniques, such as diffusion and perfusion, and then the improvement of concurrent computed tomography (CT) techniques, as well as an improved understanding of their interpretation.[4–6] Before the development of fast echo–planar imaging techniques, these types of imaging were difficult to perform because of motion artifacts. These imaging developments were at the same time accompanied by improvements in endovascular techniques for the treatment of brain ischemia.[7] The important improvements in imaging have led

---

Dr Lövblad is the recipient of a grant from the Swiss National Science Foundation on high-field stroke imaging (SNF grant 320000-121565). He is a recipient of a research grant on MR from Bayer Schering Pharma.

Division of Neuroradiology, Department of Imaging and Medical Informatics, Geneva University Hospitals HUG, 4 rue Gabrielle-Perret-Gentil, 1211 Geneva, Switzerland
* Corresponding author.
E-mail address: karl-olof.lovblad@hcuge.ch

Neuroimag Clin N Am 22 (2012) 191–205
doi:10.1016/j.nic.2012.02.002
1052-5149/12/$ – see front matter © 2012 Elsevier Inc. All rights reserved.

to the development of a model of the ischemic penumbra, or tissue at risk, that allows to triage patients for appropriate treatment[8]; this altogether has made available an extremely varied armamentarium that can help us investigate these patients. The aims of imaging should be to exclude any kind of other pathology that might simulate a stroke,[9] then establish that there is a stroke and not simply the absence of hemorrhage, demonstrate the presence of tissue that might undergo infarction, and finally in the acute setting try to demonstrate the thrombus and eventually the cause (cardiac, carotid origin).[10] Then finally the method should allow for monitoring of treatment by allowing follow-up. Although most major studies have been using CT for the initial screening, the paradigms used clinically are also changing. As stated earlier, the first initial step to be undertaken is to exclude the presence of any kind of other disease that might cause acute symptoms that might be mistaken for a stroke. This also applies to the clinical examination. Although for more than a decade scanners at 1.5 T were considered the state of the art, continuous developments in hardware and software have rendered the implementation of high-field imaging (3 T or more) possible and commercially available.[11] At the moment in the clinical neurosciences, these higher-field scanners are quickly becoming the new standard of imaging. The use of higher magnetic fields has the evident advantage of providing more signal that can be used to produce faster imaging, higher resolution, or a combination of both; also before the advent of parallel imaging techniques,[12] many MR imaging artifacts encountered at 3 T were considered a problem.[13]

IMAGING TECHNIQUES: CT VERSUS MR IMAGING

As already mentioned, the 2 main aims of neuroimaging are excluding hemorrhage and demonstrating ischemia.[9] CT has shown itself to be very sensitive

to hemorrhage and also capable of detecting signs of early ischemia in well-trained hands.[4,5] Using MR imaging, these 2 aims can be attained by using T2* images for blood detection[14] and diffusion-weighted imaging (DWI) for ischemic lesions.[15] Although initially there was a heated debate if MR could fulfill the first imaging criterion (exclusion of hemorrhage), we have now seen that this is easily feasible with MR imaging.[14,16] Although In a few select situations, such as subarachnoid hemorrhage, which usually does not mimic stroke clinically, imaging can be done with both MR imaging and CT for screening of hemorrhage; MR imaging is ideally suited for the detection of ischemia. MR imaging with diffusion has been shown to be able to detect strokes with sensitivities as high as 90% or more.[15] The reports by Kidwell and colleagues[16] and Chalela and colleagues[17] found MR imaging and CT to be equivalently suited for the detection of acute hemorrhage. Multiple studies comparing CT and MR imaging have shown that diffusion imaging is extremely sensitive to the presence of infarction.[17–22] Although CT criteria are well established and have been used with success to detect early ischemic changes, MR imaging can much better detect the presence of small subcortical and cortical infarcts.

MR imaging protocols now run for approximately 20 to 30 minutes, meaning that imaging time will not interfere to a greater degree anymore. This time allows for performance of diffusion imaging, T2* imaging, and T2 imaging, as well as MR angiography (MRA) and MR perfusion (Box 1).

Although being initially very sensitive to lesion detection, MR protocols, including diffusion imaging, have also shown themselves to provide information

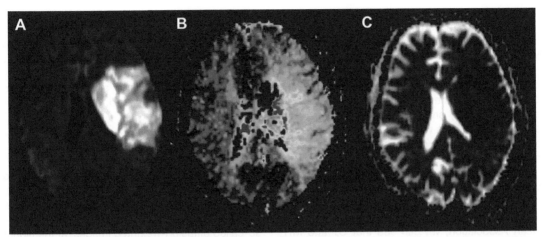

Fig. 1. Patient with right hemispheric stroke. There is a large hyperintensity in the right MCA territory on the diffusion image with maximum b value (*A*), accompanied by diminished perfusion on the MTT map (*B*) and a reduced ADC (*C*).

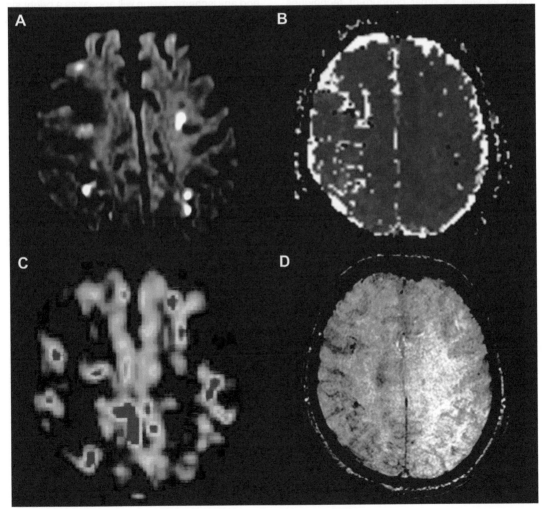

Fig. 2. Patient with embolic stroke: the diffusion image shows small lesions in the cortex (*A*). The watershed region in the right hemisphere is hypoperfused: this is seen both on the contrast-enhanced perfusion maps (*B*) and on the ASL images (*C*). No hemorrhage on the SWI images (*D*).

about outcome[23,24] and lesion progression,[25] as well as provide information about possible cause of ischemia owing to pattern differences in lesion location.[26]

MR imaging also has established itself as the post-therapeutic modality of choice. This is because DWI can be performed that is able to demonstrate very small lesions that might occur after treatment,[27] as well as demonstrate reperfusion with apparent diffusion coefficient (ADC) mapping.[28,29]

Considering all these arguments, it is obvious why MR imaging is destined to become the method of choice for stroke management.

When considering the guidelines of the American Heart Association, we can see that CT and MR imaging can be used to exclude pathology and demonstrate ischemia, that angio-MR imaging can detect the presence of occlusion as well or almost as well as other concurrent techniques, such as CT angiography or digital subtraction angiography, and that perfusion imaging, although not yet fully validated, can demonstrate the presence of hemodynamic changes that correlate well with the neurologic changes that will eventually predict outcome. Thus, the use of multimodality imaging is today necessary and this is rendered especially easy at a high field.

DIFFUSION IMAGING

To the diffusion-imaging techniques belong DWI[30] and diffusion tensor imaging.[31] DWI is mainly used for stroke and consists of a relatively simple modification of a spin-echo sequence that is sensitized to motion by diffusion gradients. This produces the so-called diffusion-weighted images; at the higher b value, early ischemia will lead to a hyperintensity on imaging that corresponds to stroke. DWIs at a high b value have an inherent strong contrast and any ischemic lesion will appear as a bright signal against a dark background (**Fig. 1**). Nowadays,

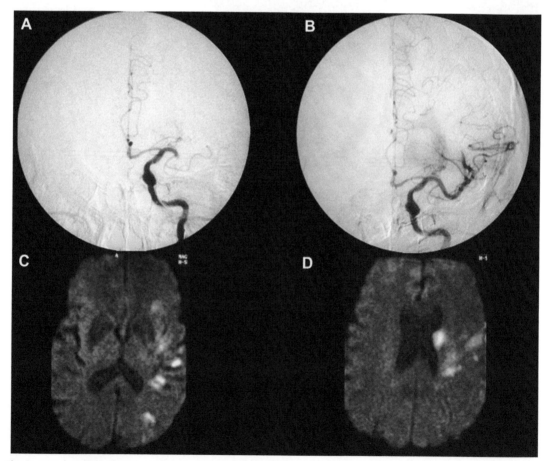

Fig. 3. Distal emboli after thrombolysis. Patient who underwent recanalization for an occlusion of the left MCA (*A, B*); afterward there are small distal subcortical lesions subcortically in the left hemisphere visible on the diffusion-weighted images (*C, D*).

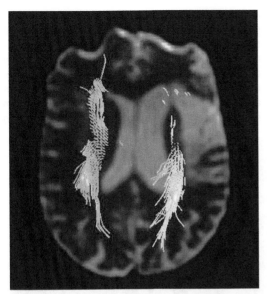

Fig. 4. Poststroke degeneration of the white matter tracts: a patient with a left-sided MCA stroke. There is a large chronic ischemic lesion visible on the T2 image in the left MCA territory. The overlaid reconstructed tractography shows a marked asymmetry of the white matter tracts.

mostly directly isotropic images are used and produced[32]: images without artifacts owing to the directionality of water motion seen when the gradients are used with different directions. Usually DWI is done at various settings of diffusion sensitivity (b values) and these various images are

then used to create the so-called maps of the ADC; whereas the DWIs are used for screening purposes and detection, the ADC maps provide an interesting way to quantify or date the ischemic event.[33] Because of their strong inherent contrast, DWIs are better suited to detect also small ischemic events, such as those caused by hemodynamic compromise or embolism (**Fig. 2**). Although the diffusion effects themselves are independent of the magnetic field, the use of a higher field will improve quality. In a study comparing DWIs at 1.5 and 3 T in 25 patients, Kuhl and colleagues[34] found an increased diagnostic confidence provided by the higher field images when compared with the standard 1.5 T images, despite the presence of higher susceptibility artifacts but principally because of higher signal-to-noise ratio (SNR). Also, diffusion imaging is ideally suited for the follow-up of patients who have undergone interventional procedures (**Fig. 3**).

Diffusion tensor imaging may at the moment have a less clearly established role in the ultra-early assessment of patients with stroke; indeed diffusion images with more directionality have a slightly lesser contrast and are often less used clinically. The maps of fractional anisotropy, which reflect directionality, have a rather low imaging resolution so they are rarely used for the diagnosis of acute stroke; however, in the follow-up after the ischemic event, the use of tractography as provided by diffusion tensor imaging could be of great interest, as it allows us to follow the impact of the stroke on connectivity (**Fig. 4**). Diffusion

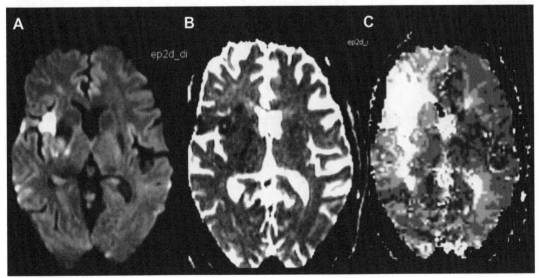

Fig. 5. Mismatch at 3 T. Patient with a small insular diffusion abnormality visible on the high b value diffusion image (*A*) with a corresponding small ADC decrease (*B*). The MTT mp at the same level (*C*) shows a lager area of hypoperfusion: there is a large mismatch zone corresponding to the functional penumbra.

tensor imaging will benefit greatly from the use of higher magnetic fields because it will increase the SNR greatly.

PERFUSION IMAGING

Brain perfusion techniques were also made possible by the development of scanners capable of fast imaging[35,36] and they now play a central role in the assessment of patients with stroke; indeed, based on the so-called diffusion perfusion mismatch model, a first easy-to-use working model of the penumbra was created. The core lesion is believed to be constituted by the diffusion lesion and this is often surrounded by a greater area of hypoperfused brain tissue; the difference between

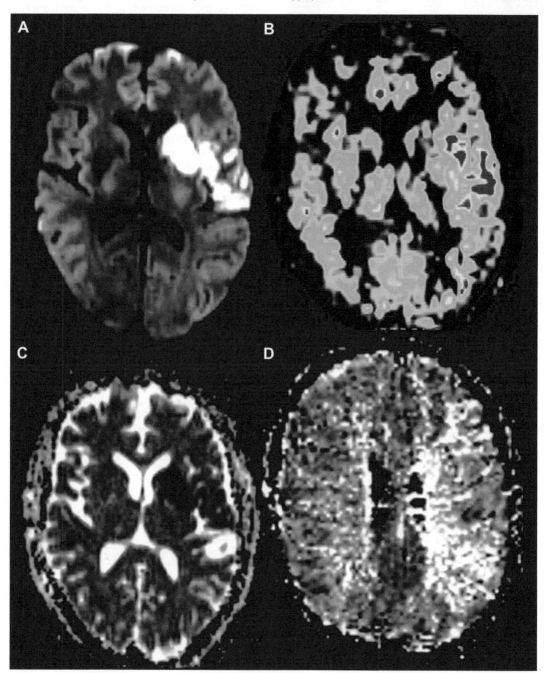

Fig. 6. ASL in stroke: patient with a left MCA lesion visible on the high b value diffusion value (*A*) with an area of hyperperfusion on ASL (*B*), despite a decrease in the ADC (*C*) and a large area of hypoperfusion on contrast-enhanced perfusion (*D*).

both constitutes the tissue at risk or so-called penumbra (Fig. 5). Although this model is somewhat different from the traditional model of the penumbra, which relied on detecting different levels of energetic failure, it has proven to be a model that helps in the patient workup. Two main types of perfusion imaging can be done with MR techniques. Perfusion using contrast material[35,36] and perfusion without contrast.[37] Perfusion with contrast or susceptibility-weighted contrast perfusion relies on T2* images to provide imaging contrast. T1-weighted images could be more reliable, but because of inherent difficulties have not been widely implemented.[38]

Arterial Spin Labeling Perfusion

Arterial spin labeling (ASL) is a noninvasive imaging technique that allows performance of perfusion imaging of the brain without the administration of contrast. It uses flowing blood as an inherent contrast material after an initial tagging has been performed. This technique has been around for more than a decade under various forms and at first was a single-slice technique[39]; however, the development of high-field scanners at 3 T and more has allowed it to become a multi-slice product that is easily implemented in the clinical setting. Although ASL has been shown to demonstrate hypoperfusion quite well in acute stroke,[40] it is also capable in some cases of demonstrating the presence of collateral flow (Fig. 6).[41,42] This, in addition to its capacity to demonstrate regional territorial flow, is what could provide a great impact in the future.[43] Also the fact that contrast material is not necessary makes ASL an interesting new possibility when confronted with elderly people whose renal function might be impaired.

Dynamic Susceptibility-Weighted Imaging Contrast

Mainly T2* imaging has been used to obtain perfusion images of the brain. After intravenous injection of a gadolinium chelate, there is a decrease in signal on images where perfusion is normal; on the raw MR images an area of hypoperfusion will thus be seen as a focus of relative hyperintensity

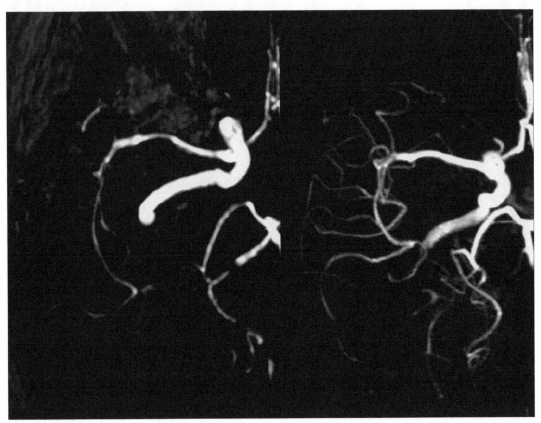

Fig. 7. TOF MRAs at 1.5 T and 3 T in the same patient. Note that the distal MCA branches are much more visible at 3 T.

(less perfusion). The use of higher magnetic fields will provide an increase in the T2* effect, thus provoking a more dramatic demonstration of any kind of altered perfusion. The use of a higher magnetic field should also allow reduction of the amount of injected contrast material, which was demonstrated by Manka and colleagues.[44]

MR ANGIOGRAPHY

The gain in signal strength has been shown to improve the quality of brain MRA to an important degree. This leads to an improvement of signal in the arteries on time-of-flight (TOF) MRA but also to a better definition of peripheral branches of the intracranial vessels (**Fig. 7**).[45] Willinek and colleagues[46] showed that the addition of sensitivity encoding was able to further improve imaging resolution and quality. Sommer and colleagues[47] found more than 35% increase in SNR in the coronaries at 3 T when compared with 1.5 T. In a study of the intracranial vessels, Willinek and colleagues[45] found an improvement in the diagnostic accuracy of TOF MRA performed at 3 T over images at 1.5 T.

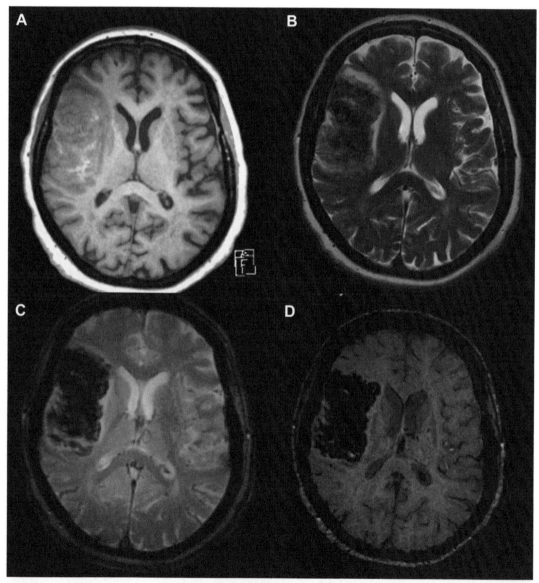

Fig. 8. Patient with a subacute right-sided MCA infarction: there is slight hyperintensity on T1 (*A*), hypointensity on T2 (*B*), and signal drop on T2* images (*C*). SWI shows an accumulation of blood after stroke even more dramatically (*D*).

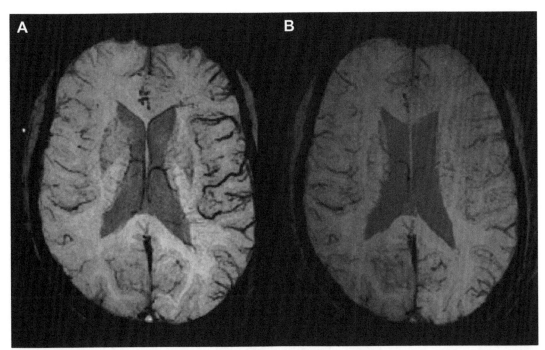

Fig. 9. Patient with a left-sided stroke who underwent successful thrombolysis: SWI before and after stroke. Before stroke there is vascular stasis (*A*) that disappears after thrombolysis (*B*).

MRA techniques have also improved to such a degree that they can reliably follow-up vessels after stenting.[48] Also, using contrast-enhanced sequences, MRA of the neck vessels has improved to a degree that it can be used with confidence to screen patients.[49]

SUSCEPTIBILITY-WEIGHTED MR IMAGING

Susceptibility-weighted MR imaging sequences offer a very strong T2* contrast but a very low tissular anatomic differentiation.[50] They have been shown to be sensitive to the presence of small hemorrhagic lesions; in the presence of intracerebral hemorrhage this can be helpful in identifying the presence of micro-bleeds (**Fig. 8**). These sequences are also capable of providing extremely high-resolution anatomic imaging of the intracranial vessels; this is mainly true for the veins. Because of its inherent sensitivity to the oxygenated/deoxygenated status of the vessels, it is also capable of demonstrating the presence of vascular stasis (**Fig. 9**), which is a known phenomenon in acute stroke and which is a predictor for

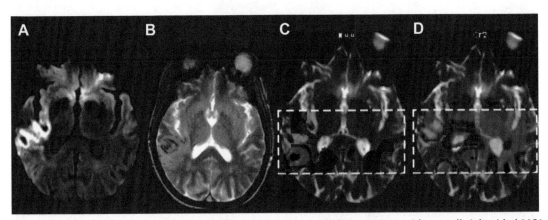

Fig. 10. Chemical shift imaging allows mapping of cerebral metabolites. Patient with a small right-sided MCA infarction: the lesion is visible in the right temporal lobe on DWI (*A*) and T2 images (*B*); on the metabolite maps there is a decrease of NAA (*C*) and CR (*D*).

hemorrhagic transformation.[51,52] In a study using 3 T perfusion imaging, Manka and colleagues[44] found that the perfusion maps were of good quality and that the distortions caused by the higher susceptibility artifacts at 3 T did not relevantly affect their clinical potential.

FUNCTIONAL MR IMAGING (ACTIVATION)

Although difficult in the early phase of infarction, functional MR imaging is of great interest for the follow-up of patients with stroke. Functional MR imaging is based on the capacity of T2* images to detect changes in local brain oxygenation. It

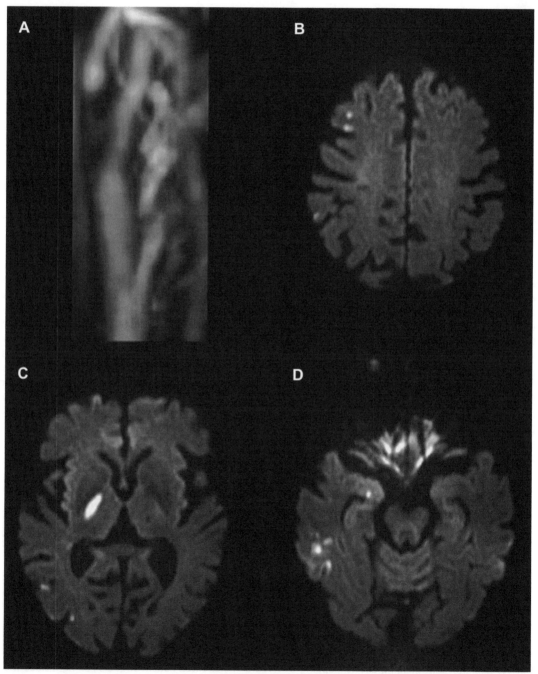

Fig. 11. Patient with a right-sided carotid stenosis (A) with distal emboli. The distal emboli are located in the watershed regions (B) as well as in the basal ganglia (C) and in the basal temporal lobe (D).

has been shown to be able to reflect functional reorganization after stroke.[53]

MR SPECTROSCOPY

Spectroscopy using MR can also provide information about alterations in brain metabolites. MR spectroscopy is used for brain tumor staging but can also be used for stroke. In the presence of ischemia there will be a decrease in N-acetyl-aspartate (NAA), which is a known neuronal marker. There will also be a concurrent decrease of lactate. Both these metabolites will be altered within the areas of altered diffusion.[54] Although MR spectroscopy has shown itself to be an important tool for the investigation of many diseases and pathologic processes, it has never gained full acceptance in clinical use for stroke; this is partly because of its complexity of use, which often necessitates postprocessing when time is critical. There is also the problem of voxel placement. High-field imaging now has made it easier to perform chemical shift imaging or multivoxel spectroscopy, where one obtains maps of metabolites. Although single-voxel spectroscopy may be more precise, multivoxel spectroscopy or chemical shift imaging has the advantage of allowing mapping of affected regions and thus one does not have to rely on one single measurement (Fig. 10). Sodium imaging may provide a further tool to improve visualization of ischemic lesions in patients with acute stroke[55] but is still under investigation and needs further validation.

TYPES OF STROKES

Using MR imaging it is possible to investigate what is the cause of stroke. Indeed, using T2 images and DWI it is now clearly possible to differentiate whether the source is cardioembolic or carotid disease (Figs. 11–13). A cardioembolic source will cause multiple emboli in both the posterior and anterior circulations on both sides, whereas a carotid unilateral source will usually affect only one defined territory. This was nicely demonstrated in a study by Baird and colleagues.[26]

Venous Ischemia

Cerebral venous thrombosis was previously believed to be a rare and severe cause of cerebral ischemia. Cerebral venous occlusive disease is more frequent than believed and, if treated early and aggressively, is not necessarily associated with a catastrophic outcome. Clinically, the initial presentation is often atypical and signs can range from typical thunderclap headache to coma with a large variety of clinical signs in-between. From a physiopathological point of view, it is important to understand that because of venous obstruction, there is at the beginning simple stasis followed by edema and eventually blood extravasation owing to vascular rupture. Venous edema will tend to be localized in the white matter and not to correspond to the classical arterial vascularization territories. On "conventional"-type MR sequences, one will often see diminished or absent flow, with absence of flow void on T2-weighted images and

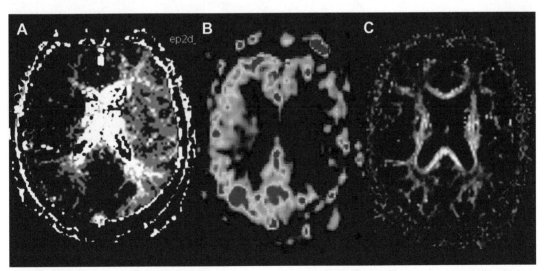

Fig. 12. Hypoperfusion demonstrated with ASL in a case of carotid stenosis. The contrast-enhanced perfusion map (A) shows a large area of hypoperfusion in the left MCA territory that can also be seen on the corresponding ASL map (B). (C) Fractional anisotropy map derived from the diffusion tensor images.

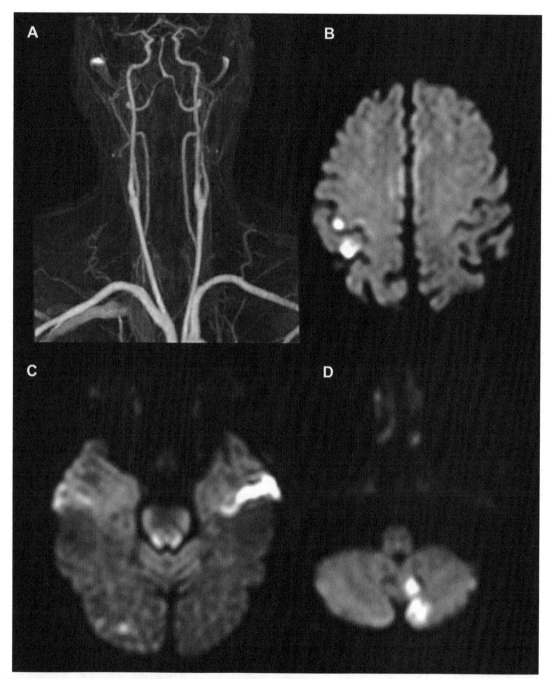

Fig. 13. Cardioembolic stroke. Multiple lesions in the supratentorial and infratentorial regions demonstrated by DWI. The head and neck MRA fails to show any stenosis (A). There are multiple ischemic lesions in the right frontal lobe (B) and in the right occipital lobe (C), as well as lesions in the left posterior inferior cerebellar artery territory (D).

hyperintensity on T1-weighted images in the presence of an intravascular occlusion. Then, by using MR phlebographic sequences, one can see the interruption of flow in the affected veins; the use of contrast-enhanced MR phlebography is strongly recommended to visualize cortical veins.[56] Diffusion can sometimes demonstrate the presence of restriction in the clot itself.[57]

Carotid Disease, Occlusion

One important underlying cause of cerebral ischemia is the presence of carotid arteriosclerotic disease. This can be fully investigated by performing contrast-enhanced MRA of the neck vessels. Contrast-enhanced MRA has replaced the more conventional TOF method and allows coverage from the aortic arch into the cerebral vasculature in much less time.

Using additional MRA sequences it is also possible to determine if a vascular dissection is underlying the ischemia.

SUMMARY

MR imaging has made great progress overall thanks to the implementation of high-field scanners and high-field imaging protocols; nowhere is this more true than in the area of stroke imaging. These new high-field units have allowed previously experimental imaging protocols to be implemented clinically. This began with the application of diffusion and perfusion techniques more than 10 years ago that revolutionized the way we visualize acute stroke lesions. Now there is a further improvement by going to higher MR fields than previously. Indeed, there is an overall gain in signal that can provide either higher resolution or imaging speed; together these 2 advantages have shown to be very helpful in acute stroke imaging. Because time is an extremely central factor in the success of stroke management, even a minimal reduction of scan time will have an extremely positive impact, we nowadays can perform either a full stroke MR protocol within 20 minutes that comprises diffusion, perfusion, angiography, and T2* images, or if time is even a more important factor, we can perform a minimal MR examination that will demonstrate or exclude ischemia with diffusion, T2* imaging, and MRA that can be performed in fewer than 10 minutes. Now that it is well established that MR imaging can reliably establish the presence or absence of hemorrhage and ischemia, the main objectives of MR and any kind of imaging will be to determine exact tissue outcome and help in selecting or excluding patients from therapy. Here, the use of perfusion with ASL can probably help because one has seen that ASL can reliably demonstrate the status of collateral flow and circulation, which was previously only reliably demonstrable with digital subtraction angiography. ASL techniques may also demonstrate areas of reperfusion or hyperperfusion that occur in the cascade of events during and after ischemia and that were difficult to assess with more conventional MR imaging methods. In addition, the use of sequences, such as susceptibility-weighted imaging, which are extremely sensitive to the presence of even small hemorrhagic deposits, should help us in assessing when it may or may not be safe to perform treatment using more conventional thrombolysis.

These developments have had a maximal impact because of their growth in parallel to modern therapies, be they pharmacologic or endovascular in nature.

REFERENCES

1. The NINDS rt-PA stroke study group tissue plasminogen activator for acute ischemic stroke. N Engl J Med 1995;333:1581–7.
2. Hacke W, Kaste M, Fieschi C, et al. Intravenous thrombolysis with recombinant tissue plasminogen activator for acute hemispheric stroke. The European Cooperative Acute Stroke Study (ECASS). JAMA 1995;274(13):1017–25.
3. Hacke W, Kaste M, Bluhmki E, et al. Thrombolysis with alteplase 3 to 4.5 hours after acute ischemic stroke. N Engl J Med 2008;359(13):1317–29.
4. Warach S, Chien D, Li W, et al. Fast magnetic resonance diffusion-weighted imaging of acute human stroke. Neurology 1992;42(9):1717–23.
5. von Kummer R, Allen KL, Holle R, et al. Acute stroke: usefulness of early CT findings before thrombolytic therapy. Radiology 1997;205(2):327–33.
6. von Kummer R, Holle R, Gizyska U, et al. Interobserver agreement in assessing early CT signs of middle cerebral artery infarction. AJNR Am J Neuroradiol 1996;17(9):1743–8.
7. Gönner F, Remonda L, Mattle H, et al. Local intra-arterial thrombolysis in acute ischemic stroke. Stroke 1998;29(9):1894–900.
8. Schlaug G, Benfield A, Baird AE, et al. The ischemic penumbra: operationally defined by diffusion and perfusion MRI. Neurology 1999;53(7):1528–37.
9. Adams HP Jr, del Zoppo G, Alberts MJ, et al, American Heart Association, American Stroke Association Stroke Council, Clinical Cardiology Council, Cardiovascular Radiology, Intervention Council, Atherosclerotic Peripheral Vascular Disease and Quality of Care Outcomes in Research Interdisciplinary Working Groups. Guidelines for the early management of adults with ischemic stroke: a guideline from the American Heart Association/American Stroke Association Stroke Council, Clinical Cardiology Council, Cardiovascular Radiology and Intervention Council, and the Atherosclerotic Peripheral Vascular Disease and Quality of Care Outcomes in Research Interdisciplinary Working Groups: the American Academy of Neurology affirms the value of this guideline as an educational tool for neurologists. Stroke 2007;38(5):1655–711.

10. Lövblad KO, Baird AE. Actual diagnostic approach to the acute stroke patient. Eur Radiol 2006;16(6): 1253–6.

11. Willinek WA, Kuhl CK. 3.0 T neuroimaging: technical considerations and clinical applications. Neuroimaging Clin N Am 2006;16(2):217–28.

12. Heidemann RM, Seiberlich N, Griswold MA, et al. Perspectives and limitations of parallel MR imaging at high field strengths. Neuroimaging Clin N Am 2006;16(2):311–20.

13. Vargas MI, Delavelle J, Kohler R, et al. Brain and spine MRI artifacts at 3 Tesla. J Neuroradiol 2009; 36(2):74–81.

14. Patel MR, Edelman RR, Warach S. Detection of hyperacute primary intraparenchymal hemorrhage by magnetic resonance imaging. Stroke 1996;27(12): 2321–4.

15. Lövblad KO, Laubach HJ, Baird AE, et al. Clinical experience with diffusion-weighted MR in patients with acute stroke. AJNR Am J Neuroradiol 1998; 19(6):1061–6.

16. Kidwell CS, Chalela JA, Saver JL, et al. Magnetic resonance imaging and computed tomography in emergency assessment of patients with suspected acute stroke: a prospective comparison. JAMA 2004;292(15):1823–30.

17. Chalela JA, Kidwell CS, Nentwich LM, et al. Magnetic resonance imaging and computed tomography in emergency assessment of patients with suspected acute stroke: a prospective comparison. Lancet 2007;369(9558):293–8.

18. Lansberg M, Albers G, Beaulieu C, et al. Comparison of diffusion-weighted MRI and CT in acute stroke. Neurology 2000;54:1557–61.

19. Barber P, Darby D, Desmond P, et al. Identification of major ischaemic change: diffusion-weighted imaging versus computed tomography. Stroke 1999;30:2059–65.

20. Mullins ME, Schafer PW, Sorensen AG, et al. CT and conventional and diffusion-weighted MR imaging in acute stroke: study in 691 patients at presentation to the emergency department. Radiology 2002; 224:353–60.

21. Fiebach JB, Schellinger PD, Jansen O, et al. CT and diffusion-weighted MR imaging in randomized order. Diffusion-weighted imaging results in higher accuracy and lower interrater variability in the diagnosis of hyperacute ischemic stroke. Stroke 2002;33: 2206–10.

22. Fiebach J, Jansen O, Schellinger P, et al. Comparison of CT with diffusion-weighted MRI in patients with hyperacute stroke. Neuroradiology 2001;43(8):628–32.

23. Lövblad KO, Baird AE, Schlaug G, et al. Ischemic lesion volumes in acute stroke by diffusion-weighted magnetic resonance imaging correlate with clinical outcome. Ann Neurol 1997;42(2):164–70.

24. Baird AE, Lovblad KO, Dashe JF, et al. Clinical correlations of diffusion and perfusion lesion volumes in acute ischemic stroke. Cerebrovasc Dis 2000;10(6): 441–8.

25. Baird AE, Benfield A, Schlaug G, et al. Enlargement of human ischemic lesion volumes measured by diffusion-weighted magnetic resonance imaging. Ann Neurol 1997;41:581–9.

26. Baird AE, Lövblad KO, Schlaug G, et al. Multiple acute stroke syndrome: marker of embolic disease? Neurology 2000;54(3):674–8.

27. Lövblad KO, Plüschke W, Remonda L, et al. Diffusion-weighted MRI for monitoring neurovascular interventions. Neuroradiology 2000;42(2):134–8.

28. Taleb M, Lövblad KO, El-Koussy M, et al. Reperfusion demonstrated by ADC mapping after intra-arterial thrombolysis for human ischemic stroke confirmed by cerebral angiography. Neuroradiology 2001;43:591–4.

29. Marks MP, Tong DC, Beaulieu C, et al. Evaluation of early reperfusion and i.v. tPA therapy using diffusion- and perfusion-weighted MRI. Neurology 1999;52(9): 1792–8.

30. Le Bihan D, Breton E, Lallemand D, et al. MR imaging of intravoxel incoherent motions: application to diffusion and perfusion in neurologic disorders. Radiology 1986;161(2):401–7.

31. Le Bihan D, Mangin JF, Poupon C, et al. Diffusion tensor imaging: concepts and applications. J Magn Reson Imaging 2001;13(4):534–46.

32. Warach S, Mosley M, Sorensen AG, et al. Time course of diffusion imaging abnormalities in human stroke. Stroke 1996;27(7):1254–6.

33. Schlaug G, Siewert B, Benfield A, et al. Time course of the apparent diffusion coefficient (ADC) abnormality in human stroke. Neurology 1997;49(1):113–9.

34. Kuhl CK, Textor J, Gieseke J, et al. Acute and subacute ischemic stroke at high-field-strength (3.0-T) diffusion-weighted MR imaging: intraindividual comparative study. Radiology 2005;234(2):509–16.

35. Rosen BR, Belliveau JW, Chien D. Perfusion imaging by nuclear magnetic resonance. Magn Reson Q 1989;5(4):263–81.

36. Lev MH, Rosen BR. Clinical applications of intracranial perfusion MR imaging. Neuroimaging Clin N Am 1999;9(2):309–31.

37. Detre JA, Wang J, Wang Z, et al. Arterial spin-labeled perfusion MRI in basic and clinical neuroscience. Curr Opin Neurol 2009;22(4):348–55.

38. Heid O. T1-gewichtete MR perfusion [dissertation]. Switzerland: University of Bern; 2000.

39. Edelman RR, Siewert B, Darby DG, et al. Qualitative mapping of cerebral blood flow and functional localization with echo-planar MR imaging and signal targeting with alternating radio frequency. Radiology 1994;192(2):513–20.

40. Viallon M, Altrichter S, Pereira VM, et al. Combined use of pulsed arterial spin-labeling and susceptibility-weighted imaging in stroke at 3T. Eur Neurol 2010; 64(5):286–96.

41. Lim CC, Petersen ET, Ng I, et al. MR regional perfusion imaging: visualizing functional collateral circulation. AJNR Am J Neuroradiol 2007;28(3):447–8.

42. Altrichter S, Kulcsar Z, Sekoranja L, et al. Arterial spin labeling demonstrates early recanalization after stroke. J Neuroradiol 2009;36(2):109–11.

43. Hendrikse J, Petersen ET, Chng SM, et al. Distribution of cerebral blood flow in the nucleus caudatus, nucleus lentiformis, and thalamus: a study of territorial arterial spin-labeling MR imaging. Radiology 2010;254(3):867–75.

44. Manka C, Träber F, Gieseke J, et al. Three-dimensional dynamic susceptibility-weighted perfusion MR imaging at 3.0 T: feasibility and contrast agent dose. Radiology 2005;234(3):869–77.

45. Willinek WA, Born M, Simon B, et al. Time-of-flight MR angiography: comparison of 3.0-T imaging and 1.5-T imaging—initial experience. Radiology 2003; 229(3):913–20.

46. Willinek WA, Gieseke J, von Falkenhausen M, et al. Sensitivity encoding (SENSE) for high spatial resolution time-of-flight MR angiography of the intracranial arteries at 3.0 T. Rofo 2004;176(1):21–6.

47. Sommer T, Hackenbroch M, Hofer U, et al. Coronary MR angiography at 3.0 T versus that at 1.5 T: initial results in patients suspected of having coronary artery disease. Radiology 2005;234(3):718–25.

48. Lövblad KO, Yilmaz H, Chouiter A, et al. Intracranial aneurysm stenting: follow-up with MR angiography. J Magn Reson Imaging 2006;24(2):418–22.

49. Debrey SM, Yu H, Lynch JK, et al. Diagnostic accuracy of magnetic resonance angiography for internal carotid artery disease: a systematic review and meta-analysis. Stroke 2008;39(8):2237–48. AJNR Am J Neuroradiol 2007;28(3):447–8.

50. Haacke EM, Mittal S, Wu Z, et al. Susceptibility-weighted imaging: technical aspects and clinical applications, part 1. AJNR Am J Neuroradiol 2009; 30(1):19–30.

51. Hermier M, Nighoghossian N, Derex L, et al. Hypointense transcerebral veins at T2*-weighted MRI: a marker of hemorrhagic transformation risk in patients treated with intravenous tissue plasminogen activator. J Cereb Blood Flow Metab 2003;23(11): 1362–70.

52. Hermier M, Nighoghossian N, Derex L, et al. Hypointense leptomeningeal vessels at T2*-weighted MRI in acute ischemic stroke. Neurology 2005; 65(4):652–3.

53. Cramer SC, Nelles G, Benson RR, et al. A functional MRI study of subjects recovered from hemiparetic stroke. Stroke 1997;28(12):2518–27.

54. Mader I, Rauer S, Gall P, et al. (1)H MR spectroscopy of inflammation, infection and ischemia of the brain. Eur J Radiol 2008;67(2):250–7.

55. Hussain MS, Stobbe RW, Bhagat YA, et al. Sodium imaging intensity increases with time after human ischemic stroke. Ann Neurol 2009;66(1):55–62.

56. Lövblad KO, Schneider J, Bassetti C, et al. Fast contrast-enhanced MR whole-brain venography. Neuroradiology 2002;44(8):681–8.

57. Lövblad KO, Bassetti C, Schneider J, et al. Diffusion-weighted MR in cerebral venous thrombosis. Cerebrovasc Dis 2001;11(3):169–76.

Vascular Disorders—Magnetic Resonance Angiography: Brain Vessels

Norbert G. Campeau, MD*, John Huston III, MD

KEYWORDS

- MRA • 3 Tesla • Aneurysm • Vascular Disorders

Key Points

- MRA obtained at 3 T is uniformly better than MRA obtained at 1.5 T, with major benefits including nearly double the SNR as well as magnetic field strength–related T1 lengthening, which improves relative background suppression.
- Parallel imaging techniques are ideally suited for high-field MRA, with advantages including faster acquisition, reduced motion artifacts, decreased blurring, less geometric distortion related to susceptibility effects, and increased spatial resolution.
- CE-MRA, and especially time-resolved CE-MRA, benefits substantially from acquisition at high magnetic field strength, with inherent competing requirements of both high spatial and temporal resolution.
- Acquisition of both unenhanced 3D-TOF and CE-MRA sequences during the same imaging session is frequently advantageous, with the diagnostic potential of the combination of techniques better than either alone, especially for evaluation of pathologic vascular entities such as AVMs, DAVFs, and coiled aneurysms.

Over the past decade, there have been substantial software and hardware improvements that improved the quality of magnetic resonance angiography (MRA), with the introduction of routine clinical 3 T imaging likely the most significant. Additional improvements include parameter optimization,[1–5] use of innovative k-space sampling schemes,[6] development of improved imaging coil arrays, incorporation of parallel imaging methods,[7–9] new gadolinium agents (eg, blood pool agents, higher relaxivity agents),[10] and improvements in radiofrequency (RF) transmission (lower power pulses, parallel RF excitation).[11] Many of these developments can be regarded as enabling technologies for high magnetic field MRA at 3 T and are essential for further development of 7 T MRA, which brings additional challenges. Parameters for commonly used MRA techniques are shown in **Tables 1–4.**

Principle clinical indications for intracranial MRA include evaluation of ischemic stroke, arterial occlusive disease, aneurysms, cerebral vascular malformations, dural arteriovenous fistula (DAVF), central nervous system vasculitis, vasospasm, and moyamoya.

MRA EVALUATION OF ISCHEMIC STROKE AND ARTERIAL OCCLUSIVE DISEASE

Causes of ischemic stroke include vascular thrombosis, cerebral embolism, hypotension, and anoxia/hypoxia. Three-dimensional time-of-flight (3D-TOF) MRA is the technique most commonly used for routine angiographic evaluation of the intracranial circulation in patients with ischemic stroke (cerebral infarction). Three-dimensional TOF MRA provides excellent depiction of the circle of Willis and its

Division of Neuroradiology, Mayo Clinic, West 2 Mayo Building, 200 First Street Southwest, Rochester, MN 55905, USA
* Corresponding author.
E-mail address: campeau.norbert@mayo.edu

Neuroimag Clin N Am 22 (2012) 207–233
doi:10.1016/j.nic.2012.02.006
1052-5149/12/$ – see front matter © 2012 Elsevier Inc. All rights reserved.

Diagnostic Checklist

Ischemic stroke and arterial occlusive disease

Aneurysm

    Aneurysm screening/follow-up of untreated aneurysm

    Aneurysm in the setting of acute subarachnoid hemorrhage

    Treated (coiled) aneurysm

    Giant/partially thrombosed aneurysm

Intracranial arterial dissection

Vascular malformations of the brain

    Arteriovenous malformation

    Capillary telangiectasia

    Cavernous angioma

    Developmental venous anomaly

Dural arteriovenous fistula

Vasculitis and vasospasm

Moyamoya

External carotid circulation pathology

---

proximal large branches. It readily depicts thrombotic vascular occlusion as well as stenosis related to arterial occlusive disease manifested by processes such as atherosclerosis and dissection. Three-dimensional TOF MRA is quite accurate for depicting widely patent normal vessels or demonstrating complete vascular occlusion, although very-slow-flow or susceptibility artifact can mimic an occlusion. Accurate assessment of partial stenosis is more precise at 3 T than 1.5 T, especially for small vessels.[2] Additional signal-to-noise ratio (SNR) available from acquisition at higher magnetic field strength in conjunction with improved multicoil arrays allows for 3D-TOF MRA with higher spatial resolution, parallel acquisition techniques with inherent reduction in acquisition time, as well as motion artifact (**Fig. 1**). Parallel imaging techniques gives rise to potentially confounding reconstruction artifacts (**Fig. 2**). In-plane saturation effects that can result in a tapered appearance of vessels because of signal dropout due to slower-moving peripheral blood are less prominent at 3 T. The combination of conventional and low-dose postgadolinium 3D-TOF MRA has been advocated to provide more robust and specific evaluation of intracranial vascular stenosis.[12,13]

Phase-contrast MRA (PC-MRA) techniques[14] are not frequently used for evaluation of stroke, except if directional flow information or velocities are desired. The phase images of PC-MRA can be used to determine direction of collateral flow about the circle of Willis. PC-MRA is useful for performing MRA after administration of intravenous gadolinium because PC-MRA benefits from acquisition with presence of intravascular gadolinium, whereas 3D-TOF MRA is typically suboptimal following full-dose gadolinium administration because of confounding overlapping vascularity due to opacified venous structures.

For specific clinical indications, gadolinium contrast–enhanced MRA (CE-MRA), including time-resolved CE-MRA, can be helpful to assess intracranial vascular patency (**Fig. 3**). High-resolution 3 T black blood MRA[15] permits high-resolution vessel wall imaging useful for assessment of intracranial atherosclerosis.

MRA EVALUATION OF ANEURYSM

A common application of intracranial MRA is evaluation of arterial aneurysms, which can be categorized morphologically as either fusiform (10%) or saccular (90%). Saccular aneurysms most commonly arise from the circle of Willis (90%) and from the vertebrobasilar system (10%) and are believed to arise from flow-related vessel wall stresses and a complex combination of genetically inherited susceptibility. The incidence of sporadic intracranial aneurysms is 1% to 2% in autopsy series. There is an approximate 10% prevalence for familial intracranial aneurysms, which typically present in younger patients compared with those

---

Recommended pulse sequence chart: 3 T magnetic resonance angiography of the brain

Ischemic stroke and arterial occlusive disease

3D-TOF MRA

Aneurysm

Aneurysm screening, follow-up of untreated aneurysm: 3D-TOF MRA

Aneurysm in setting of acute subarachnoid hemorrhage: CTA, DSA, 3D-TOF MRA (typically not first study, if obtained)

Treated (coiled) aneurysm: 3D-TOF MRA and intracranial CE-MRA

Giant/partially thrombosed aneurysm: 3D-TOF MRA, PC-MRA, CE-MRA

Intracranial arterial dissection

3D-TOF MRA, pregadolinium fat-suppressed T1 spin-echo, black blood MRA

Vascular malformations of the brain

Arteriovenous malformation: 3D-TOF MRA,[a] PC-MRA, CE-MRA, time-resolved CE-MRA

Capillary telangiectasia: GRE/SWI, postgadolinium T1 imaging[b]

Cavernous angioma: GRE/SWI, postgadolinium T1 imaging[b]

Developmental venous anomaly: CE-MRV, postgadolinium T1 imaging[b]

Dural arteriovenous fistula

3D-TOF MRA,[a] CE-MRA, time-resolved CE-MRA

Central nervous system vasculitis

3D-TOF MRA, conventional MR imaging (GRE/SWI, T2/FLAIR, pregadolinium + postgadolinium T1 imaging)

Vasospasm

3D-TOF MRA, CE-MRA, perfusion imaging

Moyamoya

3D-TOF MRA[a], CE-MRA, time-resolved CE-MRA

External carotid circulation pathology

CE-MRA, time-resolved CE-MRA

Abbreviations: 3D-TOF, three-dimensional time of flight; CE-MRA, gadolinium contrast–enhanced magnetic resonance angiography; CTA, computed tomographic angiography; DSA, digital subtraction angiography; FLAIR, fluid attenuated inversion recovery; GRE, gradient echo; MRA, magnetic resonance angiography; MRV, magnetic resonance venography; PC-MRA, phase-contrast magnetic resonance angiography; SWI, susceptibility weighted imaging.

[a] Acquisition of both unenhanced 3D-TOF and CE-MRA sequences during the same imaging session is frequently advantageous, with the diagnostic potential of the combination of techniques better than either alone, especially for evaluation of pathologic vascular entities such as arteriovenous malformations, dural arteriovenous fistulas, and coiled aneurysms.

[b] Conventional postgadolinium T1-weighted imaging (eg, SE, GRE, MP-RAGE, and so forth).

---

with sporadic aneurysms. Conditions predisposing aneurysm formation include autosomal dominant polycystic kidney disease, aortic coarctation, fibromuscular dysplasia, aberrant vascular anatomy (persistent trigeminal artery, arterial fenestration, azygous anterior cerebral artery), or connective tissue disorder (eg, Ehlers-Danlos). Aneurysms often develop on arterial feeders of an AVM; the causes of these are believed to be flow related. An additional 1% to 3% of aneurysms are related to trauma (Fig. 4) and mycotic or oncotic etiology.

Specific subindications for MRA assessment of aneurysms include screening for aneurysms in asymptomatic high-risk populations, detection of aneurysms in the setting of acute subarachnoid hemorrhage (SAH), follow-up of known untreated aneurysms, follow-up of treated endovascularly coiled aneurysms, and evaluation of giant or partially thrombosed aneurysms. The optimal MRA technique used to evaluate aneurysms in these differing settings varies with the specific indication, as discussed later.

Table 1
Comparison of 3D-TOF brain MRA techniques. Over the past decade, acquisition times for routine 3 T 3D-TOF MRA of the brain have decreased substantially, going from approximately 12 minutes to just more than 3 minutes, with comparable image quality and coverage

MR Imaging Scanner	Acquisition Time (min)	Matrix	Partitions, Thickness, Overlap	Repetition Time/Echo Time (millisecond)	Flip Angle	FOV (cm)	Bandwidth (kHz)	Imaging Options
1.5 T	11:28	256 × 224 1 NEX	145 1.4 mm –0.7 mm	36/6.9 Fr	25°	18 × 16.2	15.6	VB, MT, Z512, Z2 3-slab MOTSA
3 T, 2001 protocol, unaccelerated	12:06	384 × 224 1 NEX	145 1.4 mm –0.7 mm	38/4 Fr	25°	18 × 16.2	15.6	VB, MT, Z512, Z2 3-slab MOTSA
3 T, unaccelerated	6:08	384 × 224 1 NEX	145 1.4 mm –0.7 mm	38/4.2 Fr	25°	18 × 16.2	15.6	ED, MT, Z512, Z2 3-slab MOTSA
3 T, accelerated, sense = 2, 8 channel	3:15	384 × 224 1 NEX	145 1.4 mm –0.7 mm	25/3.9 Fr	25°	18 × 16.2	15.6	ED, MT, Z512, Z2 3-slab MOTSA
3 T, accelerated, GRAPPA = 2, 12 channel	4:24	384 × 235 2 NEX	128 0.7 mm 0 mm	21/3.69	25°	18 × 16	40.5	PFP SAT1 5-slab MOTSA

Abbreviations: ED, extended dynamic range; FOV, field of view; Fr, fractional echo; GRAPPA, generalized autocalibrating partially parallel acquisition; MOTSA, multiple overlapping thin slab acquisition[76]; MT, magnetization transfer; NEX, number of excitation; PFP, phase partial fourier; SAT1, shifting parallel presaturation, applied to single side of acquisition slice; VB, variable bandwidth.

Table 2
Parameters for first-pass intracranial CE-MRA using bolus contrast administration and elliptic centric phase encoding order to capture contrast from opacified arteries at center of k-space. Timing can be done using a small timing bolus or automated triggering software

MR Imaging Scanner	Acquisition Time (min)	Matrix	Partitions, Thickness, Overlap	Repetition Time/Echo Time (millisecond)	Flip Angle	FOV (cm)	Bandwidth (kHz)	Imaging Options
1.5 T	00:53	256 × 224 1 NEX	89 1.2 mm −0.6 mm	6.6/2.4	45°	Axial 22 × 22	31.2	ZIP 512
3 T	00:53	416 × 224 1 NEX	89 1.2 mm −0.6 mm	6.7/2.06	40°	Axial 22 × 22	31.2	ZIP 512

Abbreviations: NEX, number of excitations; ZIP, zero interpolate.

MRA Screening and MRA Observation of Untreated Aneurysms

In the nonacute setting, 3D-TOF MRA is an excellent tool for following known aneurysms and screening for aneurysms in high-risk populations,[16] such as for individuals with known autosomal dominant polycystic kidney disease[17] or aortic coarctation.[18] Superior depiction of aneurysms using 3D-TOF MRA at 3 T versus 1.5 T has been demonstrated.[19] Using 3D-TOF MRA, aneurysms as small as 2 mm can be detected with a sensitivity of 74% to 98%. More recent literature has reported the possibility of detection of aneurysms as small as 1 mm[16]; however, to date, no large study examining the sensitivity and specificity for detection of aneurysms that small has been performed. Aneurysm size[20] and location[11] influence MRA sensitivity for detection of unruptured untreated aneurysms. Recently developed inversion recovery–based MRA techniques (**Fig. 5**)[21] and CE-MRA (**Fig. 6**) are used less commonly than TOF techniques but are sensitive for detection of aneurysms.

Digital subtraction angiography (DSA) is generally a safe procedure but still has a small but nonzero risk of morbidity, including death.[22,23] A prior large review has shown an overall neurologic morbidity rate of 1.3% and a permanent neurologic complication rate of 0.5%.[24] Risk factors for DSA included advancing age (>55 years), preexisting cardiovascular disease, and longer duration of DSA procedure. For patients allergic to iodinated contrast material, DSA may be performed after pretreatment with steroids, such as in the Lasser protocol.[25]

Aneurysms in the Setting of Acute SAH

The incidence of SAH is approximately 6 to 8 per 100,000 persons per year,[26] with peak incidence occurring in the sixth decade of life. Most nontraumatic SAHs are the result of an intracranial aneurysm rupture.

MRA is typically not the first study in a patient with acute SAH. In the acute setting of SAH, conventional DSA remains the generally accepted

Table 3
CE-MRA parameters for steady state acquisition. This sequence may be acquired concomitantly with bolus contrast administration (eg, 0.1 mmol/kg standard gadolinium agent administered intravenously at 2–3 mL/s, followed by 15 to 20 mL saline at 2 mL/s). This CE-MRA technique can also be performed successfully if acquired promptly after prior intravenous gadolinium administration (eg, immediately after time-resolved CE-MRA)

MR Imaging Scanner	Acquisition Time (min)	Matrix	Partitions, Thickness	Repetition Time/Echo Time (millisecond)	Flip Angle	FOV (cm)	Bandwidth (kHz)	Imaging Options
3 T	02:40	320 × 320 1 NEX	130 1.4 mm	5.5/1.4	30°	Sagittal 25 × 25	62.5	ZIP 512, ZIP × 2, VB, ED

Abbreviations: ED, extended dynamic range; NEX, number of excitations; VB, variable bandwidth; ZIP, zero interpolate.

Table 4
Time-resolved CE-MRA parameters for commercially available TWIST and TRICKS techniques at 3 T. No timing bolus is required. For an adult with normal renal function, approximately 20 mL Multihance is administered intravenously at a rate of 3 mL/s, followed by a 20-mL saline flush given at 3 mL/s

Time-Resolved MRA Technique	Acquisition Time (min)	Matrix Orientation Partition/Thick Field of View	Repetition Time/Echo Time (millisecond)	Flip Angle	Frame Update (s)	Other
TWIST 3 T	1:15 (0:07 for mask)	192 × 192 Sagittal 120/1.4 mm 26 × 26 cm FOV	3.15/1.27	25°	2.2 (30 × 3D volumes)	32 channel coil GRAPPA 6× (Acceleration in 2 directions)
TRICKS 3 T	1:19 (0:09 for mask)	192 × 192 Sagittal 110/2.6 mm 0.75NEX 28 × 22 cm FOV	2.2/0.9	20	2.10 (36 × 3D volumes)	8 channel coil Asset 2× (Acceleration in single direction)

Abbreviations: GRAPPA, generalized autocalibrating partially parallel acquisition; TRICKS, time-resolved imaging of contrast kinetics; TWIST, time-resolved angiography with interleaved stochastic trajectories.

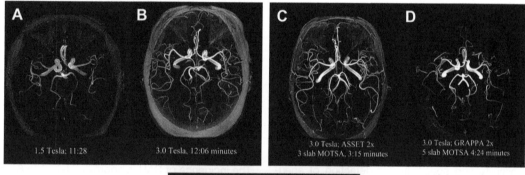

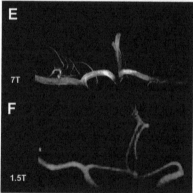

Fig. 1. Comparison of early 3 T 3D-TOF MRA with comparable 1.5 T 3D-TOF MRA, obtained using standard quadrature head coils. A decade ago, 1.5 T 3D-TOF MRA (*A*) and 3 T 3D-TOF MRA (*B*) typically required 10- to 12-minute acquisition times. Parallel acquisition techniques have been one of the most significant advances for conventional 3D-TOF MRA over the past decade, substantially reducing acquisition times. Axial maximum intensity projection (MIP) collapse from 3 T MRA using ASSET (array spatial sensitivity encoding technique) 2× acceleration acquired in 3:15 minutes using an 8-channel head coil array (*C*). Axial MIP collapse from 3 T MRA using GRAPPA (generalized autocalibrating partially parallel acquisition) 2× acceleration, acquired in 4:24 minutes using a 12-channel head coil array (*D*). An inherent benefit of acceleration techniques is reduction of patient motion artifact, principally due to decreased acquisition time. Intracranial MRA at 7 T remains primarily a research tool. Comparison of 7 T and 1.5 T 3D-TOF MRA of the anterior circle of Willis (*E, F*). Note excellent depiction of lenticulostriate arteries at 7 T, not visible on the 1.5 T MRA. (*Courtesy of* Dr Zang-Hee Cho, Neuroscience Research Institute, Gachon University of Medicine and Science.)

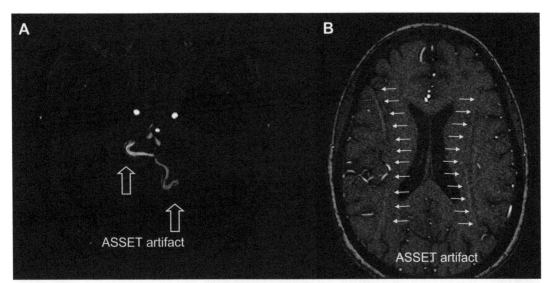

Fig. 2. Three-dimensional TOF MRA parallel acquisition artifacts. Use of parallel imaging techniques can lead to unique image artifacts, which if unrecognized could potentially lead to diagnostic misinterpretation. MRA source images should always be reviewed. (*A*, *B*) Axial 3D-TOF MRA source images depicting typical "wrap" artifacts related to ASSET (array spatial sensitivity encoding technique) parallel imaging. Patient motion is a frequent cause for these artifacts.

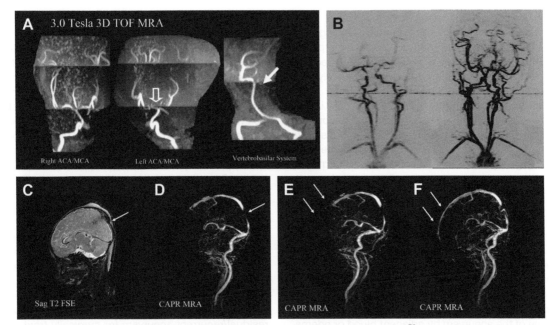

Fig. 3. Three-dimensional TOF MRA and CAPR (Cartesian projection reconstruction)[50] time-resolved CE-MRA were used to evaluate a 3-day-old infant with seizures, coagulopathy, and suspected hypoxic ischemic encephalopathy. (*A*) Conventional 3 T 3D-TOF MRA was obtained but nondiagnostic because of severe degradation by slab interface artifact as well as RF artifact arising from medication infusion pumps. The apparent intracranial stenoses noted on the 3D-TOF MRA within the left posterior cerebral artery (*solid arrow*) and left anterior and middle cerebral arteries on the 3D-TOF sequence (*open arrow*) were confirmed to represent artifact with a hand injected 1-mL CAPR time-resolved CE-MRA (*B*) that demonstrated normal patency of the intracranial vessels. (*C*) Cephalhematoma and overriding calvarial sutures (*long arrow*) identified on sagittal fast-spin echo T2-weighted image in the same patient, with clear depiction of flow defect within the superior sagittal sinus at the level of suture overlap (*long arrow*) (*D*). Sagittal venous phase MIP images from same CE-MRA shows antegrade filling of anterior superior sagittal sinus (*E*, *F*) (*double arrows*).

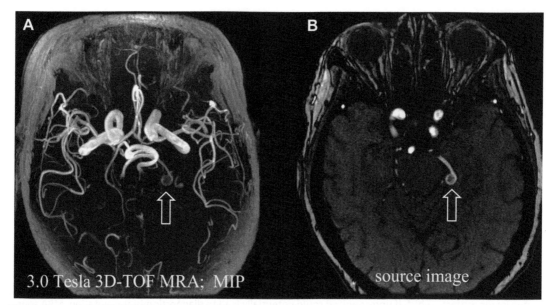

Fig. 4. Three-Tesla 3D-TOF MRA is useful for screening of aneurysms in asymptomatic individuals. Axial MIP collapse (*A*) and source image (*B*) depicting a posterior cerebral artery (PCA) aneurysm arising from the P2 segment (*arrows*). The location of this PCA aneurysm adjacent to the tentorial incisura is typical for a posttraumatic aneurysm, such as in this patient with a known history of prior severe motor vehicle accident.

gold standard for detection of intracranial aneurysms. Computed tomographic angiography (CTA) is currently playing an increasingly prominent role in the evaluation of acute SAH because it is convenient to perform CTA immediately after detection of an SAH on noncontrast head computed tomography (CT). CTA is usually immediately available, whereas magnetic resonance (MR) imaging often requires patient transfer to the MR imaging suite, which may not be near the emergency department. In addition, it is frequently necessary to summon on-call personnel necessary for MR imaging operation after routine hours. CTA has also proved quite accurate, with a reported success rate of 98% to 100% in detecting aneurysms in the setting of SAH.[27,28]

There remains a role for MRA in the setting of negative DSA examination results because false-negative rates of up to 5% to 10% are reported with DSA. It is known that vasospasm, thrombosis of the aneurysm or of the parent vessel, compression of the aneurysm by adjacent blood or edema, small aneurysm size, and limited projections may obscure a ruptured aneurysm on DSA.[26,29] In these situations, MRA has been shown to find aneurysms not identified on prior DSA.

MRA Evaluation of Treated (Coiled) Aneurysms

MRA is emerging as the technique of choice for long-term evaluation of residual or recurrent

patency of aneurysms treated with endovascular coiling.[30–35] Platinum alloy coils are designed to allow optimum visibility during endovascular treatments performed under fluoroscopic control. However, although this high attenuation is desirable during endovascular placement of the coils, the endovascular coil mass results in substantial beam hardening and streak artifact on subsequent CT and CTA examinations, degrading depiction of the aneurysm, adjacent vessels, and surrounding brain parenchyma. The susceptibility artifact arising from these platinum alloys is less at 3 T than 1.5 T predominately because of the ability to use smaller voxel sizes, usually resulting in only mild distortion of the local magnetic field and only slight loss of MRA signal intensity (**Fig. 7**). Because of these factors, MRA is favored over CTA for follow-up of coiled aneurysms. Unlike platinum coils, metallic aneurysm clips usually demonstrate substantial magnetic susceptibility artifact that usually precludes adequate MRA assessment of residual/recurrent aneurysm for surgically treated aneurysms (**Fig. 8**).

Evaluation of Giant Aneurysms and Partially Thrombosed Aneurysms

An aneurysm exceeding 2.5 cm in diameter is considered a giant aneurysm. These typically occur in the cavernous internal carotid arteries and middle cerebral artery (MCA) bifurcations. Giant aneurysms have a higher rate of rupture

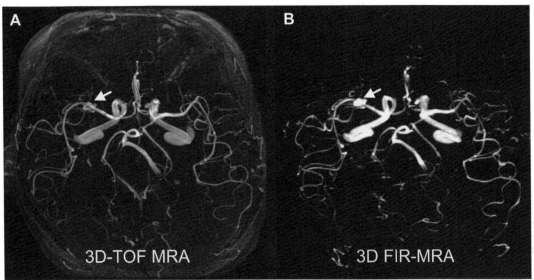

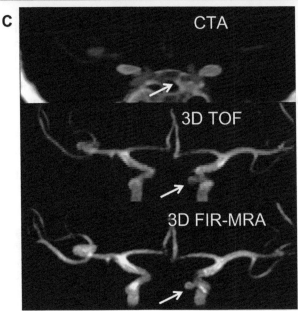

Fig. 5. Fast inversion recovery (FIR) MRA techniques combine use of inversion recovery methods and acceleration techniques made possible by 3 T MR imaging. This example demonstrates an asymptomatic right middle cerebral artery trifurcation aneurysm with unenhanced 3D-TOF MRA (*A, arrow*) and FIR-MRA (*B, arrow*). This FIR-MRA acquisition used a self-calibrated parallel imaging technique, with an acceleration factor of 2. (*C*) A second aneurysm arises from the medial aspect of the left cavernous internal carotid artery (ICA), which was not prospectively identified on CTA (*arrow, top*). This cavernous ICA aneurysm is well identified with the TOF technique (*arrow, middle*), but the cavernous region can have venous and fat signal that can confound diagnosis. Signal saturation leads to slight signal loss within the aneurysm lumen with the TOF MRA. With the FIR technique, however, the cancellation of background signal makes both aneurysms stand out (*arrow, bottom*).

than smaller saccular aneurysms.[36] Giant aneurysms are believed to enlarge from recurrent internal hemorrhage and characteristically have laminated mural hemorrhages of varying ages.

MRA evaluation of giant aneurysms is often not ideal with 3D-TOF MRA because of saturation effects on slow or recirculation internal flow (**Fig. 9**). They are typically easily identified on standard imaging and can be visualized with other MRA techniques such as CE-MRA or PC-MRA. Although less marked at 3 T, slow and/or turbulent flow within the lumen of an aneurysm may lead to

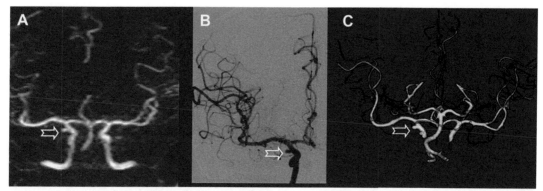

Fig. 6. Aneurysm detection with CAPR (Cartesian projection reconstruction) time-resolved CE-MRA. Although the CAPR MRA technique was primarily developed for evaluation of dynamic vascular pathology, including vascular malformations or partial stenosis, it can also detect aneurysms. CAPR CE-MRA (4× acceleration, image resolution of 0.9 mm × 1.3 mm × 2 mm, frame update rate of 2.3 seconds) depicting a 3-mm aneurysm projecting laterally from the right paraclinoid internal carotid artery (*arrow, A*). Corresponding DSA (*arrow, B*) and volume-rendered CTA images (*arrow, C*) confirming presence of the aneurysm.

dramatic signal loss on conventional 3D-TOF MRA with associated reduction in detection with this technique. Also, a thrombosed aneurysm may be harder to characterize with TOF MRA because the thrombus can be isointense. Alternatively, subacute thrombus within the wall or periphery of the aneurysm can also result in a confounding bright T1 "shine-through" signal, resulting in misinterpretation of overall patency of the aneurysm lumen. Complete clinical evaluation of a TOF MRA should include direct review of the source images, as exclusive review of the maximum

intensity projection (MIP) images alone is often diagnostically insufficient. CTA is also very useful for evaluation of giant aneurysms. Research applications of high-field PC-MRA include computational simulation of flow dynamics in a giant intracranial aneurysm.[37]

MRA EVALUATION OF INTRACRANIAL ARTERIAL DISSECTION

MRA is useful for evaluation of suspected intracranial arterial dissection.[38,39] Rarely, minor trauma is

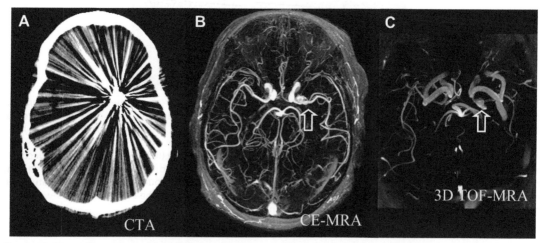

Fig. 7. Platinum alloy coils used for endovascular treatment of aneurysms are designed for optimal visibility during deployment under fluoroscopic control. The endovascular coil mass often results in substantial beam hardening and streak artifact on subsequent CT and CTA examinations (*A*), degrading depiction of the aneurysm, adjacent vessels, and surrounding brain parenchyma. (*B*) A 3 T CE-MRA MIP collapse and (*C*) a 3 T 3D-TOF MRA MIP collapse from same patient as in (*A*) depicting large aneurysm remnant (*block arrows*) of previously treated coiled aneurysm. Susceptibility artifact associated with platinum coils is relatively small, even at 3 T, usually resulting in only negligible distortion of the local magnetic field and only slight loss of MRA signal intensity.

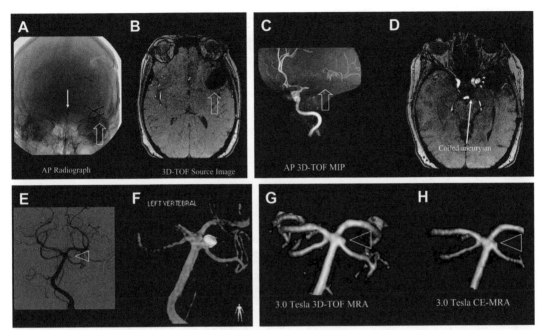

Fig. 8. Unlike platinum coils, magnetic susceptibility artifacts related to a surgically clipped aneurysm are usually quite pronounced, especially at 3 T. Anteroposterior (AP) radiograph from a DSA study (*A*) showing changes of left craniotomy with prior surgical clipping of a left middle cerebral artery aneurysm (*block arrow*, 3 clips) and endovascular coiling of a superior cerebellar artery aneurysm (*arrow*). Source image of 3D-TOF MRA (*B*) and targeted maximum intensity projection (MIP) image (*C*) from same patient showing susceptibility artifact "blowout" and corresponding loss of signal on the MIP image. Artifact related to aneurysm clips usually precludes adequate MRA assessment of residual/recurrent aneurysm. (*D*) Coiled left superior cerebellar artery aneurysm (*arrow*) has only minimal associated susceptibility artifact. Also note additional untreated aneurysm arising from the left cavernous internal carotid artery (*small arrows*). The tiny "dog-ear" aneurysm remnant (*arrowhead*) is seen on the DSA (*E*) and rotational DSA (*F*) and also on both CE TOF MRA (*G*) and CE-MRA (*H*) sequences.

sufficient to cause a dissection, or it can be spontaneous. The MRA may demonstrate complete occlusion, narrowing, or irregularity of the arterial lumen.

For evaluation of arterial dissection, 3D-TOF MRA should also be performed with conventional spin-echo images (T1 with fat suppression or proton density with fat suppression if imaging follows intravascular gadolinium administration) because they are very sensitive for detecting the intramural hemorrhage. The typical appearance of a crescent hyperintensity with an eccentrically situated flow void may be more convincing of a dissection than the MRA findings. Black blood MRA techniques[21,40] are also useful for evaluating arterial dissection and should be considered for evaluation of suspected dissection (**Fig. 10**). MRA also plays a very useful role in the follow-up imaging of dissection, determining if there is recanalization of a previously complete occlusion or depicting resolution of the vascular compromise caused by the intramural thrombus.

MRA EVALUATION OF VASCULAR MALFORMATIONS OF THE BRAIN

Vascular malformations of the brain are categorized into 4 distinct subtypes[41]: arteriovenous malformations (AVM), developmental venous anomaly (DVA), capillary telangiectasia, and cavernous malformation. Time-resolved MRA, which is best acquired at 3 T versus 1.5 T because of competing SNR requirements for both high spatial and temporal resolution, is playing an increasingly greater role in the evaluation of AVM and DAVF.

MRA Evaluation of AVM

An AVM is defined as a cerebral vascular malformation with arteriovenous shunting, without intervening capillary bed.[41] An AVM has 3 angiogenic components, including enlarged supplying arteries, a nidus of tightly packed vessels, and rapidly filling draining veins due to arteriovenous shunting. Arterial supply is usually from pial vessels; however, approximately 30% of AVMs (more common in larger AVMs) have

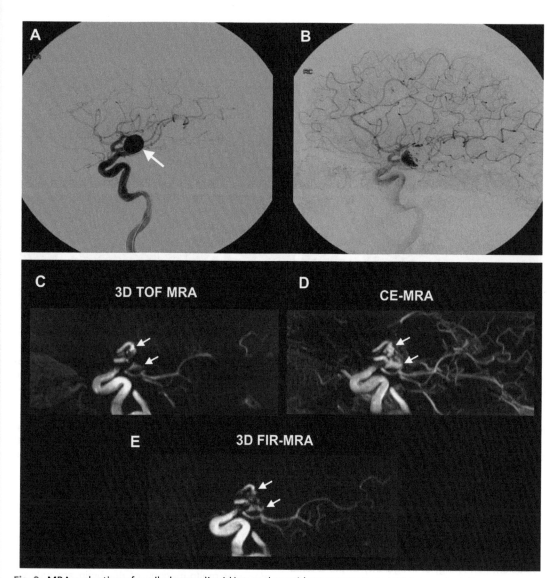

Fig. 9. MRA evaluation of a coiled supraclinoid internal carotid artery aneurysm. DSA image depicting an aneurysm before treatment (*A*) and later DSA image following endovascular coiling (*B*). A 3-month follow-up MRA was performed: 25 mm thick sagittal maximum intensity projections are shown on (*C*) 3D-TOF MRA, (*D*) CE-MRA, (*E*) and fast inversion recovery (FIR)-MRA. CE-MRA shows the upper and lower aneurysm remnants (*arrows*) better than TOF MRA. The appearance of the remnant on FIR-MRA is nearly as good as on the CE-MRA. Also, note that vessel conspicuity in FIR-MRA is superior to that in TOF MRA in this 76-year-old patient. Note that the platinum coils do not result in substantial susceptibility artifact on the MRA acquisitions, even though acquired at 3 T.

a dual arterial supply from both pial and dural vessels. The size of AVMs can range from a few millimeters to many centimeters. About 98% of AVMs are solitary and sporadic. Approximately 85% of AVMs are supratentorial in location and 15% infratentorial. Clinical presentation is typically severe headache with hemorrhage in a young adult. Peak ages for symptomatic presentation are between 20 and 40 years; however, approximately 25% of AVMs present before age 15 years. Most symptomatic AVMs range in diameter from 3 to 6 cm.

Angiographic assessment of AVMs characteristically includes determining the location, identification of arterial feeders, venous drainage pattern, and any other associated vascular anomalies, such as presence of feeding pedicle or intranidal aneurysms.[41] AVMs are typically graded according to the Spetzler-Martin grading system,[42] which is useful for predicting surgical risk if an attempt at surgical resection is made. Parameters included in the Spetzler-Martin grading system include largest diameter of the nidus that is graded as small

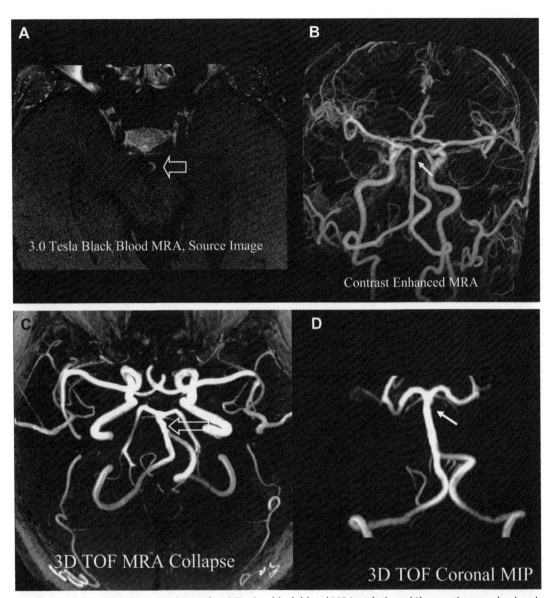

Fig. 10. Vertebrobasilar dissection imaged at 3 T using black blood MRA technique (*A*), non–time-resolved gado-linium bolus CE-MRA technique (*B*), and 3D-TOF MRA (*C, D*). Note the excellent conspicuity of the hyperintense crescent in the vessel wall of the upper basilar artery (*block arrow* [*A*]), representing site of basilar artery dissec-tion. The MIP images from (*B–D*) demonstrate only a small focal irregularity in the caliber of the vessel at the site of dissection (*arrow* [*B, D*]; *block arrow* [*C*]).

(<3 cm), medium (3–6 cm), and large (>6 cm); eloquence/noneloquence of adjacent brain (eloquent areas include sensorimotor, language, visual, thal-amus, hypothalamus, internal capsule, brain stem, cerebellar peduncles, and deep cerebellar nuclei); and pattern of venous drainage, which is considered superficial only if all drainage is via the cortical drainage system and not if there is presence of a deep venous component. There is a high correla-tion of Spetzler-Martin grade determined from MRA and DSA modalities.[43–45]

The current gold standard for imaging intracra-nial AVMs remains intra-arterial DSA. Patients with AVM usually require multiple DSA examina-tions over the course of their diagnostic evaluation and therapeutic care, resulting in increased expo-sure to DSA-related procedural morbidity (vascular injury, thromboembolic complications, radiation exposure, nephrotoxicity/allergic reaction related to iodinated contrast dye administration), which is low but not insignificant.[22–24] Consequently, there is an increasing interest for a high-quality noninvasive imaging method such as time-resolved MRA to both supplement and decrease the amount of required DSA examinations, leading to improved patient care and outcome. The major disadvantage of MRA relative to DSA is lack of sufficient spatial and temporal resolution required for adequate separation of arterial, capillary, and venous phases. Although CTA has the ability to demonstrate the AVM nidus, it has substantially less spatial resolution and dynamic information compared with DSA. In addition, exposure to ionizing radiation and iodinated contrast agents are other factors that make use of CTA less desirable than MRA. A major advantage of MR imaging/MRA compared with CTA or DSA includes better visualization of the surrounding cerebral structures. Functional MR imaging can assist in treatment planning by defining the functionality of adjacent brain.

Many MRA techniques have been studied for evaluation of AVM. Three-dimensional TOF MRA is a good first sequence, especially for demonstrating feeding arteries; however, because it relies on the physiologic properties of blood flow, the quality of 3D-TOF MRA is often degraded (less so at 3 T) from spin dephasing that occurs in complex or turbulent flow patterns commonly present in the nidus of the AVMs as well as from signal saturation in areas of slow flow. Nevertheless such flow-related signal changes on conventional 3D-TOF MRA do provide important assessment of the high-flow AVM hemodynamics.

CE-MRA overcomes some of the limitations inherent to the 3D-TOF technique, relying on the T1 shortening of administered intravascular gadolinium, which permits shorter acquisition times with increased SNR and consequently better depiction of the nidus and draining veins with improved whole head coverage (Fig. 11), better visualization of nidus and draining veins (Fig. 12), and improved detection of smaller vascular malformations obscured by hemorrhage (Fig. 13). Time-resolved CE-MRA sequences (eg, TRICKS [time-resolved imaging of contrast kinetics],[46] TREAT [time-resolved echo-shared angiographic technique],[47] TWIST [time-resolved angiography with interleaved stochastic trajectories],[48] HYPR [highly constrained back-projection],[49] CAPR [Cartesian projection reconstruction][50]) have been developed with sufficiently high temporal resolution to allow the acquisition of diagnostic quality images at a high enough temporal resolution such that the phases of intracranial circulation are adequately separated. Because of competing SNR requirements of temporal and spatial resolution, time-resolved MRA is universally superior when acquired at 3 T than at 1.5 T. Time-resolved CE-MRA is superior to other MRA techniques for depicting the AVM nidus and assessing AVM vascular architecture and hemodynamics[45,51–53] but still falls short of the gold standard set by conventional DSA. A combination of MR imaging techniques (eg, 3D-TOF MRA, inversion recovery MRA, and CE-MRA) is frequently advantageous

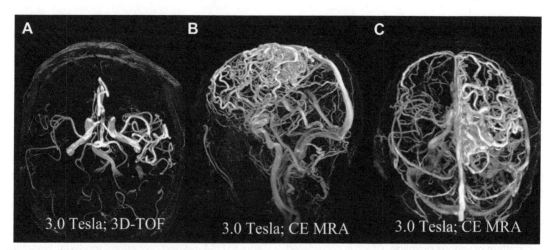

Fig. 11. Left frontal-temporal AVM evaluated using 3D-TOF MRA and 3D CE-MRA techniques. Axial MIP 3D-TOF MRA collapse (A) and sagittal and axial MIP collapse images (B, C) from a non–time-resolved 3D CE-MRA of the brain obtained at 3 T using bolus intravenous injection of gadolinium. A small test bolus of gadolinium is used to determine appropriate timing for the CE-MRA sequence. Anatomic coverage of the TOF MRA is limited compared with the whole head coverage of the CE-MRA. This CE-MRA is not time resolved and provides simultaneous opacification of the arteries and veins.

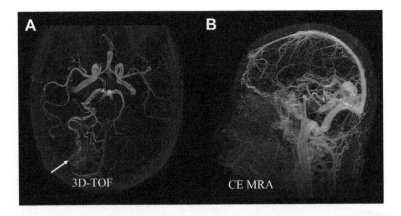

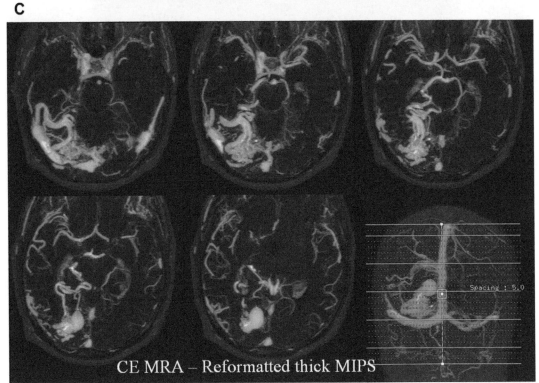

Fig. 12. Right occipital AVM evaluated using a combination of 3D-TOF MRA (*A*), and non–time-resolved CE-MRA (*B*). Review of the 3D CE-MRA is best performed using an independent workstation that allows interactive segmentation and multiplanar display to reduce confounding overlap of vessels (*C*). The CE-MRA technique (*B*, *C*) results in opacification of the arterial feeders, AVM nidus, and draining veins, whereas TOF shows principally the arterial vessels and nidus (*arrow*, [*A*]). When evaluated in combination, these 2 techniques can provide more specific and confident evaluation of the AVM components and can usually depict all features necessary for Spetzler-Martin grading of the AVM, including diameter of the nidus, eloquence of adjacent brain (eloquent areas include sensorimotor, language, visual, thalamus, hypothalamus, internal capsule, brain stem, cerebellar peduncles, and deep cerebellar nuclei), and pattern of venous drainage (considered superficial only if all drainage is via the cortical drainage system and not if there is presence of a deep venous component).

for evaluation of AVM, with the diagnostic potential of the combination of techniques better than either alone (**Fig. 14**). Continued MRA improvements, such as new PC HYPRFlow[54] technique (**Fig. 15**), enable better detection of residual nidus or early draining veins for treated AVMs and minimize the number of DSA procedures required. Novel methods of displaying 4-dimensional time-resolved MRA datasets are currently being developed, which use color overlays (**Fig. 16**)[55] to encode temporal/hemodynamic information.

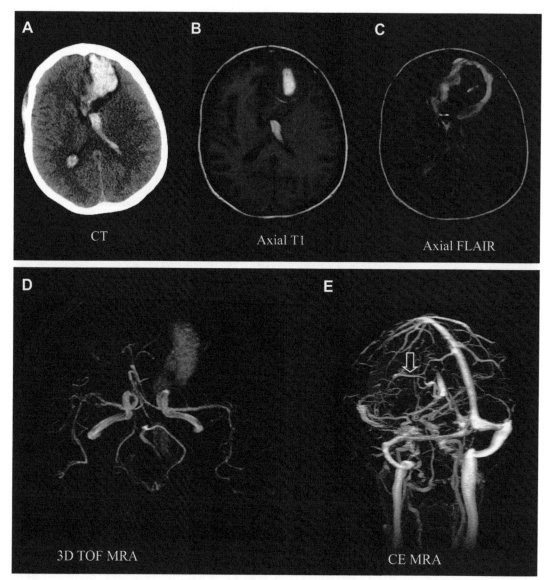

Fig. 13. AVM imaged with axial CT (*A*), axial T1 (*B*) and FLAIR (*C*) MR imaging, axial 3D-TOF MRA (*D*), and CE-MRA (*E*). Active bleeding into a brain parenchymal hematoma can be identified on CE-MRA and DSA. This smaller AVM is better depicted on CE-MRA (*arrow, E*) than on TOF. Furthermore, TOF MRA is more susceptible to degradation from bright T1 signal related to surrounding hemorrhage.

MRA Evaluation of DVA

A DVA is the most commonly identified cerebral vascular malformation at autopsy (60% of all cerebral vascular malformations) and have a population incidence of approximately 2% to 4%.[56] DVA is generally considered as a nonpathologic congenital variant of venous drainage.[57,58] The term venous angioma is often used as a synonym for DVA but is misleading because the term angioma suggests a more ominous entity with risk of bleeding. As such, the term DVA is currently preferred.

The pathogenesis of DVA is largely unknown. Histologically, most (80%) DVAs consist of only histologically mature venous elements, with some (20%) having mixed histology, including cavernous elements that typically appear as a co-existing cavernous malformation–like abnormality within the drainage field of the DVA. These cavernoma-like lesions may be acquired, related to hemorrhage within the drainage field of the DVA, rather than presence of a true congenital cavernous malformation.[59] DVAs are not surgically resected because they drain functional brain

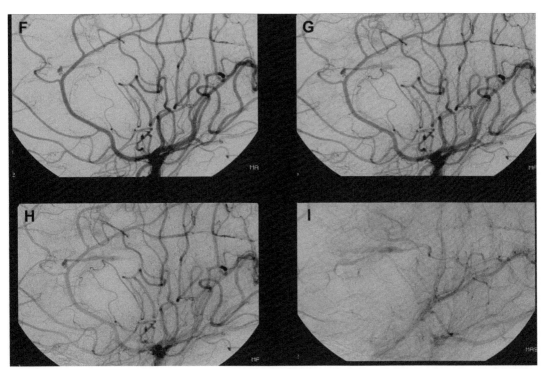

Fig. 13. AVM imaged with conventional DSA (*F–I*). Active bleeding into a brain parenchymal hematoma can be identified on CE-MRA and DSA. This smaller AVM is better depicted on CE-MRA (*arrow, E*) than on TOF. Furthermore, TOF MRA is more susceptible to degradation from bright T1 signal related to surrounding hemorrhage.

tissue and are believed to have a low risk of hemorrhage.

A DVA is typically not seen on 3D-TOF or PC-MRA. DVA is identified most reliably with contrast-enhanced MRA techniques or simply postgadolinium T1-weighted imaging. Susceptibility weighted imaging[60] (SWI) helps to identify DVA and associated cavernoma-like abnormality.

MRA Evaluation of Cavernous Malformations

Cavernous malformations (cavernous angioma, cavernoma) represent benign vascular hamartoma, containing masses of closely juxtaposed immature blood vessels, without intervening neural tissue.[41] Most cavernous malformations (75%) occur as solitary sporadic lesions. There is a familial form of cavernous malformations (10%–30%) in which lesions are often multiple and prone to repeated spontaneous hemorrhages.

Cavernous malformations are slow-flow lesions that are not conspicuous using conventional MRA sequences, except for susceptibility changes on source images. Gradient echo imaging and SWI are best for detection of these lesions, with SWI especially useful for detection of multiple lesions that are often small.[60,61]

MRA Evaluation of Capillary Telangiectasia

Capillary telangiectasia is a small slow-flow vascular malformation that is typically asymptomatic and usually occult on MRA.[62] It can be seen as a contrast blush on T1-weighted imaging, occurring in characteristic locations, most often in the central pons. SWI has recently been reported to be helpful in depicting the microvascular characteristics of capillary telangiectasia,[63] thereby confirming the lesion and eliminating more ominous differential considerations. SWI[60] relies on blood oxygen level dependent effect for contrast, the effect of which increases as the square of the main magnetic field strength.

MRA EVALUATION OF CRANIAL DAVF

Intracranial DAVF is an additional type of vascular malformation that is supplied by dural arteries and drains directly into meningeal veins or dural venous sinuses without intervening nidus.[41] DAVF accounts for approximately 10% to 15% of all intracranial vascular malformations.[64] The clinical features of DAVFs range from mild complaints such as headache, vertigo, or tinnitus to disabling neurologic deficits or a life-threatening intracranial hemorrhage. The cause of DAVF remains unknown,

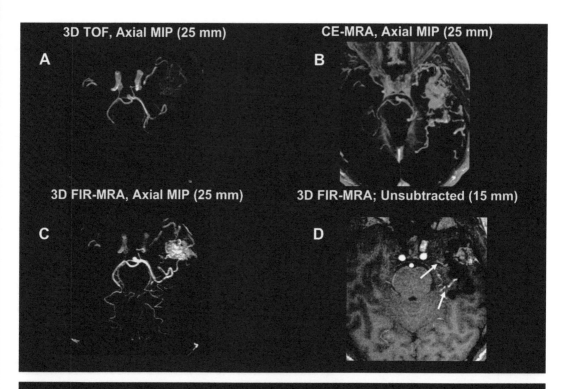

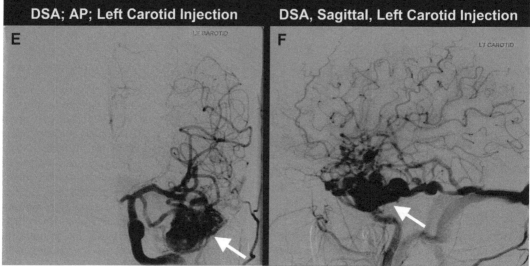

Fig. 14. Comparison of 3D fast inversion recovery (FIR)-MRA, 3D-TOF MRA, and CE-MRA for evaluation of a left temporal lobe AVM with a diameter of approximately 3 cm. Targeted 25 mm axial thick MIP images at the same location obtained at 3 T using (*A*) 3D-TOF MRA, (*B*) bolus gadolinium CE-MRA, (*C*) FIR-MRA subtraction image, (*D*) FIR-MRA bright blood image, and (*E*) sagittal and (*F*) lateral DSA images of the same AVM (*arrow* [*E, F*]). Of the MRA techniques, the unsubtracted FIR-MRA image (*D*) provides best depiction of the small hyperintense feeding arteries (*arrows* [*D*]) next to the larger hypointense draining veins. The combination of these MRA techniques, when evaluated together, can be better than either technique alone.

but the condition may be predisposed by trauma or vascular thrombosis.

Intracranial DAVF is usually categorized into 2 principal groups based on location, with one group including DAVF involving the cavernous sinus and one that does not. Cavernous sinus DAVFs are further subdivided into 2 groups, direct and indirect, depending on whether the fistula directly shunts into the cavernous sinus or indirect if the fistula shunts via meningeal vessels located

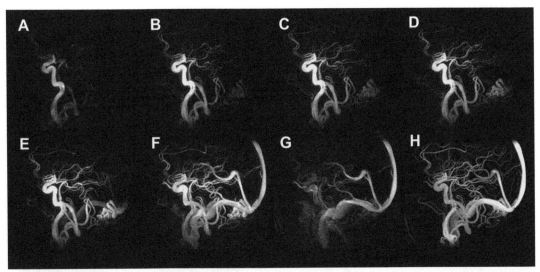

Fig. 15. PC HYPRFlow[54] images of a posterior fossa AVM. Five frames from a 60-frame acquisition are displayed (*A–G*). A 3D whole head acquisition is acquired every 500 millisecond during the first pass of contrast using an undersampled 3D radial technique. Following the dynamic series, a 3D phase-contrast scan (*H*) is obtained also using undersampled 3D radial methods. The total scan time is 360 seconds. Each time frame is constrained (essentially multiplied) by the 3D phase contrast improving the SNR and resolution of the dynamic series. The phase-contrast velocity data can be used to calculate volume flow and estimate hemodynamic parameters. (*Courtesy of* Dr Patrick Turski. Department of Radiology, University of Wisconsin.)

remotely from the cavernous sinus. Typical clinical symptoms of cavernous sinus DAVF include proptosis and chemosis that may be associated with orbital pain. Although DSA is the preferred method for evaluating cavernous sinus DAVF, 3D-TOF MRA is often the first-line angiographic examination technique used for evaluation of cavernous sinus DAVF,[64,65] with MRA findings including demonstration of prominent extracranial vessels feeding the fistula or draining venous structures resulting from flow-related enhancement. Three-dimensional TOF MRA must be obtained before administration of gadolinium because distinguishing subtle pathologic flow differences within the cavernous sinuses from normal slow cavernous sinus blood flow following the administration of contrast may be quite difficult. CE-MRA (**Fig. 17**) and newer faster time-resolved MRA techniques (**Fig. 18**) are promising for evaluation of carotid-cavernous DAVF.[65]

Noncavernous sinus DAVFs are most commonly located in the transverse and sigmoid sinuses with other sites including the superior sagittal sinus, tentorium, petrosal sinuses, and dura of the anterior cranial fossa. DAVFs occurring in the lateral and transverse sinuses often present clinically with pulsatile tinnitus. The Borden classification organizes noncavernous sinus intracranial DAVF malformations into 3 groups based on their venous drainage[66]: type I DAVFs drain directly into dural venous sinuses or meningeal veins; type II DAVFs drain into dural sinuses or meningeal veins, including retrograde drainage into subarachnoid veins; and type III DAVFs drain into subarachnoid veins without dural sinus or meningeal venous drainage. Type I dural fistulas are often asymptomatic, do not have a high risk of bleeding, and do not necessarily need to be treated. Type II and type III DAVFs need to be treated.[67] Elevated pressure within a type II DAVF results in retrograde flow of blood into subarachnoid veins, which normally drain into the sinus, usually as a result of the development of sinus outflow obstruction. Such draining veins can form venous varices or aneurysms, which are predisposed to hemorrhage. Various modalities are used to treat DAVF, including endovascular, surgical, radiation, or combined approaches. With the advent of improved interventional devices and techniques during the past decade, endovascular therapy is generally becoming the first treatment modality of choice. Treatment of type II fistulas includes embolization of the draining sinus as well as clipping or embolization of the draining veins. Type III DAVFs drain directly into subarachnoid veins, which can form aneurysms and bleed. Treatment of type III DAVFs can be as simple as clipping the draining vein at the site of the dural sinus. Embolization of type III

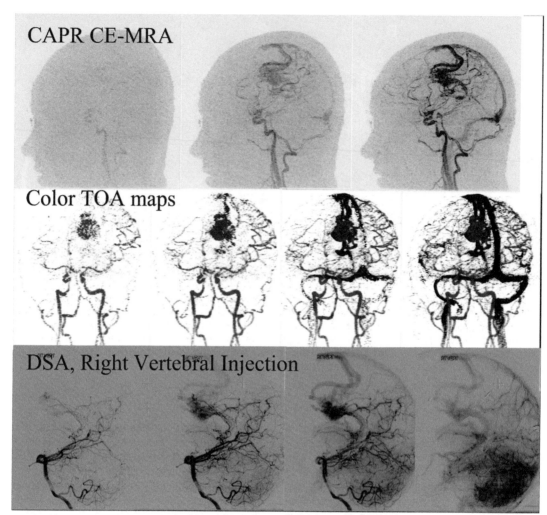

Fig. 16. Color time-of-arrival (TOA) mapping. Color encoding may be used to concisely display temporal vascular flow information from multiple time frames of a time-resolved 3D MRA on a single image. Three sagittal MIP images from individual time frames of a time-resolved CAPR[50] CE-MRA acquisition (*top row*) performed for evaluation of new hemorrhage associated with a previously treated pericallosal AVM. Data from the same CAPR MRA acquisition shown with colorized TOA display (*middle row*). There are many ways to color encode temporal information. Color TOA mapping can be useful to visually separate arterial and venous components of the AVM. Selected time frames from corresponding right vertebral artery injection DSA in the same patient (*bottom row*).

DAVF is only successful if the glue traverses the actual fistula and at least to some extent occludes the draining vein.[68]

Important imaging features to characterize DAVF include location, size, arterial supply, and presence or absence of cortical venous reflux. The presence of cortical venous reflux correlates with a more aggressive clinical course of DAVF and hence an increased propensity for more aggressive treatment of these DAVFs. It may be difficult to diagnose DAVFs at an early stage in clinical practice because of its nonspecific clinical and imaging findings. The diagnosis or confirmation of DAVFs usually requires the high spatial and high temporal resolution of DSA. DAVF is a treatable disease but is difficult to detect in many cases, eventually leading to irreversible morbidity because of the diagnostic delay.

MR imaging findings of DAVF are variable, ranging from no demonstrable lesion to identifiable fistula, venous flow-related enhancement, prominent extracranial vessels, intracranial hemorrhage, or venous infarction.[69–71] A high index of suspicion is needed to successfully diagnose DAVFs. MR images should be closely scrutinized, as well as any flow void cluster or flow-related enhancement, which are the most common MR imaging and MRA findings, respectively. If enlarged leptomeningeal

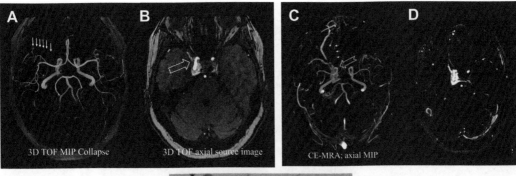

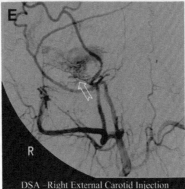

Fig. 17. Cavernous-carotid fistula evaluated at 3 T with 3D-TOF MRA (*small arrows* [*A*]) (*open arrow* [*B*]) and CE-MRA (*C, D*). The CE-MRA axial MIP collapse (*C*) shows abnormally increased blood flow within the right cavernous sinus, prominence of the right ophthalmic vein, and asymmetrically prominent small dural based vessels (*3 small arrows and single longer tailed arrow* [*C*]) along the floor of the anterior cranial fossa on source images. Reformatted axial CE-MRA image delineates the right internal carotid artery from the cavernous sinus (*open notched arrow* [*C*]) but not as well as on the TOF MRA (*B*). Right external carotid artery injection DSA (*E*) confirms presence of the indirect cavernous-carotid fistula (*open notched arrow*).

or medullary vessels are identified or if there are prominent areas of vascular enhancement noted on MR images, further evaluation, including MRA and/or conventional DSA, is indicated. A low threshold for performing conventional DSA is needed because diagnosis of DAVF often requires the high spatial and temporal resolution of DSA. It is better to detect and treat DAVF before aggressive symptoms manifest and the possibility of permanent morbidity is less.

The role of MRA in the evaluation of DAVFs is to help with early diagnosis including noninvasive screening, evaluate therapeutic success, and then monitor for recurrence. The use of 3 T time-resolved CE-MRA[70] has been shown to be useful for screening of DAVF and for surveillance of treated DAVF. Assessment of venous drainage patterns with MRA can be helpful.[71] PC-MRA can provide an effective way of assessing venous flow reversal. Concomitant MR imaging is useful to assess for complications of DAVF, such as venous infarction, parenchymal hemorrhage or signal change, hydrocephalus, and dilated cortical veins.

MRA IN THE EVALUATION OF VASCULITIS AND VASOSPASM

Intracranial vasculitis can be evaluated to an extent using MRA, but at least part of the advantage of using MRA is the possibility of performing concomitant MR imaging evaluation of the brain during the same session. The role of MRA in the evaluation of intracranial vasculitis remains unclear. When characteristic segmental vascular caliber changes are identified on MRA (Fig. 19), the diagnosis can be suggested[72]; however, a negative study result is insufficient to exclude vasculitis. Nevertheless, 3D-TOF MRA is often requested for this indication. Because MR imaging evaluation of vasculitis typically includes gadolinium-enhanced images, it can be convenient to administer the gadolinium contrast as part of a CE-MRA sequence.

MRA, especially when performed at a high magnetic field strength, can play a role in the assessment of vasospasm.[73] Complementary MR imaging diffusion and perfusion imaging can be obtained during the same imaging session.

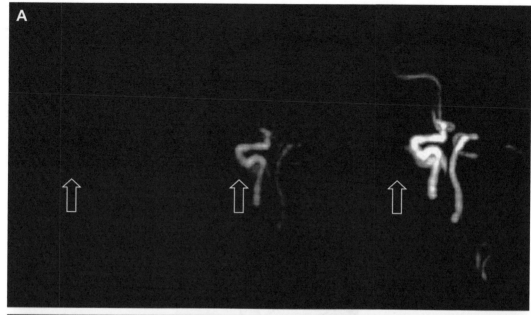

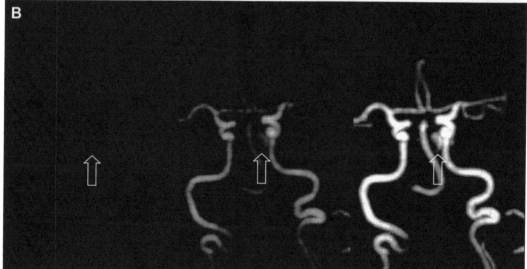

Fig. 18. Time-resolved CE-MRA of carotid-cavernous fistula obtained at 3 T using TWIST technique (parameters shown in Table 4) and 32-channel head coil and total acceleration factor of 6 (2 directions, 3 × 2). Pixel size was 1.4 mm isotropic, frame update time was 2.56 seconds, temporal footprint was 7.1 seconds, and acquisition time was 75 seconds. No timing bolus is necessary. Three sagittal MIP (A) and 3 AP MIP (B) images of the intra-cranial circulation from consecutive frames demonstrating early arrival of gadolinium contrast within the left cavernous sinus in this 85-year-old patient with an indirect carotid-cavernous fistula (open arrows).

DSA remains the gold standard and continues to be used, especially because endovascular therapy is often used to treat vasospasm (balloon angioplasty, intra-arterial administration of vasodilators). Doppler ultrasonography is still commonly used to assess for vasospasm in the anterior circulation, with best results for the MCA, with the transducer positioned over the thin temporal window. CTA, often coupled with perfusion CT, is also commonly used.

MRA Evaluation of Moyamoya Disease

MRA evaluation of moyamoya disease and moyamoya syndrome[74] is best performed using a combination of 3D-TOF and CE-MRA. Angiographic

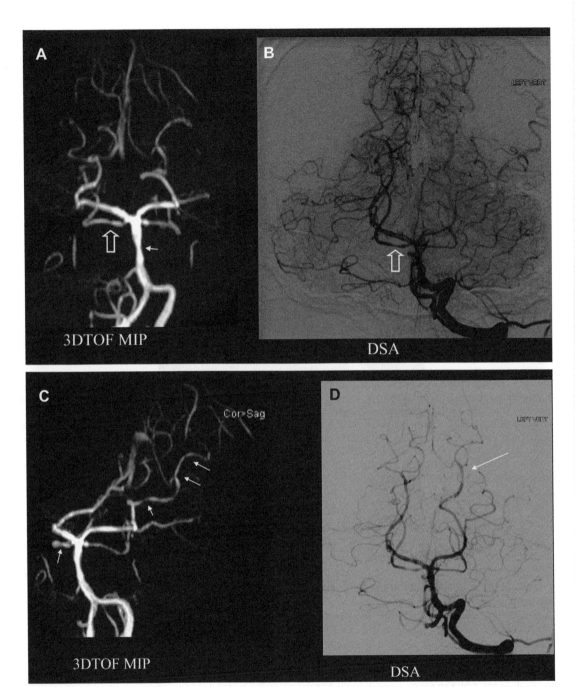

Fig. 19. Evaluation of central nervous system vasculitis related to cocaine and marijuana abuse evaluated with 3D-TOF MRA and DSA. Targeted MIP images of the posterior circulation from 3D-TOF MRA (*A, C*) and corresponding DSA images (*B, D*). There are multiple segmental and focal areas of luminal narrowing seen on both the TOF and DSA studies in a pattern and distribution compatible with vasculitis (*short and long arrows, open arrows*). The diagnosis of vasculitis can be suggested when segmental caliber changes are noted on MRA; however, a negative MRA study is generally considered insufficient to exclude vasculitis.

findings of moyamoya disease include occlusion of cervical arteries and proximal large intracranial arteries, typically the internal carotid arteries, with development of innumerable small collaterals.

Moyamoya disease is believed to be inherited and is more common in young women and children. Moyamoya syndrome results in a similar pattern of occlusion as moyamoya disease and

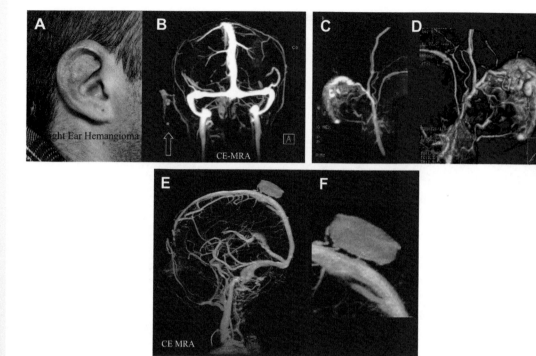

Fig. 20. Evaluation of the external carotid circulation may be effectively performed with CE-MRA techniques. Three-dimensional TOF MRA does not image the external carotid branches well. Soft tissue hemangioma involving the right ear (*A*) was evaluated using non–time-resolved CE-MRA technique. Coronal MIP collapse of the head (*B, open arrow* depicts hemangioma), targeted MIP of the right ear (*C*), and volume-rendered image of the right ear (*D*). Additional example showing the utility of CE-MRA for evaluation of a vascular scalp mass in a 7-month-old child (*E*). Targeted MIP of the mass from the same study shows only few small vascular branches connected to this mass, without invasion/involvement of the superior sagittal sinus (*F*). The mass was resected based on this MRA without performing DSA and shown to represent a subcutaneous capillary hemangioma.

can be the result of advanced atherosclerosis (smokers, diabetics) or associated with Down syndrome, neurofibromatosis, or sickle cell disease. After disease onset, moyamoya typically progresses to complete occlusion of involved vessels and collaterals.

DSA is the preferred technique for diagnosis with the characteristic angiographic finding of "puff of smoke," which is a loose translation of the Japanese word moyamoya. The moyamoya collaterals are better depicted with CE-MRA techniques than 3D-TOF MRA.[3] Concomitant brain MR imaging is useful for depiction of collateral vessels and complications of moyamoya, such as cerebral infarction and hemorrhage.

Treatment of moyamoya is surgical; the treatment of choice is the STA-MCA procedure in which the superficial temporal artery is directly sutured to the MCA. Encephalo-duro-arterio-synangiosis is a procedure in which a scalp artery is dissected free and then sutured to the meninges of the brain. The encephalomyosynangiosis procedure harvests the temporalis muscle, which is then placed onto the surface of the brain. MRA evaluation of the patency of an STA-MCA bypass or synangiosis procedure is preferably performed at 3 T using a CE-MRA technique[75] (steady state or time resolved).

MRA EVALUATION OF THE EXTRACRANIAL CIRCULATION

Evaluation of extracranial vascular masses, such as nasopharyngeal angiofibroma, sinonasal hemangiopericytoma, and soft tissue hemangioma, can be effectively performed using CE-MRA techniques (**Fig. 20**). Such pathologic processes typically derive their blood supply from external carotid artery branches for which evaluation using conventional 3D-TOF MRA techniques is often inadequate.

SUMMARY

MRA techniques play a substantial role for angiographic assessment of the brain, and its clinical importance continues to increase, especially with continued development of high magnetic field imaging. Although MRA at 3 T is well established, MRA at 7 T and higher remains early in development. Continued breakthroughs in enabling technologies, such as parallel imaging, innovative k-space sampling schemes, new gadolinium agents (eg, blood pool agents, higher relaxivity agents),[10] improved RF excitation methods, and novel image reconstruction methods (eg, HYPR, compressed sensing), will expand the utility of MRA to diagnose and monitor intracranial vascular disease.

REFERENCES

1. Soher BJ, Dale BM, Merkle EM. A review of MR physics: 3T versus 1.5T. Magn Reson Imaging Clin N Am 2007;15(3):277–90, v.

2. Willinek WA, Born M, Simon B, et al. Time-of-flight MR angiography: comparison of 3.0-T imaging and 1.5-T imaging—initial experience. Radiology 2003; 229(3):913–20.

3. Ozsarlak O, Van Goethem JW, Maes M, et al. MR angiography of the intracranial vessels: technical aspects and clinical applications. Neuroradiology 2004;46(12):955–72.

4. Campeau NG, Huston J 3rd, Bernstein MA, et al. Magnetic resonance angiography at 3.0 Tesla: initial clinical experience. Top Magn Reson Imaging 2001; 12(3):183–204.

5. Bernstein MA, Huston J 3rd, Lin C, et al. High-resolution intracranial and cervical MRA at 3.0T: technical considerations and initial experience. Magn Reson Med 2001;46(5):955–62.

6. Wilman AH, Riederer SJ. Performance of an elliptical centric view order for signal enhancement and motion artifact suppression in breath-hold three-dimensional gradient echo imaging. Magn Reson Med 1997;38(5):793–802.

7. Sodickson DK, Manning WJ. Simultaneous acquisition of spatial harmonics (SMASH): fast imaging with radiofrequency coil arrays. Magn Reson Med 1997;38(4):591–603.

8. Pruessmann KP, Weiger M, Scheidegger MB, et al. SENSE: sensitivity encoding for fast MRI. Magn Reson Med 1999;42(5):952–62.

9. Griswold MA, Jakob PM, Heidemann RM, et al. Generalized autocalibrating partially parallel acquisitions (GRAPPA). Magn Reson Med 2002;47(6): 1202–10.

10. Bock J, Frydrychowicz A, Stalder AF, et al. 4D phase contrast MRI at 3 T: effect of standard and blood-pool contrast agents on SNR, PC-MRA, and blood flow visualization. Magn Reson Med 2010;63(2): 330–8.

11. Setsompop K, Wald LL, Alagappan V, et al. Parallel RF transmission with eight channels at 3 Tesla. Magn Reson Med 2006;56(5):1163–71.

12. Sohn CH, Sevick RJ, Frayne R. Contrast-enhanced MR angiography of the intracranial circulation. Magn Reson Imaging Clin N Am 2003;11(4):599–614.

13. Villablanca JP, Nael K, Habibi R, et al. 3 T contrast-enhanced magnetic resonance angiography for evaluation of the intracranial arteries: comparison with time-of-flight magnetic resonance angiography and multislice computed tomography angiography. Invest Radiol 2006;41(11):799–805.

14. Dumoulin CL. Phase contrast MR angiography techniques. Magn Reson Imaging Clin N Am 1995;3(3): 399–411.

15. Qiao Y, Steinman DA, Qin Q, et al. Intracranial arterial wall imaging using three-dimensional high isotropic resolution black blood MRI at 3.0 Tesla. J Magn Reson Imaging 2011;34(1):22–30.

16. Tang PH, Hui F, Sitoh YY. Intracranial aneurysm detection with 3T magnetic resonance angiography. Ann Acad Med Singapore 2007;36(6):388–93.

17. Gibbs GF, Huston J 3rd, Qian Q, et al. Follow-up of intracranial aneurysms in autosomal-dominant polycystic kidney disease. Kidney Int 2004;65(5):1621–7.

18. Connolly HM, Huston J 3rd, Brown RD Jr, et al. Intracranial aneurysms in patients with coarctation of the aorta: a prospective magnetic resonance angiographic study of 100 patients. Mayo Clin Proc 2003;78(12):1491–9.

19. Gibbs GF, Huston J 3rd, Bernstein MA, et al. Improved image quality of intracranial aneurysms: 3.0-T versus 1.5-T time-of-flight MR angiography. AJNR Am J Neuroradiol 2004;25(1):84–7.

20. Huston J 3rd, Nichols DA, Luetmer PH, et al. Blinded prospective evaluation of sensitivity of MR angiography to known intracranial aneurysms: importance of aneurysm size. AJNR Am J Neuroradiol 1994; 15(9):1607–14.

21. Tan ET, Huston J 3rd, Campeau NG, et al. Fast inversion recovery magnetic resonance angiography of the intracranial arteries. Magn Reson Med 2010; 63(6):1648–58.

22. Kaufmann TJ, Huston J 3rd, Mandrekar JN, et al. Complications of diagnostic cerebral angiography: evaluation of 19,826 consecutive patients. Radiology 2007;243(3):812–9.

23. Cloft HJ, Joseph GJ, Dion JE. Risk of cerebral angiography in patients with subarachnoid hemorrhage, cerebral aneurysm, and arteriovenous malformation: a meta-analysis. Stroke 1999;30(2):317–20.

24. Willinsky RA, Taylor SM, TerBrugge K, et al. Neurologic complications of cerebral angiography: prospective analysis of 2,899 procedures and review of the literature. Radiology 2003;227(2):522–8.

25. Lasser EC, Berry CC, Mishkin MM, et al. Pretreatment with corticosteroids to prevent adverse

reactions to nonionic contrast media. AJR Am J Roentgenol 1994;162(3):523–6.

26. van Gijn J, Rinkel GJ. Subarachnoid haemorrhage: diagnosis, causes and management. Brain 2001; 124(Pt 2):249–78.

27. Villablanca JP, Hooshi P, Martin N, et al. Three-dimensional helical computerized tomography angiography in the diagnosis, characterization, and management of middle cerebral artery aneurysms: comparison with conventional angiography and intraoperative findings. J Neurosurg 2002;97(6):1322–32.

28. Villablanca JP, Jahan R, Hooshi P, et al. Detection and characterization of very small cerebral aneurysms by using 2D and 3D helical CT angiography. AJNR Am J Neuroradiol 2002;23(7):1187–98.

29. Greenberg E, Janardhan V, Katz JM, et al. Disappearance and reappearance of a cerebral aneurysm: a case report. Surg Neurol 2007;67(2):186–8 [discussion: 188–9].

30. Anzalone N, Righi C, Simionato F, et al. Three-dimensional time-of-flight MR angiography in the evaluation of intracranial aneurysms treated with Guglielmi detachable coils. AJNR Am J Neuroradiol 2000;21(4):746–52.

31. Anzalone N, Scomazzoni F, Cirillo M, et al. Follow-up of coiled cerebral aneurysms at 3T: comparison of 3D time-of-flight MR angiography and contrast-enhanced MR angiography. AJNR Am J Neuroradiol 2008;29(8):1530–6.

32. Farb RI, Nag S, Scott JN, et al. Surveillance of intracranial aneurysms treated with detachable coils: a comparison of MRA techniques. Neuroradiology 2005;47(7):507–15.

33. Kaufmann TJ, Huston J 3rd, Cloft HJ, et al. A prospective trial of 3T and 1.5T time-of-flight and contrast-enhanced MR angiography in the follow-up of coiled intracranial aneurysms. AJNR Am J Neuroradiol 2010;31(5):912–8.

34. Pierot L, Delcourt C, Bouquigny F, et al. Follow-up of intracranial aneurysms selectively treated with coils: prospective evaluation of contrast-enhanced MR angiography. AJNR Am J Neuroradiol 2006;27(4): 744–9.

35. Nael K, Villablanca JP, Saleh R, et al. Contrast-enhanced MR angiography at 3T in the evaluation of intracranial aneurysms: a comparison with time-of-flight MR angiography. AJNR Am J Neuroradiol 2006;27(10):2118–21.

36. Investigators ISoUIA. Unruptured intracranial aneurysms—risk of rupture and risks of surgical intervention. International Study of Unruptured Intracranial Aneurysms Investigators. N Engl J Med 1998; 339(24):1725–33.

37. Steinman DA, Milner JS, Norley CJ, et al. Image-based computational simulation of flow dynamics in a giant intracranial aneurysm. AJNR Am J Neuroradiol 2003;24(4):559–66.

38. Hosoya T, Adachi M, Yamaguchi K, et al. Clinical and neuroradiological features of intracranial vertebrobasilar artery dissection. Stroke 1999;30(5):1083–90.

39. Lee JS, Bang OY, Lee PH, et al. Two cases of spontaneous middle cerebral arterial dissection causing ischemic stroke. J Neurol Sci 2006;250(1–2):162–6.

40. Liu K, Margosian P. Multiple contrast fast spin-echo approach to black-blood intracranial MRA: use of complementary and supplementary information. Magn Reson Imaging 2001;19(9):1173–81.

41. Forsting M, Wanke I. Intracranial vascular malformations and aneurysms: from diagnostic work-up to endovascular therapy. 2nd edition. Berlin: Springer; 2008.

42. Spetzler RF, Winestock D, Newton HT, et al. Disappearance and reappearance of cerebral aneurysm in serial arteriograms. Case report. J Neurosurg 1974;41(4):508–10.

43. Oleaga L, Dalal SS, Weigele JB, et al. The role of time-resolved 3D contrast-enhanced MR angiography in the assessment and grading of cerebral arteriovenous malformations. Eur J Radiol 2010; 74(3):e117–21.

44. Hadizadeh DR, von Falkenhausen M, Gieseke J, et al. Cerebral arteriovenous malformation: Spetzler-Martin classification at subsecond-temporal-resolution four-dimensional MR angiography compared with that at DSA. Radiology 2008;246(1):205–13.

45. Eddleman CS, Jeong HJ, Hurley MC, et al. 4D radial acquisition contrast-enhanced MR angiography and intracranial arteriovenous malformations: quickly approaching digital subtraction angiography. Stroke 2009;40(8):2749–53.

46. Korosec FR, Frayne R, Grist TM, et al. Time-resolved contrast-enhanced 3D MR angiography. Magn Reson Med 1996;36(3):345–51.

47. Fink C, Ley S, Kroeker R, et al. Time-resolved contrast-enhanced three-dimensional magnetic resonance angiography of the chest: combination of parallel imaging with view sharing (TREAT). Invest Radiol 2005;40(1):40–8.

48. Lim SD, Park HC, Kim BY. Twist effect on spectral properties of two-mode fiber acousto-optic filters. Opt Express 2008;16(17):13042–51.

49. Mistretta CA, Wieben O, Velikina J, et al. Highly constrained backprojection for time-resolved MRI. Magn Reson Med 2006;55(1):30–40.

50. Haider CR, Hu HH, Campeau NG, et al. 3D high temporal and spatial resolution contrast-enhanced MR angiography of the whole brain. Magn Reson Med 2008;60(3):749–60.

51. Krings T, Hans F. New developments in MRA: time-resolved MRA. Neuroradiology 2004;46(Suppl 2): s214–22.

52. Farb RI, McGregor C, Kim JK, et al. Intracranial arteriovenous malformations: real-time auto-triggered elliptic centric-ordered 3D gadolinium-enhanced

MR angiography—initial assessment. Radiology 2001;220(1):244–51.

53. Petkova M, Gauvrit JY, Trystram D, et al. Three-dimensional dynamic time-resolved contrast-enhanced MRA using parallel imaging and a variable rate k-space sampling strategy in intracranial arteriovenous malformations. J Magn Reson Imaging 2009;29(1):7–12.

54. Chang W, Landgraf B, Johnson KM, et al. Velocity measurements in the middle cerebral arteries of healthy volunteers using 3D radial phase-contrast HYPRFlow: comparison with transcranial Doppler sonography and 2D phase-contrast MR imaging. AJNR Am J Neuroradiol 2011;32(1):54–9.

55. Riederer SJ, Haider CR, Borisch EA. Time-of-arrival mapping at three-dimensional time-resolved contrast-enhanced MR angiography. Radiology 2009;253(2): 532–42.

56. Sarwar M, McCormick WF. Intracerebral venous angioma. Case report and review. Arch Neurol 1978;35(5):323–5.

57. Truwit CL. Venous angioma of the brain: history, significance, and imaging findings. AJR Am J Roentgenol 1992;159(6):1299–307.

58. Ostertun B, Solymosi L. Magnetic resonance angiography of cerebral developmental venous anomalies: its role in differential diagnosis. Neuroradiology 1993;35(2):97–104.

59. Campeau NG, Lane JI. De novo development of a lesion with the appearance of a cavernous malformation adjacent to an existing developmental venous anomaly. AJNR Am J Neuroradiol 2005;26(1):156–9.

60. Haacke EM, Mittal S, Wu Z, et al. Susceptibility-weighted imaging: technical aspects and clinical applications, part 1. AJNR Am J Neuroradiol 2009; 30(1):19–30.

61. de Souza JM, Domingues RC, Cruz LC Jr, et al. Susceptibility-weighted imaging for the evaluation of patients with familial cerebral cavernous malformations: a comparison with t2-weighted fast spin-echo and gradient-echo sequences. AJNR Am J Neuroradiol 2008;29(1):154–8.

62. Barr RM, Dillon WP, Wilson CB. Slow-flow vascular malformations of the pons: capillary telangiectasias? AJNR Am J Neuroradiol 1996;17(1):71–8.

63. Yoshida Y, Terae S, Kudo K, et al. Capillary telangiectasia of the brain stem diagnosed by susceptibility-weighted imaging. J Comput Assist Tomogr 2006; 30(6):980–2.

64. Panasci DJ, Nelson PK. MR imaging and MR angiography in the diagnosis of dural arteriovenous fistulas. Magn Reson Imaging Clin N Am 1995; 3(3):493–508.

65. Sakamoto S, Shibukawa M, Kiura Y, et al. Evaluation of dural arteriovenous fistulas of cavernous sinus before and after endovascular treatment using time-resolved MR angiography. Neurosurg Rev 2010;33(2):217–22 [discussion: 222–3].

66. Borden JA, Wu JK, Shucart WA. A proposed classification for spinal and cranial dural arteriovenous fistulous malformations and implications for treatment. J Neurosurg 1995;82(2):166–79.

67. Kiyosue H, Hori Y, Okahara M, et al. Treatment of intracranial dural arteriovenous fistulas: current strategies based on location and hemodynamics, and alternative techniques of transcatheter embolization. Radiographics 2004;24(6):1637–53.

68. Carlson AP, Taylor CL, Yonas H. Treatment of dural arteriovenous fistula using ethylene vinyl alcohol (onyx) arterial embolization as the primary modality: short-term results. J Neurosurg 2007;107(6): 1120–5.

69. De Marco JK, Dillon WP, Halback VV, et al. Dural arteriovenous fistulas: evaluation with MR imaging. Radiology 1990;175(1):193–9.

70. Farb RI, Agid R, Willinsky RA, et al. Cranial dural arteriovenous fistula: diagnosis and classification with time-resolved MR angiography at 3T. AJNR Am J Neuroradiol 2009;30(8):1546–51.

71. Kwon BJ, Han MH, Kang HS, et al. MR imaging findings of intracranial dural arteriovenous fistulas: relations with venous drainage patterns. AJNR Am J Neuroradiol 2005;26(10):2500–7.

72. Demaerel P, De Ruyter N, Maes F, et al. Magnetic resonance angiography in suspected cerebral vasculitis. Eur Radiol 2004;14(6):1005–12.

73. Heiserman JE. MR angiography for the diagnosis of vasospasm after subarachnoid hemorrhage. Is it accurate? Is it safe? AJNR Am J Neuroradiol 2000; 21(9):1571–2.

74. Scott RM, Smith ER. Moyamoya disease and moyamoya syndrome. N Engl J Med 2009;360(12): 1226–37.

75. Tsuchiya K, Honya K, Fujikawa A, et al. Postoperative assessment of extracranial-intracranial bypass by time-resolved 3D contrast-enhanced MR angiography using parallel imaging. AJNR Am J Neuroradiol 2005;26(9):2243–7.

76. Blatter DD, Parker DL, Ahn SS, et al. Cerebral MR angiography with multiple overlapping thin slab acquisition. Part II. Early clinical experience. Radiology 1992;183(2):379–89.

Current State-of-the-Art 1.5 T and 3 T Extracranial Carotid Contrast-Enhanced Magnetic Resonance Angiography

J. Kevin DeMarco, MD[a,*], Winfried A. Willinek, MD[b],
J. Paul Finn, MD[c], John Huston III, MD[d]

KEYWORDS

- Carotid MR angiography
- Gadolinium-based contrast agent
- Time-resolved carotid MR angiography

Key Points

- Time-resolved carotid MR angiography with a small test bolus of GBCA provides:
  - A good estimation of the GBCA arrival for accurate timing of first-pass CE MR angiography
  - Useful dynamic vascular assessment and functional information in the head and neck region
- Consistently, good-quality, high-resolution, first-pass CE carotid MR angiography is possible; however:
  - At 1.5 T, strive for resolution of 0.71 mm^3 or less in carotid CE MR angiography
  - At 3 T, strive for resolution of 0.54 mm^3 or less in carotid CE MR angiography, perhaps with decreased GBCA
- Be aware of potential pitfalls when developing and implementing carotid CE MR angiography protocols:
  - Understand how phase resolution and slice resolution are displayed by your MR manufacturer
  - Understand the advantages/disadvantages of methods to acceleration CE MR angiography:
    - Partial k_y/k_z and percent sampling
    - Parallel imaging
    - Bandwidth

---

[a] Department of Radiology, Michigan State University, 184 Radiology Building, East Lansing, MI 48824, USA
[b] Department of Radiology, University of Bonn, Sigmund-Freund-Str. 25, D-53105, Bonn, Germany
[c] Department of Radiology, David Geffen School of Medicine at UCLA, Peter V. Ueberroth Building, Suite 3371, 10945 LeConte Avenue, Los Angeles, CA 90095-7206, USA
[d] Department of Radiology, Mayo Clinic, 200 1st Street SW, Rochester, MN 55905, USA
* Corresponding author.
E-mail address: jkd@rad.msu.edu

Neuroimag Clin N Am 22 (2012) 235–257
doi:10.1016/j.nic.2012.02.007
1052-5149/12/$ – see front matter © 2012 Elsevier Inc. All rights reserved.

Diagnostic Checklist

- Use time-resolved magnetic resonance (MR) angiography with a small test bolus of gadolinium-based contrast agent (GBCA) to identify the individual bolus arrival time and obtain additional useful information about vascular kinetics in the head and neck.

- With attention to specific imaging parameters, resolution of 0.7 mm^3 or less can be obtained consistently with first-pass contrast-enhanced (CE), MR angiography of the head and neck at 1.5 T with even higher spatial resolution possible with a smaller dose of GBCA at 3 T.

- Be aware of pitfalls in prescribing first-pass CE carotid MR angiography, as well as the potentially confusing annotations, especially regarding resolution in the phase direction and slice thickness with three-dimensional (3D) sequences.

- Strong collaboration between the MR technologist and radiologist in understanding the specific techniques used by each MR manufacturer when prescribing CE carotid MR angiography can lead to consistently good image quality.

The American College of Cardiology Foundation (ACCF) and the American Heart Association (AHA) have jointly written new guidelines on the management of patients with extracranial carotid and vertebral artery disease.[1] The writing committee assigned by the ACCF-AHA Task Force on Practice Guidelines has developed several recommendations based on expert review of evidence-based methodologies. In this document, the Task Force specifically recommends the use of MR angiography or computed tomography (CT) angiography to detect carotid stenosis when sonography either cannot be obtained or yields equivocal or otherwise nondiagnostic results. When intervention for significant carotid stenosis detected by sonography is planned, the Task Force also concluded that MR angiography, CT angiography, or catheter-based contrast angiography could be useful to evaluate the severity of carotid stenosis. It is clear from these recommendations that high-quality carotid MR angiography that can accurately and reproducibly detect extracranial carotid stenosis is necessary. This article reviews the technical factors necessary to obtain high-quality extracranial carotid MR angiography.

In the 1990s, time-of-flight (TOF) MR angiography was reported to have good sensitivity and specificity in detecting internal carotid artery (ICA) stenosis greater than 70% using North American Symptomatic Carotid Endarterectomy Trial (NASCET) criteria identified on digital subtraction angiography.[2–5] CE MR angiography offered the opportunity to cover more of the carotid artery distribution in a fraction of the time that TOF MR angiography required.[6] There has been much work presented on various techniques for time-resolved extracranial carotid CE MR angiography.[7,8] Although there are new techniques that hold much promise for improving spatial resolution of time-resolved CE MR angiography

while maintaining adequate temporal resolution,[9] currently available clinical time-resolved CE MR angiography techniques cannot achieve the spatial resolution of less than 1 mm that is probably necessary for accurate depiction of extracranial severe carotid stenosis. The advent of elliptical-centric phase reordering and effective timing of the gadolinium contrast bolus moved first-pass CE MR angiography from research into routine clinical practice at the Mayo Clinic.[10,11] Other workers reported success with breath-held CE MR angiography, which included the great vessel origins at the aortic arch.[12] Some, but not all, of the literature from 2000 to 2005 concluded that first-pass carotid CE MR angiography is superior to TOF MR angiography in the detection of severe extracranial carotid stenosis.[13,14] This may in part be because of the effect of spatial resolution of extracranial carotid CE MR angiography.[15] In the past 5 years, as submillimeter-resolution first-pass CE MR angiography has become more routine, a general consensus has emerged that CE MR angiography is accurate in the measurement of extracranial carotid stenosis.[16–18] In this article, the discussion of carotid CE MR angiography is restricted to the first-pass extracranial carotid CE MR angiography technique. Improvements in the technique that have allowed the routine clinical acquisition of submillimeter-resolution carotid CE MR angiography are reviewed. Specifically, the imaging parameter details that provide submillimeter resolution while speeding up the CE MR angiography acquisition are discussed and both the amount and type of GBCA that is required to support such high-resolution CE MR angiography acquisitions are reviewed, taking into account concerns about nephrogenic systemic fibrosis (NSF) in susceptible populations. Various techniques for adequate timing of the GBCA arrival are also reviewed. In addition, vendor-specific protocols at both 1.5 T and 3 T MR are provided to help obtain consistently high-quality extracranial carotid CE MR angiography.

RESOLUTION AND SCAN TIME

Hinatiuk and colleagues[16] recently reviewed the effect of increased spatial resolution in depicting carotid stenosis as seen on CE MR angiography at 1.5 T. In patients with carotid artery stenosis, decreasing the voxel volume from 0.9 mm^3 to 0.53 mm^3 by increasing the scan matrix and while keeping the field of view (FOV) constant caused the scan time to increase from 21 to 40 seconds. The resulting extracranial carotid CE MR angiography with improved resolution resulted in sharper depiction of the carotid stenosis. With modern gradient systems, repetition times (TR) for 3D gradient-echo acquisitions are approximately half what they were during the early work on carotid CE MR angiography. The investigators made use of the 50% reduction in TR to nearly double the spatial resolution of elliptical-centric carotid CE MR angiography compared with the initial 0.8-mm^3 to 1.0-mm^3 voxel size while maintaining an imaging time of 40 seconds. This reduction in voxel volume to 0.53 mm^3 resulted in a better depiction of the carotid stenosis. Further decreases in voxel volume at 1.5 T, by extending the acquisition time to 50 to 60 seconds, did not improve the vessel depiction because of both a reduction in signal-to-noise ratio (SNR) and sharpness losses, possibly from motion. Recently, the resolution of large FOV first-pass carotid CE MR angiography has been extended to 0.44 to 0.49 mm^3 by making use of the extra SNR at 3 T.[17,18] Further reductions in voxel size to 0.28 mm^3 have been made possible by combining dedicated carotid surface coils with 3 T MR imaging.[19]

With modern MR scanners and high-performing gradients, it is possible to achieve a resolution of 1 mm or less in all 3 primary axes with first-pass CE MR angiography. Despite the plethora of articles that show the usefulness of first-pass CE MR angiography with a resolution of 1 mm or less, many centers do not routinely obtain this high resolution. One reason may be confusion about the multiple imaging parameters that affect the final CE MR angiography resolution. This article therefore discusses the potential pitfalls and sources of confusion when attempting to prescribe a CE MR angiography protocol with a resolution of 1 mm or less.

Percent Phase FOV

What happens when a partial or asymmetrical FOV is prescribed? In our example of coronally acquired CE MR angiography, we typically use an FOV of 28 to 40 cm in the superior-inferior direction, which is also the direction of the frequency-encoding gradient. Rarely is such a large FOV needed in the right-left direction. Most modern large FOV clamshell-style neurovascular coils or integrated head and neck coils have the ability to turn off elements far laterally near the shoulders. The wraparound artifact from the shoulders is thereby diminished so that typically only an FOV of around 20 to 27 cm is needed, depending on what other acceleration factors such as parallel imaging are being used. Take for example 28-cm FOV, CE, MR angiography with a prescribed matrix of 384 × 220. If a 0.8 rectangular FOV (80% phase FOV) is chosen, the FOV in the y direction (right-left) is decreased to 22.4 cm and the number of phase-encoding steps is decreased to 176. This choice diminishes the total acquisition time, but increases the size of the voxel in the y direction to greater than 1-mm resolution. Depending on the MR manufacturer, the annotation of the final image may say 28 × 22 cm FOV with 384 × 220 matrix. failure to understand what a specific MR vendor is acquiring may result in failure to achieve the desired resolution. This annotation could be interpreted to mean that an acquired matrix of 0.73 × 1.0 mm has been obtained, which would not be true. To maintain resolution at 1 mm or less in the example, a 28-cm FOV with a matrix of 384 × 288 may be needed. Using a 0.8 rectangular FOV, the MR scanner will then obtain a 28 × 22 cm FOV, CE, MR angiogram with an acquired matrix of 384 × 220 with a pixel size of 0.73 × 0.97 mm while decreasing scan time by 20% compared with the scan time without using an asymmetric or partial FOV. The specifics of 3 MR manufactures (GE, Philips, Siemens) are reviewed later in this article to detail with screen shots from their individual software interfaces to help decrease any potential for confusion or misunderstanding.

Partial k_y/k_z and Percent Sampling

Another way the radiologist can speed up the scan time of CE MR angiography and maintain resolution at 1 mm or less is to use partial Fourier schemes which enables faster imaging but at the expense of SNR. Only a portion of k-space in the phase encoding direction (ky) or in the slice direction (kz) can be obtained. In addition, only a partial number of averages can be acquired to speed up image acquisition. This technique takes advantage of the inherent symmetry in k-space. Instead of obtaining all of the phase-encoding lines in k-space in either/both the y direction or z direction, most of them can be obtained and technique called conjugate synthesis used to intelligently guess what the remaining lines would have looked like. Number of averages is also called number of excitations (NEX), and represents the number of times the same lines of k-space are acquired, which is done to increase the SNR or to average out motion artifact. When the MR technologist requests a partial NEX, it is the same as doing partial k_y. Instead of not obtaining specific sections of k_y or k_z, some MR manufactures allow radiologists to not obtain the corners of 3D k-space. This method is sometimes called the k-space filter or percent sampling. The potential effects on the resolution of the lumen of vessels coursing obliquely through the 3D imaging slab when applying either/both partial k_y and k_z or cutting the corners of 3D k-space is beyond the scope of this article. Suffice it to say that, if the corners are not cut too much, good image quality can be maintained. Many investigators suggest that, as long as at least 75% to 80% of k_y and k_z are obtained, or at least 75% to 80% sampling, any deleterious effects on the depiction of the lumen are probably minimal and acceptable. The radiologist therefore needs to know what values of partial k_y and k_z or percent sampling are being using in the CE MR angiography prescription. The specific recommendations for GE, Philips, and Siemens are discussed later.

Zero Interpolation

Zero interpolation means expanding the k-space matrix beyond what was acquired by assigning zeroes to the outer (nonacquired) parts, before performing image reconstruction by the Fourier transform. This technique was originally described in 1994 as a way to decrease partial volume artifacts, especially in small vessels in MR angiography.[20] It can improve image quality, especially if the acquired k-space data are asymmetric, and it can be applied in all 3 primary axes. A version of this technique has been applied by most MR manufactures. Again, it is important for radiologists to understand whether the matrix values displayed on their MR angiography images are the acquired resolution or the interpolated resolution. Although zero interpolation helps decrease partial volume artifacts and is useful, when discussing the optimal voxel resolution for CE MR angiography, this article refers specifically to the acquired resolution. The potential for misunderstanding zero interpolation is especially a problem when reviewing the number of slices and slice thickness of a CE MR angiography. Many MR manufactures display the number of interpolated coronal slices and the spacing between these

interpolated slices. For instance, if a 60-mm thick coronal CE MR angiography slab in the anterior-posterior (AP) direction is prescribed and 44 slices are requested, a set of images each with 1.4-mm thickness is obtained. The annotation can read that 88 slices were obtained with a thickness of 0.7 mm, which represented the interpolated number of slices and the distance between each slice. Although this is accurate, it can lead radiologists to interpret that they have achieved a resolution of 1 mm or less. In this example, the radiologist needs to prescribe at least 60 slices to achieve 1 mm or better resolution in the slice direction with a 60-mm thick CE MR angiography coronal slab acquisition.

Parallel Imaging

Parallel imaging is a major advance in CE MR angiography. It has allowed acquisition to speed up and helped support higher acquired matrices with better resolution. Parallel imaging techniques take advantage of the signal originating from a given location in the body being detected with different sensitivity by various surface coil elements, depending on where the elements are located relative to the structure generating the signal. In this way, surface coils contain spatial information that is used to substitute for lines in k-space, saving time. Depending on the specific arrangement of the coils and patient anatomy, it might be possible to skip every second line, 2 out of every 3 lines, 3 out of every 4 lines, or even more. By skipping lines in k-space, the distance between adjacent acquired lines is increased (by a factor equal to the acceleration factor), and this effectively reduces the FOV by the same factor. An acceleration factor of 4 in a specified phase-encoding direction reduces the FOV in that direction by a factor of 4. Without accurate surface coil calibration, the resulting wraparound artifact would be disastrous, but accurate coil sensitivity information can be used to completely unwrap the signal. The price that is paid for the accelerated performance is in SNR. As discussed later, there are ways to mitigate the SNR loss from parallel imaging by judicious use of GBCA as well as accurate timing of the GBCA bolus arrival. There are 2 main types of parallel imaging: sensitivity encoding (SENSE) and SMASH (SiMultaneous Acquisition of Spatial Harmonics). These original sequence names morphed into a plethora of specific names as they were adopted for use by most MR manufactures. Variants of 1 or both are used in modern CE MR angiography sequences by MR manufactures. SENSE techniques acquire a separate scan to obtain sensitivity maps for each coil in the FOV and the unwrapping is performed in the image domain (after image reconstruction), whereas SMASH techniques have a calibration scan built into the CE MR angiography sequence and the unwrapping is performed in the k-space domain (before image reconstruction). For any parallel imaging technique to work well, whether image space–based or k-space–based, coils separated in space along the acceleration direction are needed. In the typical 1-directional (1D) acceleration of CE MR angiography using parallel imaging, the right-left direction is used. Multiple coils are needed along the right and left lateral aspects of the head and neck. If 2 direction (2D) acceleration of CE MR angiography with parallel imaging is required, multiple coils along the AP direction and right-left directions are needed. Many MR manufactures now have new multi-channel large FOV coils designed to do this. The better-designed coils minimize the signal loss caused by the position of these various elements. The signal loss can be quantified by measuring the geometry factor (G factor), also known as the noise amplification factor. The optimal 1D or 2D acceleration with parallel imaging depends on many factors, such as the coil design, MR field strength, and gradient performance. Specific recommendations for GE, Philips, and Siemens at 1.5 T and 3 T are given later in this article.

Bandwidth

Another way to speed up the CE MR angiography acquisition while maintaining a resolution of 1 mm or less is to increase the bandwidth (BW). Increasing BW allows shorter repetition time (TR) and shorter echo times (TE). For conventional MR imaging, increasing bandwidth is associated with lower SNR but, for CE MR angiography, this is generally not the case. The added signal available with very short echo times and with condensing the acquisition window into the peak of the contrast bolus can, up to a point, compensate for SNR lost with increased bandwidth. As with parallel imaging, judicious increases in BW can decrease total acquisition time of CE MR angiography while supporting resolution of 1 mm or less with acceptable overall SNR and image quality. In general, higher BW along with more aggressive parallel imaging acceleration is possible at 3 T compared with 1.5 T because of the inherently higher SNR at 3 T.[18,21] The shorter TR and higher acceleration factors allow more phase encoding in the y direction and z direction as well as more frequency-encoding steps, which results in higher spatial resolution and smaller

voxel sizes with CE MR angiography at 3 T MR compared with 1.5 T MR scans.

GBCA

Now that the various technical components to obtaining CE MR angiography with resolution of 1 mm or less have been introduced, the GBCA should be discussed. Workers differ in their approach to how best to coordinate image acquisition with the GBCA contrast bolus. An ideal image acquisition would take advantage of the first pass encompassing the high arterial concentration of GBCA There is more debate about how important the later phases of GBCA distribution are to quality CE MR angiography. Carotid CE MR angiography can be extended to take advantage of the large residual of the initial bolus of contrast injection caused by recirculation. The blood-brain barrier and rapid return of gadolinium contrast through the brain parenchyma and jugular vein back to the heart makes carotid CE MR angiography especially capable of longer acquisitions and potentially higher resolutions. By modeling the elliptical-centric technique, Fain and colleagues[10] showed that there is sufficient contrast for high resolution with increased acquisition time of carotid CE MR angiography. Initial experience with the use of elliptical-centric phase reordering in combination with a bolus arrival scan or fluoroscopic triggering allowed carotid CE MR angiography with voxel size of 1 mm^3 or less with good intra-arterial contrast and little venous contamination.[11] Other workers have focused exclusively on the first arterial peak within a breath-hold acquisition at 1.5 T, also with excellent results.[12]

As with most MR sequence parameters, the choice of GBCA agent and dose varies by MR field strength. In the past 10 years, most investigators achieving CE MR angiography with the desired resolution of 1 mm or less at 1.5 T have used more than a single dose of a variety of the original extracellular GBCA.[11,13,15,16] A high T1 relaxivity GBCA, gadobenate dimeglumine (Multihance, Bracco Diagnostic, Inc.), was recently introduced. Intraindividual crossover comparison of 2 GBCAs showed superior depiction of arterial lumen with a single dose of gadobenate dimeglumine (Multihance, Bracco Diagnostic, Inc.) compared with gadopentetate dimeglumine (Magnevist, Bayer HealthCare Pharmaceuticals) at 1.5 T.[22] Recent work showed that a single dose of gadobenate dimeglumine (Multihance, Bracco Diagnostic, Inc.) can provide similar image quality of CE MR angiography compared with a double dose of other extracellular GBCAs.[23] The use of high

T1 relativity GBCA such as gadobenate dimeglumine (Multihance, Bracco Diagnostic, Inc.), gadofosveset (Ablavar, Lantheus Medical Imaging) and gadobutrol (Gadavist, Bayer HealthCare Pharmaceuticals) helps to minimize the total dose of GBCA administration while supporting sufficient SNR to produce carotid CE MR angiography with high image quality. Typically, a single dose (0.1 mmol/kg) of gadobenate dimeglumine is sufficient to maintain high SNR and image quality with a resolution of 0.8-mm^3 or less for carotid CE MR angiography at 1.5 T.[15]

At 3 T, similar intraindividual crossover studies have shown the superiority of gadobenate dimeglumine (Multihance, Bracco Diagnostic, Inc.) compared with other extracellular GBCA in CE MR angiography when using a single dose.[24] Although the initial work on carotid CE MR angiography at 3 T MR used a double dose (0.2 mmol/kg) of GBCA,[17] subsequent dose reduction studies showed that lower doses of GBCA could still support the desired CE MR angiography with resolution of 1 mm or less.[25] There was sufficient SNR with 0.05 mmol/kg of GBCA (half dose) at 3 T in one large study of carotid CE MR angiography.[21] The trade-off in arterial signal when reducing the contrast dose is less noticeable at 3 T. Because of the higher intrinsic blood-to-tissue signal available at 3 T compared with at 1.5 T, half-dose CE MR angiography is particularly successful at 3 T.

The final image quality on carotid CE MR angiography depends in part on the choice of GBCA, the dose of GBCA, and the field strength and configuration of the MR scanner used. The concern of NSF in connection with GBCA injections also needs to be considered. US Food and Drug Administration (FDA) guidelines currently recommend caution when injecting GBCA in patients with severe or end-stage chronic kidney disease (glomerular filtration rate [GFR] <30 mL/min/1.73 m^2) and in patients with acute renal or hepatic failure. These symptoms are uncommon in outpatients presenting with carotid stenosis. The risk/benefit ratio of GBCA in outpatients with moderate chronic kidney disease (GFR 30–59 mL/min/1.73 m^2) is unclear, but no proven cases of NSF have occurred in patients with GFR greater than 30 mL/min/1.73 m^2, other than in the context of acutely deteriorating renal function. Although practice guidelines continue to evolve in the light of accumulating clinical data, the need to use the minimum established dose of GBCA to achieve consistently good image quality of carotid CE MR angiography needs to be balanced with the need to minimize the risk of NSF according to the FDA guidelines.

Optimal Flip Angle

The flip angle that will result in the highest SNR for carotid CE MR angiography depends on the amount of T1 shortening achieved during the first pass of GBCA, and this is called the Ernst angle. The optimal flip angle to use with carotid CE MR angiography varies with the choice of GBCA, the field strength of the MR scanner, and the TR. As described earlier, gadobenate dimeglumine (Multihance), gadofosveset (Ablavar, Lantheus Medical Imaging), and gadobutrol (Gadavist, Bayer HealthCare Pharmaceuticals) have higher T1 relativity GBCA. Therefore, the Ernst angle or optimal flip angle for first-pass carotid CE MR angiography with, for example, gadobenate dimeglumine (Multihance) is higher than with any of the original extracellular GBCAs. At 3 T, high flip angles may not be possible because of specific absorption ratio (SAR) limits exceeding FDA limits for potential heating. Given the longer T1 times at 3 T compared with 1.5 T, the Ernst angle is smaller at 3 T. As noted earlier, the higher SNR at 3 T allows the radiologist to chose to use less GBCA, which results in slightly longer T1 times for CE MR angiography. The optimal flip angle for carotid CE MR angiography therefore varies with the choice of GBCA, field strength, and TR. **Table 1** lists specific recommendations. In general, the flip angle should be as large as is allowed by the SAR monitor on the MR scanner.

GBCA ARRIVAL

It is not enough simply to prescribe a sufficient amount of GBCA to achieve good SNR while maintaining a resolution of 1 mm or less. The timing of the GBCA bolus arrival to match the filling of the center of 3D k-space during the CE MR angiography is also critical. If the GBCA arrives after part of the center of 3D k-space is filled, there will be an apparent flow void in the middle of large arteries such as the common carotid arteries (CCAs). The edges will be well defined because the more peripheral part of k-space was acquired when there was plenty of GBCA. This situation causes the so-called high pass filter artifact, because only the high spatial frequencies are passed through. This artifact may be less apparent on smaller arteries such as distal ICAs because the contrast enhancement of 2 edges of the lumen may blend together. If the edge of the arterial lumen is well depicted for 2 mm, then a 4-mm lumen of the distal ICA may appear normal even if the GBCA arrives too late. In the study in which the GBCA arrives too late, the ringing artifact will be apparent in the 8-mm

CCA where the 2-mm peripheral aspects of the lumen will now be separated by a 4-mm gap in the center of the CCA lumen. If the CE MR angiography sequence begins long after the initial bolus arrival of GBCA in the neck, it is possible that contrast will arrive in the neck veins during the acquisition of the center of 3D k-space. In this case, there will be extensive contrast enhancement in both the neck arteries and veins that can partially obscure arterial depiction of maximum intensity pixel projections (MIP). There may also be less enhancement in the neck arteries because of less than maximal concentration of GBCA in the arteries after the bolus arrival. Of these 2 pitfalls of GBCA arrival timing, the latter may be interpretable (with more work), whereas the former may be nondiagnostic. All major MR manufactures now offer an option in which the absolute center of 3D k-space is recessed slightly. Instead of beginning the CE MR angiography acquisition exactly at the center of 3D k-space, the near-center portion of k-space is acquired in the first few seconds, with the absolute center then acquired a predefined number of seconds later. This method decreases the risk of high pass filtering if the CE MR angiography acquisition is centered too early. The risk of venous contamination is also lessened by judicious use of parallel imaging, higher bandwidth, partial k_y/k_z, and partial FOV to decrease the total acquisition time and thereby decrease the amount of time it takes to cover the center of k-space. A good general rule is that the central portion of k-space that is responsible for much of the contrast portion of the final images with elliptical-centric CE MR angiography is about 10% of the total acquisition time. Therefore, for an elliptical-centric CE MR angiography acquisition of 20 to 40 seconds, it is only necessary to time the beginning of the sequence such that there is no significant contrast in the neck veins for the first 2 to 4 seconds of the scan.

How can the GBCA arrival be timed such that the single-pass elliptical-centric CE MR angiography acquisition is acquired with mostly arterial enhancement? There are 2 commercially available techniques. One technique uses a timing bolus. A small dose of GBCA (usually 1–2 mL) is injected with a saline flush using injection rates identical to that planned for the full-dose GBCA injection. Images of the neck are obtained usually with a time frame of approximately 1 second. As originally described, this resulted in a series of single axial images through the distal CCA.[6] A multiple-image region of interest analysis could then quickly identify the time of arrival of the GBCA bolus. This technique was recently expanded to include time-resolved MR angiography with just 2 mL of GBCA at 3 T.[26] The radiologist cannot only accurately time the beginning of the CE MR angiography sequence to the bolus arrival of the full dose of GBCA, but now also has access to temporal information about the flow in the neck vessels. Fluoroscopic imaging to visualize the arrival of the full dose of GBCA and rapidly switch to the acquisition of the CE MR angiography is also available from most MR manufactures.[27] This technique has the advantage of simplicity; only 1 GBCA injection and 1 sequence to acquire. The disadvantages are the time it takes to accurately prescribe the fluoroscopic plane to visualize the aortic arch and carotid arteries, and that occasionally it is difficult to accurately visualize the GBCA arrival in the carotid arteries, especially in patients with poor cardiac output. Although, with a timing bolus, the shape and exact timing of the main bolus can be accurately predicted, fluoroscopic triggering detects the leading edge of the bolus and, in general, accurate matching of the bolus peak and k-space center is more challenging. Either technique can result in a high percentage (>95%) of diagnostic carotid CE MR angiography studies, but the bolus timing approach allows for more accurate planning. The final decision of which technique to use rests on clinical experience and individual site preferences.

VENDOR-SPECIFIC RECOMMENDATION FOR CAROTID CE MR ANGIOGRAPHY AT 1.5 AND 3 T
General Electric

The concept of elliptical-centric phase reordering for first-pass CE MR angiography and fluoroscopic triggering was first developed by Steve Riederer.[27] This technique was then applied to carotid CE MR angiography, verifying the high sensitivity and specificity of carotid CE MR angiography using a 1.5 T MR scanner to detect more than 70%, as confirmed on digital subtraction angiography in 2001.[11] Carotid CE MR angiography underwent further improvements with the addition of parallel imaging, higher-performing gradients, and higher channel neurovascular coils. With these improvements, radiologists can now routinely obtain 1.5 T carotid CE MR angiography with higher resolution, more coverage, and less scan time compared with the initial experience in 2001. More recently, the availability of commercial 3 T MR scanners has allowed radiologists to push the resolution of carotid CE MR angiography even further. Despite these improvements, there are many MR imaging centers that are not producing optimal carotid

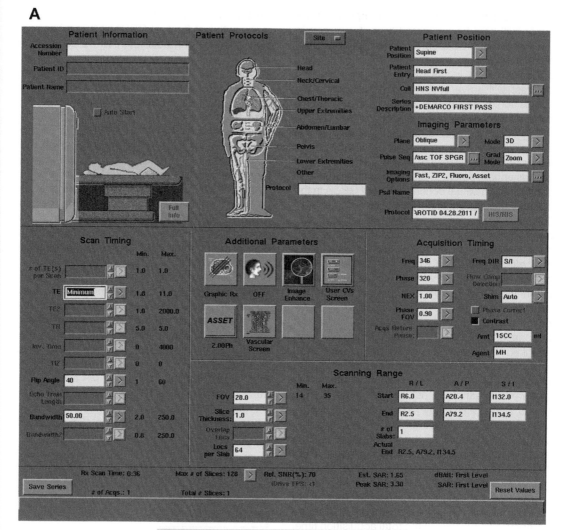

Fig. 1. First-pass delayed elliptical-centric CE carotid 1.5 T MR (*A*) The 15× software presents the user with multiple variables to optimize the MR angiography acquisition. Note that the frequency and phase matrix allows for submillimeter in-plane resolution with a 28-cm FOV CE MR angiogram.angiography. (*B*) Advanced settings such as delayed elliptical-centric phase ordering and Turbo mode 2 can be found under the User CVs (control variables) screen.

CE MR angiography studies. This omission may be caused in part by an incomplete understanding of the trade-offs in the multitude of imaging parameters that are part of a modern carotid CE MR angiography study. Each of these parameters is introduced earlier in this article. This article presents a review of the specifics of each of these parameters because GE has implemented them in their commercial carotid CE MR angiography product at 1.5 T and 3 T. GE has not reviewed or endorsed the protocols described here.

At 1.5 T, high-performing gradients with an MR scanner with both a 60-cm and 70-cm bore are commercially available. With 12-channel or higher neurovascular coils, the Array Spatial Sensitivity Encoding Technique (ASSET) is the GE implementation of 1D parallel imaging that is compatible with elliptical-centric phase-encoding carotid CE MR angiography. This 1-directional parallel imaging

makes use of the separations of receiver coils in the right-left direction to speed up the total acquisition time. In our recommendations, the ASSET factor is set at 2.0 (Fig. 1, Table 1). Next, we prescribe a 75% scan, which means that 25% of the corners of k-space are not acquired. Lastly, we prescribe a 0.90 phase FOV to further speed up the acquisition time. Instead of using all 280 mm of the FOV that are needed in the superior-inferior direction to capture arteries from the aortic arch through the circle of Willis, only 90% of that FOV are needed in the right-left direction. We then image 252 mm in the right-left direction. As long as there is little signal in the region of the distal clavicles and shoulders, we have minimal effects of the distal left subclavian artery wrapping over the proximal right subclavian artery and innominate artery. It is important for the radiologist to understand the coil configurations of their particular

Table 1
Imaging parameters for CE MR angiography of the extracranial carotid arteries

	1.5 T			3 T		
	Avanto	Intera	HDx	TIM Trio	Achieva	HD750
TR (ms)	2.6	4.8	5.0	3.0	4.8	4.4
TE (ms)	1.2	1.5	1.4	1.2	1.61	1.3
Flip angle (degrees)	25	40	35	20	25	25
BW	440 Hz/pixel	434 Hz/pixel	±50 kHz	720 Hz/pixel	768 Hz/pixel	±90.9 kHz
FOV (cm)	41	35	28	45	35	30
Matrix	512 × 457	432 × 432	346 × 320	640 × 461	584 × 560	376 × 352
RFOV	0.75	0.5	0.9	0.6	1	0.75
Actual FOV	410 × 305	350 × 175	280 × 252	450 × 270	350 × 350	300 × 225
Rx matrix	512 × 340	432 × 260	346 × 288	640 × 346	640 × 640	376 × 264
Slab thickness	108	65	66	102	252	70
No. of slices	120	65	66	128	360	88
Pixel size	0.80 × 0.90	0.81 × 0.81	0.80 × 0.88	0.70 × 0.78	0.6 × 0.62	0.80 × 0.85
Slice thickness (mm)	0.9	1.0	1.0	0.8	1.4	0.8
Voxel volume (mm³)	0.65	0.66	0.71	0.44	0.52	0.54
Parallel image	3×	0	2×	4×	16×	2×
Partial k_y	0.75	1.0	1.0	0.75	1.0	1.0
Partial k_z	0.75	1.0.	1.0	0.75	1.0	1.0
Percent scan	No	78	75	No	No	75
Scan time (s)	24	71	36	20	67	40

Sonata BW = 440 Hz/pixel × 512 pixel/1000 = 225.3 kHz or ±112.6 kHz.
Interia BW = 434 Hz/pixel × 432 pixel/1000 = 187.5 kHz or ±93.7 kHz.
GE HD × BW = ±50 kHz or 100,000 Hz/346 = 289 Hz/pixel.
Trio BW = 720 Hz/pixel × 640 pixel/1000 = 460.8 kHz or ±230.4 kHz.
Achieva BW = 768 Hz/pixel × 584 pixel/1000 = 448.5 kHz or ±224.3 kHz.
GE MR750 BW = ±90.9 kHz or 181,800 Hz/376 pixel = 484 Hx/pixel.
Abbreviations: FOV, field of view; RFOV, rectangular field of view; Rx, prescribed.

neurovascular multichannel coil to optimally visualize the head and neck arteries without unwanted vessel wrapping. For example, the GE head/neck/spine (HNS) coil has a configuration file named NV Full, which includes the anterior chest plate coils, anterior/posterior neck coils, and head coils while turning off coils laterally over the distal clavicle and shoulder regions. In our recommendations for first-pass elliptical-centric carotid CE MR angiography, we prescribe a 28-cm FOV, 346 × 320 matrix, with 66 locations per slab with each location 1 mm thick. If there were no techniques to speed up this acquisition, the total scan time would be 106 seconds, assuming a minimum TR of 5.0 milliseconds. By using a 0.90 phase FOV, an ASSET of 2, and a slice resolution of 75%, the total scan time

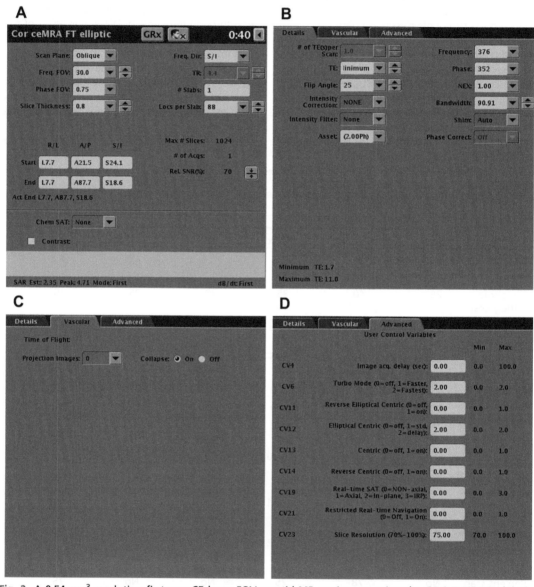

Fig. 2. A 0.54-mm³ resolution first-pass CE large FOV carotid MR angiogram using the GE 3 T MR750. (A) The summary page from the new 20× software presents the imaging parameters that may need to be modified based on patient body habitus. Note the 0.8-mm slice thickness of this higher resolution MR angiography technique compared with 1.5 T MR angiography. (B) Selecting the button in the upper right hand corner of the Summary page can expose the Details page. Note the higher spatial resolution matrix at 3 T compared with the 1.5 T MR protocol. (C) In the Vascular tab, the user can prescribe how many global maximum intensity projections to automatically generate. (D) Under the Advanced tab, the user has easy access to many important CVs, such as the method of phase reordering. We have found that delayed elliptical-centric phase reordering works best for first-pass CE carotid MR angiography.

is reduced to 36 seconds. With this scan time, we have acquired a resolution of $0.80 \times 0.88 \times 1.00$ mm for carotid CE MR angiography with a total voxel volume of 0.71 mm^3. **Fig. 1** details the parameters for this recommended 1.5 T carotid CE MR angiography. If enough GBCA and a modern multi-channel coil with a good G factor for head/neck imaging are used, there will be enough SNR to

support this -resolution of less than 1 mm and it will result in a good overall image quality in the carotid CE MR angiogram.

With both 1.5 T and 3 T MR angiography, we recommend using delayed elliptical-centric phase ordering. This modification of the original description of elliptical-centric phase ordering is more robust to slight variations in the predicted

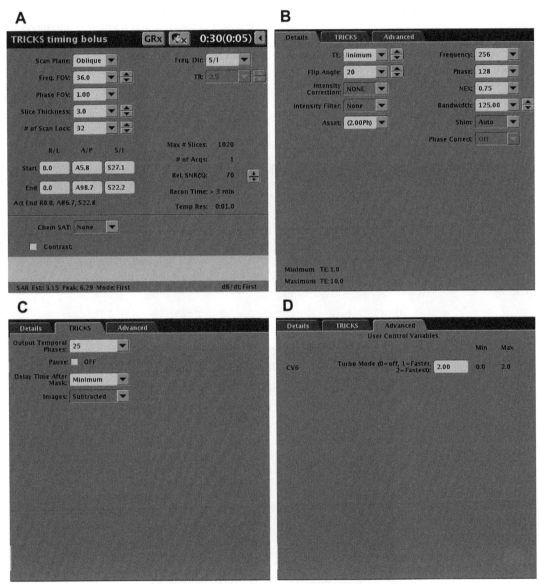

Fig. 3. A 3D time-resolved CE carotid MR angiogram using TRICKS on GE 3 T MR750. (*A*) On the Summary page, note that the 3D MR angiography slab is more than 90 mm thick in the AP direction, with a temporal resolution of 1 second and a TR of 2.5 milliseconds. (*B*) The Detail tab is where the imaging matrix, bandwidth, and partial NEX are inputted. (*C*) On the TRICKS tab, the user can prescribe the number of time phases to be acquired. Here it is set for 25 time points that are obtained with a temporal resolution of 1 second. This tab can be set for 30 or greater if there is the clinical suspicion of delayed gadolinium arrival, as can occur in sick inpatients as shown in **Fig. 4.** Also note that reconstruction of subtracted images is chosen. We have not found reconstructing unsubtracted images to be useful. (*D*) Under the Advanced tab, the user can prescribe the Turbo Mode. In general, Turbo Mode 2 works well to accelerate the acquisition without significant artifacts.

gadolinium bolus arrival time. The ringing artifact described earlier is less likely with delayed elliptical-centric phase ordering and, in our experience, there is little increase in venous contamination. GE provides the user with 3 versions of Turbo mode. Turbo mode 2 minimizes the TR with only a slight degradation in the excitation slab profile, which is optimal for carotid CE carotid MR angiography in which there is a minimal TR to capture the pass of gadolinium into the carotid arteries.

At 3 T, there is more SNR compared with 1.5 T MR imaging. This extra SNR can be used to generate even higher-resolution carotid CE MR angiography with the same amount (or potentially less) GBCA. One way to use this extra SNR is to increase the bandwidth from ±50 kHz to ±90.91

kHz. This results in a lower minimum TR and TE that allows the matrix to be increased from 346 × 320 to 376 × 352. The thickness of each slice (location) within the slab is decreased from 1.0 mm to 0.8 mm and the total number of locations in the slab is now 88 with a scan time of 40 seconds. The resulting resolution of the 3 T carotid CE MR angiography is now 0.80 × 0.85 × 0.80 mm with a total voxel volume of 0.54 mm^3 compared with 0.71 mm^3 at 1.5 T. If further coverage in the AP direction is needed, the number of locations per slab can be increased from 88 to 120, which would increase the slab thickness to 96 mm and increase the imaging time from 40 seconds to 53 seconds. **Fig. 2** details the parameters for this recommended 3 T carotid CE MR angiography. Again, with a well-designed multichannel coil, there is enough

A

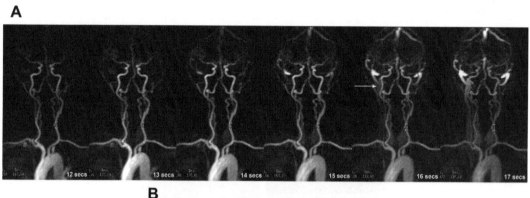

B

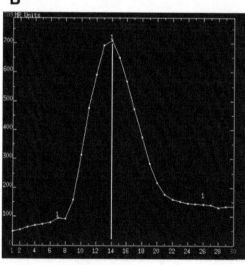

Fig. 4. Estimation of gadolinium bolus contrast agent arrival in the carotid artery using TRICKS. (*A*) Montage of multiple time points after intravenous gadolinium contrast agent injection at 12 to 17 seconds. The carotid arteries appear equally well enhanced at 13, 14, and 15 seconds. Note the first visualization of the right internal jugular vein in the upper neck especially on the right at 16 seconds (*arrow*). Given that the peak arterial enhancement is usually 2 seconds before the early appearance of upper neck veins, this visual inspection of the TRICKS suggests that the peak arterial gadolinium bolus arrival is at 14 seconds. There is a small region of interest in the mid–left CCA (please go to www.neuroimaging.theclinics.com to view an animated version of this image). (*B*) The dedicated MIROI confirms the peak arrival time in the mid–left CCA at 14 seconds.

SNR at 3 T MR to support this improved resolution of carotid CE MR angiography.

We recently began to use time-resolved intravascular contrast kinetics (TRICKS) to generate 1-second temporal resolution 3D scans of the head and neck during bolus administration of 2 mL of GBCA with spatial resolution of 1 × 2 × 3 mm. The specifics of the protocol are included in **Fig. 3**. By using a high bandwidth (±125 kHz) and ASSET factor of 2, we can prescribe a slab with a 36-cm FOV with a thickness of 96 mm in the A-P direction from the aortic arch through the circle of Willis based on a quick 3 plane localizer. The extended coverage in the AP direction virtually guarantees that all neck vessels will be included. The resulting 1-second temporal resolution images make it easy to identify the bolus arrival time of the GBCA and give the radiologist additional useful information about flow in the carotid and vertebral arteries.

The MR technologist can chose to complete the 3D TRICKS noncontrast mask, which takes 5 seconds, and then begin the injection of GBCA, which has the advantage that the time frame equals the bolus arrival time, but requires more 3D TRICKS datasets to be reconstructed. As an alternative, the MR technologist can begin the

GBCA intravenous injection at the beginning of the TRICKS acquisition. In this case, the first 5 seconds of the acquisition are used to generate the mask. The first time point from the TRICKS acquisition corresponds with 6 seconds after intravenous injection. This injection technique has the advantage of simplifying the acquisition by beginning the sequence and the injection at the same time, but has the disadvantage of requiring the MR technologist to add 5 seconds to the time frame to arrive at the correct bolus arrival time. The choice of injection protocol is site specific.

We compared the estimation of bolus arrival time using the originally described single axial image through the CCA with the bolus arrival time identified using TRICKS. The peak of the bolus arrival curve as generated on a multiple-image region of interest (MIROI) occurred at the same time with the 2 timing techniques. It is frequently difficult to identify the peak arterial contrast on TRICKS and there are usually 3 or 4 time points that appear equally well opacified. MIROI can easily identify the peak arrival time (**Fig. 4**B) but is tedious to generate. We have found that estimating peak arterial contrast based on the bolus arrival of GBCA in the upper neck veins works well. We typically identify the first appearance of

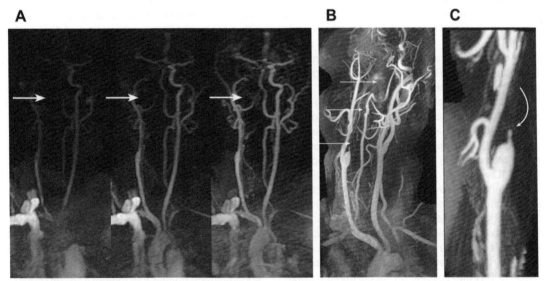

Fig. 5. Complete occlusion of right ICA. (*A*) Three time points from the 30 time-resolved 3D TRICKS MR angiography during the bolus administration of 2 mL of GBCA. By 18 and 20 seconds after gadolinium injection, both CCAs and left ICA are beginning to opacify in this sick inpatient. The peak carotid artery contrast was at 29 seconds after antecubital injection. Note that there is still no opacification of the right ICA (*straight arrows*). (*B*) Maximum intensity projection of the 0.54 mm³-resolution CE MR angiogram confirms complete occlusion of the right ICA (*straight arrows*) as well as sharp depiction of both remainder of carotid arteries and vertebral artery lumens. The left subclavian artery origin was not included on the high-resolution MR angiogram, but was shown to be normal on the TRICKS timing sequence. (*C*) Targeted magnified right carotid bifurcation maximum intensity projections of the 0.54-mm³ resolution CE MR angiogram confirms complete occlusion with excellent visualization of the right ICA stump (*curved arrow*).

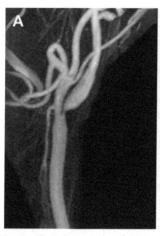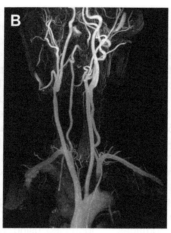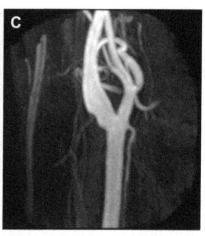

Fig. 6. Clinical example of 0.54-mm³ resolution 3 T carotid CE MR angiography. (*A*) A 58-year-old white woman with recent onset of left body weakness and numbness. The magnified targeted maximum intensity projection image of the right carotid bifurcation shows severe narrowing of the proximal right ICA, estimated to be a 91% diameter stenosis by NASCET criteria. Note the sharp depiction of the carotid lumen. (*B*) The large FOV, 0.54-mm³ resolution, carotid CE MR angiography shows excellent visualization of the distribution of both carotid arteries from the aortic arch to the circle of Willis. (*C*) Magnified targeted maximum intensity projection images of the left carotid bifurcation show only minimal indentation on the posterior lateral wall of the left carotid bulb.

contrast in the upper neck (arrow in **Fig. 4**A) and go back 2 earlier time points. We then look at that time frame and confirm visually that no adjacent time frame shows greater arterial contrast enhancement. As described earlier, the final GBCA arrival time is a combination of the time frame (in this case 14 seconds) and the 5 seconds needed to acquire the mask. The GBCA arrival time used to generate the first-pass high-resolution carotid CE MR angiography in this patient (see **Fig. 4**) was therefore 19 seconds.

Fig. 5 is an example of complete occlusion of the right ICA on the time-resolved MR angiography as well as the high-spatial-resolution single-pass carotid CE MR angiography detailing the residual right ICA stump. **Fig. 6** shows a severe stenosis of the left ICA.

In summary, an overview is provided of current state-of-the-art carotid CE MR angiography using GE 1.5 T and 3 T MR scanners running 15× and 20× software. **Table 1** and the specific screenshots help translate the general discussion about the important imaging parameters that affect final image quality into specific protocols that are applicable across a large number of the installed bases of GE 1.5 T and 3 T MR scanners.

Philips

A technique for CE MR angiographic data acquisition with random segmentation of the central k-space (CE timing robust angiography [CENTRA]) was first introduced by Willinek and colleagues[28]

in 2002 and applied to carotid MR angiography covering the supraaortic arteries from the aortic arch up to the circle of Willis with very high spatial resolution. To randomize sampling points in the middle of k-space where contrast material concentration is not maximal at the time of acquisition, a stochastic segmentation of the central disk is used in CENTRA. In this k-space ordering, the central contrast giving phase-encoding views are randomly sampled during the arterial phase. In the implementation of the stochastic segmentation, it is prohibited for the central points in k-space to be acquired first to avoid ringing artifacts if the arterial opacification has not been fully realized. The segmentation of the central sphere in k-space makes it possible to start the acquisition during the upslope of the contrast-time curve. Despite the short arterial time window in the carotid arteries and different circulation times, the CENTRA technique allows a high degree of venous suppression with barely visible, or absent, internal jugular vein signal in the most cases and avoids artifacts, especially the typical edge-enhancement artifact that occurs if CE MR angiography is begun too early; cases suggest that the random method of central k-space acquisition minimizes any artifact caused by instable contrast material concentration.

A study that compared 0.66-mm³ resolution CENTRA MR angiography of the supraaortic arteries including the origins at the aortic arch and the circle of Willis at 1.5 T prospectively with digital subtraction angiography as the standard of reference in a total of 833 arteries of 50 consecutive patients found a good agreement between the 2 techniques. Independent readings of 2 radiologists and assessment according to the NASCET criteria yielded the following results: CENTRA MR angiography had a sensitivity of 100% (73/73), a specificity of 99.3% (760/765), a positive predictive value (PPV) of 93.6% (73/78), and a negative predictive value (NPV) of 100% (760/760) by using a 70% to 99% threshold of arterial diameter stenosis.[13] For detection of occlusion, the sensitivity, specificity, PPV, and NPV of CENTRA MR angiography were 100%, respectively.[13] The investigators concluded that noninvasive, 0.66-mm³ resolution, CE MR angiography with CENTRA is suited to replace diagnostic digital subtraction angiography for the detection of steno-occlusive disease of the supraaortic arteries.[13]

Philips has not reviewed or endorsed the protocols described in this article.

1.5 T

At 1.5 T, we recommend a large FOV with 350-mm coverage and a noninterpolated voxel size of 0.66 mm³ with a multielement neurovascular coil (eg, 16-channel neurovascular coil) (see Table 1). On the Geometry page, the coil selection button allows the selection of coil elements. We recommend selection of the HNACPC combination (head, neck, anterior coil, and posterior coil elements). We use a scan of 80% with a 432 matrix to yield an acquisition time of 59 seconds. Previous studies showed that the CENTRA approach enables expansion of the acquisition time beyond 2 minutes while providing arterial phase imaging at even higher spatial resolution without venous overlay. This ability might, in part, be a product of recirculation of the contrast agent that still accounts for more than 40% of peak contrast of the contrast-over-time curve. We recommend a bolus of a GBCA at single

dose administered at a flow rate of 2 to 3 mL per second, depending on the concentration of the agent, followed by a saline flush of 25 mL. **Fig. 7** shows the scan parameters. The recommended protocol is feasible with any standard 1.5 T magnet and is robust and reliable in daily clinical practice.

3 T

The signal gain at 3 T allows modification of the 1.5 T protocol for spatial resolution and coverage or a combination of both. We investigated the feasibility of several CE MR angiography protocols at 3 T that were modified from a 3D gradient-echo pulse sequence with parallel imaging (SENSE) using parallel imaging factors (PIF) ranging from 1 to 16.[18] The 3 T MR angiography protocols using parallel imaging in a single direction were based on the standard protocol for supraaortic MR angiography at 1.5 T (see Table 1).

At higher field strength, we recommend a standardized, automatic bolus injection of a single dose of GBCA at a slightly lower flow rate of 1.5 ml per second compared with 1.5 T, followed by a saline solution flush.

When real-time fluoroscopy reveals that the bolus of contrast material reaches the aortic arch, the angiographic pulse sequence is started manually with a delay of 1 second (**Fig. 8**). To minimize motion artifacts, we ask patients to hold their breath during the initial 15 seconds of data acquisition.

Our results showed that, with a parallel imaging factor of 16, a 760 × 700 matrix is feasible over a 350-mm FOV with thin sagittal slices of 365 × 0.98 mm (0.49 mm more than contiguous) yielding a submillimetric spatial resolution of 0.46 × 0.46 × 0.98 mm³ (before interpolation). However, acquisition time of this protocol is long at 1 minute and 27 seconds.[18] To reduce acquisition while maintaining the anatomic coverage of the head and neck, we prefer, for clinical routine, a matrix of 640 × 640

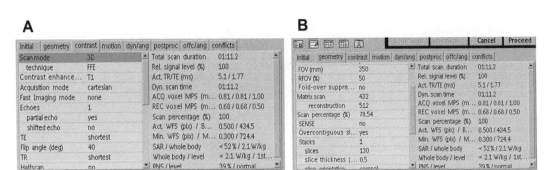

Fig. 7. Using the Philips 1.5 Intera MR scanner for 0.66-mm³ resolution, first-pass CE large FOV carotid MR angiography. (*A*) The Contrast tab shows the choices of fast field echo with T1 weighting as well as shortest TR and TE. (*B*) The Geometry tab is where imaging options such as FOV, rectangular FOV, matrix size, and scan percentage can be modified. Also note that SENSE is not used at 1.5 T with this protocol.

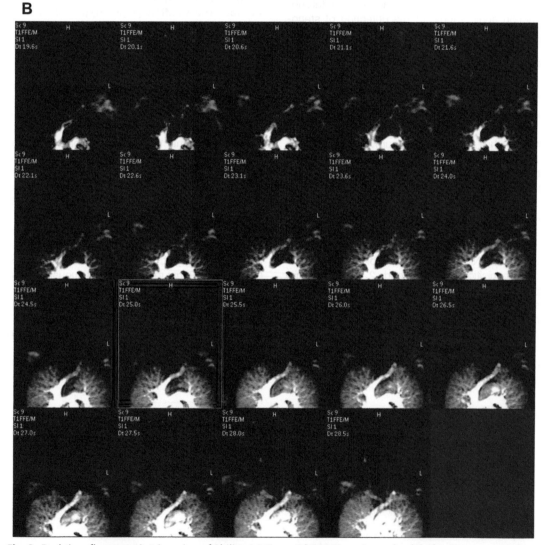

Fig. 8. Real-time fluoroscopic triggering of Philips 1.5 T carotid CE MR angiography. (*A*) The Geometry tab from the fluoroscopic triggering prescription shows the use of a 450-mm FOV and a slab thickness of 50 mm to include the upper heart as well as the aortic arch and carotid arteries. (*B*) This screenshot of the fluoroscopic triggering shows the contrast arrival in the chest and later in the neck. Note that the CE MR angiography sequence is initiated manually when the bolus leaves the left ventricle. Temporal resolution is 0.5 seconds.

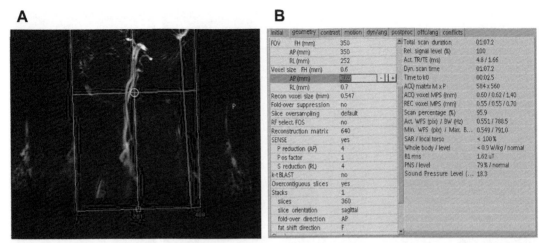

Fig. 9. Using the Philips 3 T Achieva MR scanner for 0.52-mm³ resolution first-pass CE large FOV carotid MR angiography. (*A*) Note how the large coverage in the AP direction simplifies prescription of the carotid CE MR angiography without the need for additional MR angiography localizers. (*B*) The Geometry tab details the use of 2D SENSE to achieve a 16-fold acceleration and allow for submillimeter in-plane resolution with the extended A-P coverage in a scan time of 1:07 minutes.

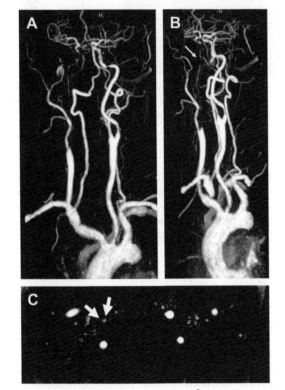

Fig. 10. Clinical example of 0.66-mm³ resolution, 1.5 T, carotid CE MR angiography. (*A*) A 70 year-old man with ischemic stroke. The maximum intensity projection of the 0.66-mm³ resolution, CE, MR angiogram shows a tight stenosis of the right ICA. (*B*) Oblique enlarged view confirms opacification of the distal ICA with string sign (ie, pseudoocclusion (*arrow*). (*C*) Axial MPR of 3D CE MR angiogram confirms the central opacification of the distal ICA at the C2/3 level (*arrows*). MPR, multiplanar reformations.

with 360 slices of 1.4-mm thickness yielding a voxel size of 0.52 mm³ (see **Table 1**). The increased anatomic coverage (compared with the protocol at 1.5 T) simplifies the positioning of the scan volume because it includes the head and neck and may not need adjustment for the individual anatomy of different patients. Therefore, additional TOF or phase contrast angiography (PCA) surveys for planning are no longer required, which in turn reduces overall acquisition time and gives more reliable results (**Fig. 9**). This high-resolution, 3 T, CE MR angiography technique provides wide coverage as well as excellent depiction of carotid stenosis (**Fig. 10**).

In summary, an overview of current state-of-the-art imaging protocols is provided for Philips 1.5 T and 3 T systems running standard software releases. With more advanced software capabilities, these protocols can be fine-tuned according to the individual clinical needs (**Fig. 11**). However, this article provides screenshots of imaging parameters that are applicable across a large number of Philips installations.

Siemens

At UCLA, we base our high-resolution carotid CE MR angiography acquisition on a bolus timing study with syngo 3D TWIST. We perform most of our carotid CE MR angiography at 3 T, although we have comparable protocols at 1.5 T in case 3 T is not available.

Carotid CE MR angiography 1.5 T

Note that the protocols described in this article are specific to the Siemens 32-channel Magnetom

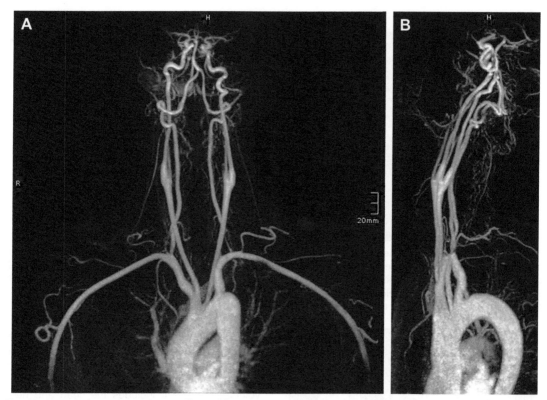

Fig. 11. Extended coverage to image all possible vascular supply to a recently diagnosed neck tumor. (*A*) CE 3 T MR angiogram in the sagittal plane was acquired with a parallel imaging factor of 9. (*B*) Note the excellent coverage of the upper chest and entire neck including the internal mammary arteries, thyrocervical trunk, and branches of the external carotid artery in this patient with a known neck tumor.

TIM Avanto, but are implemented at UCLA based on clinical practice. Siemens has not reviewed or endorsed the protocols described here.

Contrast preparation: 1.5 T

At 1.5 T, we aim for a GBCA dose of about 0.1 mmol/kg for high-resolution CE MR angiography (ie, 17 mL of a standard 0.5 mmol/L GBCA solution). We initially perform the 3D TWIST timing run with 2 mL of GBCA, for a total dose of 20 mL. To maintain consistency in injection rates, we first dilute the native GBCA solution by a factor of 2 with normal saline. Therefore, 20 mL of 0.5 M GBCA solution are drawn into the contrast syringe and then 20 mL of saline are drawn into the same syringe and the dilute solution is allowed to mix while the syringe is orientated horizontally. The saline syringe and the injection tubing are primed with normal saline, as is usual. In total, we inject 40 mL of half-strength GBCA solution at a rate of 2 mL/s. The first injection is 6 mL at 2 mL/s for the 3D TWIST (timing) acquisition, followed by a 20-mL saline flush. The second injection is 34 mL at 2 mL/s for the high-resolution 3D

CE MR angiography. Immediately following the high-resolution (breath-held) arterial study, we acquire a full 3D (non–breath-held) cerebral venogram without additional GBCA injection. The parameters for all 3 acquisitions are summarized later.

3D syngo TWIST

The technique is similar to that described for 3 T MR, except that the acceleration (GRAPPA) factor is 4.

High-resolution CE MR angiography

Activated coil elements are the same as for the TWIST acquisition. The primary orientation is coronal with an FOV of 410 mm (head-foot) × 305 (R-L) × 110 mm (AP). The matrix is 512 (frequency) × 340 (phase) × 120 (slice), yielding voxels of 0.8 × 0.9 × 0.9 mm. The TR/TE is 2.6/1.16 milliseconds and the acceleration (GRAPPA) factor is 3 (R-L). The time from the beginning of the acquisition to the center of k-space is freely selectable and is generally chosen as 6 seconds (**Fig. 12**).

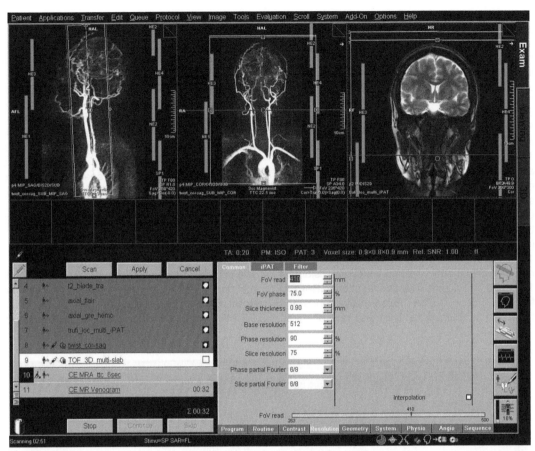

Fig. 12. Using the Siemens 32 channel Magnetom TIM Avanto for 0.65-mm³ resolution, first-pass CE large FOV carotid 1.5 T MR angiography. The imaging parameters for the 1.5 T first-pass high-resolution CE MR angiography are shown on the Resolution tab. The acceleration factors and spatial resolution are not as aggressive as their 3 T MR counterparts.

Once the appropriate timing for the contrast bolus is noted, the injection is initialized and breathing instructions are timed to coincide with bolus arrival. Thirty-four milliliters of half-strength GBCA solution are injected at 2 mL/s, followed by 20 mL of saline at 2 mL/s.

Venographic acquisition

Immediately following the arterial phase CE MR angiography, a 3D cerebral venographic study is initiated while the patient breathes normally. This acquisition is focused on the head and neck, takes approximately 30 seconds, and uses an acceleration (GRAPPA) factor of 4.

Carotid CE MR angiography 3 T

Note that the protocols described are specific to the Siemens 32-channel Magnetom TIM Trio, but are implemented at UCLA based on clinical practice. Siemens has not reviewed or endorsed the protocols described here.

Contrast preparation: 3 T

At 3 T, we aim for a GBCA dose of about 0.05 mmol/kg for high-resolution, CE MR angiography (ie, 8 mL of a standard 0.5 mmol/L GBCA solution).[21] We initially perform the 3D TWIST timing run with 2 mL of GBCA, for a total dose of 10 mL. Because, at this low dose level, the small volumes of the native GBCA formulation would limit our injection rates, we first dilute the native GBCA solution by a factor of 4 with normal saline. Therefore, 10 mL of 0.5 M GBCA solution are drawn into the contrast syringe and then 30 mL of saline are drawn into the same syringe and the dilute solution is allowed to mix while the syringe is orientated horizontally. The saline syringe and the injection tubing are primed with normal saline, as is usual. In total, we inject 40 mL of quarter-strength GBCA solution at a rate of 2 mL/s. The first injection is 8 mL at 2 mL/s for the 3D TWIST (timing) acquisition, followed by a 20-mL saline flush. The second injection is 32 mL at 2 mL/s for high-resolution 3D CE MR angiography. Immediately following the high-resolution (breath-held) arterial study, we acquire a full 3D (non–breath-held) cerebral venogram without additional GBCA injection. The parameters for all 3 acquisitions are summarized later.

3D syngo TWIST

Following initial scout sequences, we prescribe a 425 mm (head-foot) × 290 mm (A-P) FOV 3D TWIST acquisition encompassing the head, neck, and upper thorax (**Fig. 13**). Elements from the head coil (12), neck coil (6), and spine coil (1) are activated for this acquisition. The primary orientation is sagittal, the in-plane phase-encoding direction is AP and the through-plane phase-encoding (slice) direction is right to left (R-L). We acquire 176 partitions (slices) with a slice thickness of 1.5 mm on a 326 matrix, yielding voxel dimensions of 1.7 × 1.3 × 1.5 mm. The acceleration (GRAPPA) factor is 6 (2 × 3). The TR is 2 milliseconds and the TE is 1.1 milliseconds. The mask set is acquired

in approximately 5 seconds and the TWIST 3D data are updated approximately once every 1.5 seconds. The sequence is set to run repeatedly for about 50 seconds, starting with the injection of the 8-mL, quarter-strength gadolinium solution while the patient breathes quietly. On completion of the TWIST acquisition, the mask image is automatically subtracted from the remaining 3D data-sets and full-thickness coronal and sagittal MIP projects are calculated and displayed with a time stamp denoting the time from the start of the sequence (injection) to each specific frame. The first frame, which optimally shows the arch and carotids, is used to define the delay from the main injection to the start of the high-resolution 3D acquisition.

High-resolution CE MR angiography

The coronal and sagittal projections from the optimal phase TWIST acquisition are used for precise positioning of the 3D slab for the high-resolution CE MR angiography run (**Fig. 14**). Depending on

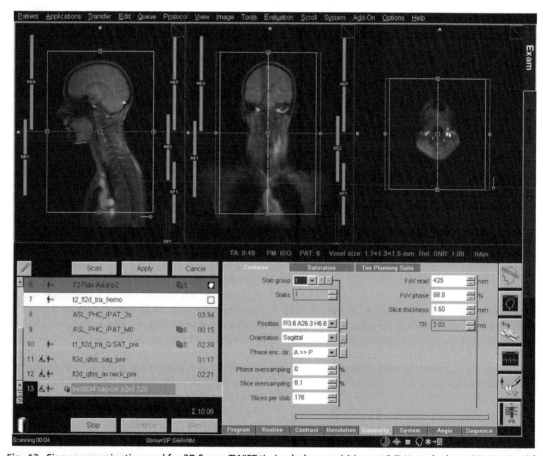

Fig. 13. Siemens examination card for 3D Syngo TWIST timing bolus acquisitions at 3 T. Note the large FOV to simplify placement of the imaging volume and the sagittal plane of acquisition. Some of the image parameters are listed on the Geometry tab, which is highlighted. Full details of all the pertinent image parameters are given in the text.

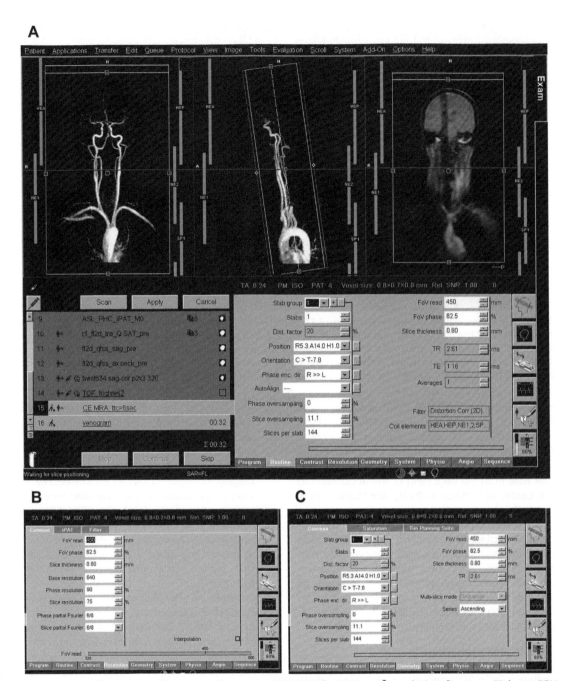

Fig. 14. Using the Siemens 32 channel Magnetom TIM Trio for 0.44-mm³ resolution first-pass CE large FOV carotid, 3 T MR angiography. (*A*) Note the large FOV and wide coverage to simply the placement of the 3D prescription. The excellent opacification of the aortic arch, great vessels, carotid artery, and vertebral artery also ensures that all these vessels are included in the high-resolution, first-pass CE MR angiogram. (*B*) The Resolution tab details many of the imaging parameters required to achieve the 0.44-mm³ voxel size. (*C*) The Geometry tab specifies the FOV, percent phase FOV, slice thickness, and slices per slab.

patient-specific anatomy, the acquisition time is 22 to 24 seconds, and patients are requested to hold their breath as best they can for this time. The goal is to encompass the aortic arch and great

vessel origins, the subclavians, carotids, and vertebrals from their origins to the vertex of the skull.

Activated coil elements are the same as for the TWIST acquisition. The primary orientation is

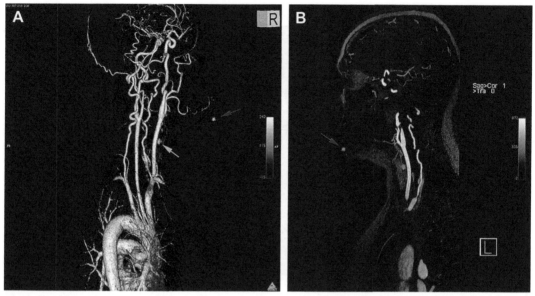

Fig. 15. Clinical example of 0.44 mm³ resolution 3 T carotid contrast-enhanced MRA using the Siemens 32 channel Magnetom TIM Trio. (*A*) On the high-resolution 3D Volume Reformations of the 0.44 mm³ resolution contrast-enhanced MRA shows an enhancing hemangioma (*red arrow*) involving the soft tissue structures against to the right mandible. Also note the enhancing right thyroid nodule (*blue arrow*). (*B*) Selective multiplanar reformation of the right neck confirm the enhancing hemangioma (*red arrow*) and thyroid nodule.

coronal with an FOV of 450 mm (head-foot) × 280 (R-L) × 115 mm (AP). The matrix is 640 (frequency) × 350 (phase) × 144 (slice), yielding 0.7 × 0.8 × 0.8 mm voxels. The TR/TE is 2.6/1.16 milliseconds and the acceleration (GRAPPA) factor is 4 (R-L). The time from the beginning of the acquisition to the center of k-space is freely selectable and is generally chosen as 6 seconds.

Once the appropriate timing for the contrast bolus is noted, the injection is initialized and breathing instructions are timed to coincide with bolus arrival. Thirty-two milliliters of quarter-strength gadolinium solution are injected at 2 mL/s, followed by 20 mL of saline at 2 mL/s. Routine high resolution CEMRA is consistently generated with this technique (**Fig. 15**).

Venographic acquisition
Immediately following the arterial phase CE MR angiography, a 3D cerebral venographic study is initiated while the patient breathes normally.[29] This acquisition is focused on the head and neck, takes approximately 30 seconds, and uses an acceleration (GRAPPA) factor of 6 (2 × 3).

REFERENCES

1. Brott TG, Halperin JL, Abbara S, et al. 2011 guideline on the management of patients with extracranial carotid and vertebral artery disease: executive summary. J Am Coll Cardiol 2011;57(8):1002–44.

2. Anderson CM, Lee RE, Levin DL, et al. Measurement of internal carotid artery stenosis from source MR angiograms. Radiology 1994;193(1): 219–26.

3. Kent KC, Kuntz KM, Patel MR, et al. Perioperative imaging strategies for carotid endarterectomy. An analysis of morbidity and cost-effectiveness in symptomatic patients. JAMA 1995;274(11):888–93.

4. Patel MR, Kuntz KM, Klufas RA, et al. Preoperative assessment of the carotid bifurcation. Can magnetic resonance angiography and duplex ultrasonography replace contrast arteriography? Stroke 1995; 26(10):1753–8.

5. Demarco JK, Nesbit GM, Wesbey GE, et al. Prospective comparison of extracranial carotid stenosis with intraarterial angiography versus MR angiography using maximum-intensity projections and multiplanar reformations. AJR Am J Roentgenol 1994;163:1205–12.

6. De Marco JK, Schonfeld S, Keller I, et al. Contrast-enhanced carotid MR angiography with commercially available triggering mechanisms and elliptic centric phase encoding. AJR Am J Roentgenol 2001;176(1):221–7.

7. Turski PA, Korosec FR, Carroll TJ, et al. Contrast-enhanced magnetic resonance angiography of the carotid bifurcation using the time-resolved imaging of contrast kinetics (TRICKS) technique. Top Magn Reson Imaging 2001;12(3):175–81.

8. Yang CW, Carr JC, Futterer SF, et al. Contrast-enhanced MR angiography of the carotid and

vertebrobasilar circulations. AJNR Am J Neuroradiol 2005;26(8):2095–101.

9. Mistretta CA. Undersampled radial MR acquisition and highly constrained back projection (HYPR) reconstruction: potential medical imaging applications in the post-Nyquist era. J Magn Reson Imaging 2009;29(3):501–16.

10. Fain SB, Riederer SJ, Bernstein MA, et al. Theoretical limits of spatial resolution in elliptical-centric contrast-enhanced 3D-MRA. Magn Reson Med 1999;42(6):1106–16.

11. Huston J, Fain SB, Wald JT, et al. Carotid artery: elliptic centric contrast-enhanced MR angiography compared with conventional angiography. Radiology 2001;218(1):138–43.

12. Carr JC, Ma J, Desphande V, et al. High-resolution breath-hold contrast-enhanced MR angiography of the entire carotid circulation. AJR Am J Roentgenol 2002;178(3):543–9.

13. Willinek WA, von Falkenhausen M, Born M, et al. Noninvasive detection of steno-occlusive disease of the supra-aortic arteries with three-dimensional contrast-enhanced magnetic resonance angiography: a prospective, intra-individual comparative analysis with digital subtraction angiography. Stroke 2005;36(1):38–43.

14. Fellner C, Lang W, Janka R, et al. Magnetic resonance angiography of the carotid arteries using three different techniques: accuracy compared with intra-arterial x-ray angiography and endarterectomy specimens. J Magn Reson Imaging 2005;21(4):424–31.

15. DeMarco JK, Huston J, Nash AK. Extracranial carotid MR imaging at 3T. Magn Reson Imaging Clin N Am 2006;14(1):109–21.

16. Hnatiuk B, Emery DJ, Wilman AH. Effects of doubling and tripling the spatial resolution in standard 3D contrast-enhanced magnetic resonance angiography of carotid artery disease. J Magn Reson Imaging 2008;27(1):71–7.

17. Nael K, Villablanca JP, Pope WB, et al. Supraaortic arteries: contrast-enhanced MR angiography at 3.0 T–highly accelerated parallel acquisition for improved spatial resolution over an extended field of view. Radiology 2007;242(2):600–9.

18. Kukuk GM, Hadizadeh DR, Gieseke J, et al. Highly undersampled supraaortic MRA at 3.0 T: initial results with parallel imaging in two directions using a 16-channel neurovascular coil and parallel imaging factors up to 16. Magn Reson Imaging 2010;28(9):1311–8.

19. Demarco JK, Ota H, Underhill HR, et al. MR carotid plaque imaging and contrast-enhanced MR angiography identifies lesions associated with recent ipsilateral thromboembolic symptoms: an in vivo study at 3T. AJNR Am J Neuroradiol 2010;31(8):1395–402.

20. Du YP, Parker DL, Davis WL, et al. Reduction of partial-volume artifacts with zero-filled interpolation in three-dimensional MR angiography. J Magn Reson Imaging 1994;4(5):733–41.

21. Tomasian A, Salamon N, Lohan DG, et al. Supra-aortic arteries: contrast material dose reduction at 3.0-T high-spatial-resolution MR angiography—feasibility study. Radiology 2008;249(3):980–90.

22. Knopp MV, Giesel FL, von Tengg-Kobligk H, et al. Contrast-enhanced MR angiography of the run-off vasculature: intraindividual comparison of gadobenate dimeglumine with gadopentetate dimeglumine. J Magn Reson Imaging 2003;17(6):694–702.

23. Pediconi F, Fraioli F, Catalano C, et al. Gadobenate dimeglumine (Gd-DTPA) vs gadopentetate dimeglumine (Gd-BOPTA) for contrast-enhanced magnetic resonance angiography (MRA): improvement in intravascular signal intensity and contrast to noise ratio. Radiol Med 2003;106(1–2):87–93.

24. Bueltmann E, Erb G, Kirchin MA, et al. Intra-individual crossover comparison of gadobenate dimeglumine and gadopentetate dimeglumine for contrast-enhanced magnetic resonance angiography of the supraaortic vessels at 3 Tesla. Invest Radiol 2008;43(10):695–702.

25. Habibi R, Krishnam MS, Lohan DG, et al. High-spatial-resolution lower extremity MR angiography at 3.0 T: contrast agent dose comparison study. Radiology 2008;248(2):680–92.

26. Lohan DG, Tomasian A, Saleh RS, et al. Ultra-low-dose, time-resolved contrast-enhanced magnetic resonance angiography of the carotid arteries at 3.0 tesla. Invest Radiol 2009;44(4):207–17.

27. Riederer SJ, Bernstein MA, Breen JF, et al. Three-dimensional contrast-enhanced MR angiography with real-time fluoroscopic triggering: design specifications and technical reliability in 330 patient studies. Radiology 2000;215(2):584–93.

28. Willinek WA, Gieseke J, Conrad R, et al. Randomly segmented central k-space ordering in high-spatial-resolution contrast-enhanced MR angiography of the supraaortic arteries: initial experience. Radiology 2002;225(2):583–8.

29. Nael K, Fenchel M, Salamon N, et al. Three-dimensional cerebral contrast-enhanced magnetic resonance venography at 3.0 Tesla: initial results using highly accelerated parallel acquisition. Invest Radiol 2006;41(10):763–8.

Vascular Disorders: Insights from Arterial Spin Labeling

Jeroen Hendrikse, MD, PhD[a],*, Esben Thade Petersen, PhD[a],
Xavier Golay, PhD[b]

KEYWORDS

• Arterial spin labeling • Cerebrovascular diseases • Stroke

Key Points

• ASL provides additional information in cerebrovascular diseases
• ASL is easy to implement and quick to perform
• ASL is nowadays available from all vendors
• ASL is recommended especially at high-fields ($\geq$3 T)

Cerebral blood flow (CBF) has been measured since the early pioneers Kety and Schmidt[1] did their first studies using inhalation of nitrous oxide as a freely diffusible tracer, accompanied by both arterial and venous blood sampling. These early studies only revealed the mean CBF of the brain without any spatial information or separation between tissue types. Nevertheless, the methodology serves as a basis for the more advanced perfusion imaging methods used today, based on modalities such as single-photon emission computed tomography (SPECT), positron emission tomography (PET), X-ray computed tomography (CT), or magnetic resonance (MR) imaging. Despite the important diagnostic and pathophysiologic information that they provide, such perfusion imaging methods are rarely used and have only a small role in radiology. There are many reasons for this, including the cost and time needed for these studies, with $H_2{}^{15}O$–positron emission tomography (PET) being the most expensive because of the requirement of an on-site cyclotron. In addition, all methods listed earlier (with 1 notable exception) require the injection of a contrast medium for the assessment of perfusion, with the additional burden of radiation for nuclear medicine and CT-based methods. MR perfusion imaging involves the use of a gadolinium-based contrast agent, which can be contraindicated in certain diseases such as kidney failure.[2] However, recent advances in MR imaging hardware, especially the introduction of high-field systems (3 T) in the clinics, have made another approach a viable clinical alternative: ASL. The method was first published in 1991 and is based on the direct magnetic labeling of blood water protons as an endogenous tracer, without the need of exogenous contrast agent.[3] Higher field strength usually comes with an increase in the signal/noise ratio (SNR) in all MR imaging methods, but ASL in particular benefits from the higher field strength[4] because of the additional

Financial disclosures: Esben Thade Petersen and Xavier Golay received consultation honoraria from Philips Medical Systems.
[a] Department of Radiology, University Medical Center Utrecht, Room E01.132, PO Box 85500, 3508 GA Utrecht, The Netherlands
[b] UCL Institute of Neurology, National Hospital for Neurology & Neurosurgery, Queen Square, London WC1N 3BG, UK
* Corresponding author.
E-mail address: J.Hendrikse@umcutrecht.nl

neuroimaging.theclinics.com

Diagnostic Checklist

- Vascular disorders in general: add global arterial spin labeling (ASL; eg, 3 minutes pulsed ASL [PASL]/ pseudo continuous arterial spin labeling [pCASL] with background suppression) to the standard clinical protocol if possible
- In large vessel stenosis or occlusion, an additional acquisition after vascular challenge should be considered
- Experimentally, territorial ASL can also be considered in large vessel disease, but the sequence is still not clinically available from the vendors

---

prolongation of blood longitudinal relaxation time (T_1), which makes the labeled bolus last longer.

This article reviews the basic principles of ASL, their implementations, and what information can be obtained in addition to CBF using such methods. The main clinical applications of ASL in vascular disorders are reviewed, in particular chronic cerebrovascular disease, stroke, moyamoya disease, arteriovenous malformation (AVM), and neurodegenerative diseases of potential vascular origin, such as vascular dementia. In addition, pulse sequence recommendations are given in Table 1.

ASL

Two main implementations of ASL exist. The first approach uses continuous labeling of the blood water during its passage through a label plane typically labeling extracranial arteries close to, or at, the cerebromedular junction (continuous ASL [CASL]). Labeling is typically performed continuously for 1 to 2 seconds, after which a postlabeling delay is inserted before imaging. This delay allows the labeled blood to reach the region of interest in the brain and lets it clear from the feeding arteries. The second approach is based on a single inversion pulse that spatially labels the blood over an extended region in the neck (pulsed ASL [PASL]).

Again, a postlabeling delay is inserted before imaging, for the same reasons. To get a perfusion-weighted image, a control experiment needs to be performed without any labeling of the blood, and it is the subtraction of the 2 (control minus label) that gives the perfusion-weighted image (Fig. 1). The signal differences for normal CBF levels are in the order of 0.5% to 2.0% of the full tissue signal and therefore several control-label pairs need to be acquired and averaged to achieve sufficient SNR in the perfusion-weighted images.

Until recently, PASL was the preferred method because of its ease of implementation and minimal hardware requirements. CASL necessitated special labeling coils or the use of a transmit/receive head coil, which is now obsolete in clinical practice because of the introduction of parallel imaging using large arrays of receiver coils used in combination with the quadrature body coil as the transmit coil. This method has changed with the recent alternative implementation of CASL called pseudo-CASL,[5] which has gained popularity because of minimal hardware requirements and superior SNR, compared with PASL.

There are several aspects to consider when interpreting or quantifying ASL data. This article focuses on the main aspects of clinical interest, whereas a more complete description can be found elsewhere (for example, see Ref.[6]). The main strength

---

Table 1
Recommended pulse sequences in cerebrovascular diseases

Sequence	TR (s)	Readout	Bolus Definition	TI/PLD	Special
QUASAR/ITS-FAIR	3–4	EPI	500–600 ms	100–3000 ms	Saturation pulse
Multi-TI	TI+1	3D-GRASE	500–600 ms	100–3000 ms	Background suppression
CASL/pCASL	4–5	EPI or GRASE or Spiral	1.8 s	1.2 s	Background suppression

Abbreviations: 3D-GRASE, 3 dimensional gradient and spin echo imaging; CASL, continuous ASL; EPI, echo planar imaging; ITS-FAIR, inflow turbo-sampling EPI-FAIR; PLD, post labeling delay; pCASL, pseudo continuous ASL; QUASAR, quantitative STAR labeling of arterial regions; TI, inversion time; TR, recovery time.

Pulsed-base multi-TI sequences are preferable to CASL/pCASL in neurovascular diseases. All the sequences in the table can be combined with methods for labeling each artery selectively and independently. PASL methods (the first 2 rows in the table), use additional radiofrequency pulses for defining the bolus, whereas the bolus definition is intrinsic in CASL/pCASL.

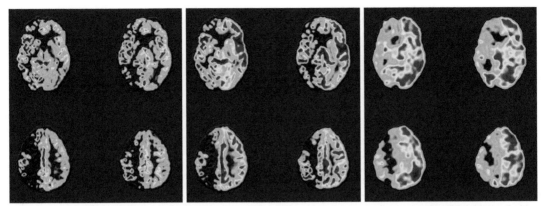

Fig. 1. A patient with a right-sided carotid artery occlusion and transient ischemic attacks. ASL perfusion at rest (*left*) shows a clear decreased perfusion of the right hemisphere. After the acetazolamide injection, the ASL perfusion image (*middle*) shows a clearer asymmetry with a decreased perfusion of the right hemisphere. The reactivity image (*right*) shows impaired autoregulation in the right hemisphere.

of ASL is its noninvasiveness, which allows the performance of repeated perfusion studies such as in neuroscience, pharmacologic, or patient follow-up studies, but it also makes it an ideal choice for the pediatric population or patients with contraindications for contrast injections.[2] However, the same noninvasive use of the blood water as an endogenous contrast bolus also becomes its main clinical disadvantage, because the magnetically labeled bolus decays with the T_1 of blood, and therefore has a limited lifespan. Regions to which the travel time of the blood from the labeling area exceeds ∼2 seconds are hard to get perfusion information from. Because of their location, such areas experience slow flow because of a stenosis or long collateral pathways making the CBF map appear dark, suggesting no or little flow, whereas it could be late-arriving flow. This error is intrinsic to the method and cannot be overcome.

In addition to being a potential problem, information on the transit time of the blood might have significant diagnostic usefulness, just as in other perfusion measurement methods (eg, dynamic susceptibility-based MR imaging and perfusion CT). In ASL, there are several ways to gather information about the transit time, with the most common ones making use of repeated experiments at different postlabeling delays or inversion times (TI). This method allows assessment of the arterial travel time (ATT) from the labeling region to the tissue of interest, which improves quantification and helps guide the interpretation of the ASL data. However, it does not solve the problem of late-arriving blood beyond the sensitivity limits of ASL in which the bolus disappears with the T_1 relaxation of blood. Therefore, clinical experience is needed to be aware of it and possibly interpret the result in other ways than

just as a quantitative CBF measure. As already mentioned, delayed perfusion is a predictor of bad outcome (eg, in stroke).[7]

Another issue common to all perfusion modalities is related to motion artifacts during acquisition. The need for several control-label pairs makes ASL acquisition last typically 2 to 5 minutes, and it is therefore prone to motion artifacts in uncooperative patients. Background-suppressed ASL methods[8] minimize this effect, but motion can still affect the resulting perfusion map and interpretation has to be done with care in these cases.

However, ASL has the unique advantage of being capable of labeling single vessels independently, and therefore it is able to assess the extent of different perfusion territories from all major vessels supplying the brain, thereby including important clinical information on collateral perfusion (**Fig. 2**).[9,10] In addition, vascular reactivity can easily be assessed using an acetazolamide challenge together with ASL,[11] and both methods used together make ASL an ideal tool for assessment of vascular disorders, especially because they can be combined with quantitative measurement of CBF. In addition, ASL perfusion measurements may be used in evaluation of the effectiveness of medication treatments in patients with cerebrovascular disease.[12]

CHRONIC CEREBROVASCULAR DISEASE

The most obvious example of chronic cerebrovascular disease is a stenosis or occlusion of one of the brain feeding arteries. The most well-known example of extracranial stenoses is the stenosis at the origin of the internal carotid artery (ICA). Patients with recent symptoms on the side of an

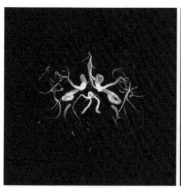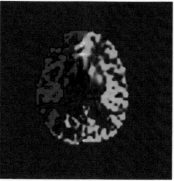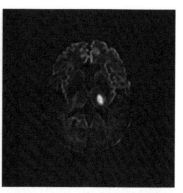

Fig. 2. A patient with a left-sided posterior cerebral artery (PCA) occlusion as seen on time-of-flight imaging (*left*). Territorial ASL reveals the leptomeningeal collateral flow to the left PCA territory (*middle*), although it is not sufficient to avoid infarct, as seen on diffusion-weighted imaging (*right*).

ICA stenosis are considered for carotid surgery if the stenosis has a certain severity, typically greater than 70%. However, this procedure only prevents recurrent ischemic stroke in less than 20% of patients,[13] meaning that most of the patients currently being operated on would not have experienced any future stroke if they had not had the surgery. In addition, the operation has a risk of causing an ischemic event and it would therefore be beneficial to improve patient selection to carotid endarterectomy. ASL may be helpful to select patients for carotid surgery in 2 ways. First, perfusion imaging at rest can discriminate between brain tissue that is underperfused and brain tissue with a normal perfusion. Patients with severely decreased perfusion on the side of the carotid artery stenosis may benefit most from carotid endarterectomy compared with patients with intact perfusion collaterals, for instance via the circle of Willis, which thereby compensates for the stenosis. Most strokes from a carotid artery stenosis are considered to be thromboembolic. The presence of a vulnerable plaque and therefore high risk of thromboembolism in combination with hypoperfusion (eg, measured with ASL) increases the patient's risk of a recurrent stroke, according to the washout hypothesis introduced by Caplan and Hennerici.[14] In these patients, the low perfusion decreases the ability of the vasculature to wash out small emboli.

Nevertheless, the presence of normal perfusion in a resting condition does not always mean that the vasculature is not compromised. The first-line compensation mechanism for a decrease in perfusion pressure is dilation of the arterioles, resulting in lower resistance and higher flow, thereby maintaining a constant CBF. However, in some patients this autoregulatory ability is compromised because it reaches its maximum diameter to recruit flow (eg, via collaterals). Further vascular events with an accompanying reduction in perfusion pressure could cause ischemia.

The advantage of MR imaging is that, within the same scan session, carotid plaque imaging, perfusion imaging, and a vascular reactivity challenge can be performed using, for example, acetazolamide and ASL, allowing assessment of plaque rupture risk, baseline perfusion status, and the ability to compensate in future vascular events. Autoregulation status can be assessed by combining a baseline or rest perfusion scan with a perfusion measurement after a vasodilatory challenge. Cerebrovascular reserve capacity (CVR) is then defined as the percentage CBF change between baseline and vasodilatation. ASL is advantageous for such measurements because of its noninvasiveness, which allows repeated perfusion measurements before and after the vasodilatory challenge after a short time span. In comparison, the use of SPECT for the same type of examination would take place over several days, with the baseline scan typically performed after the challenge scan. When using ASL, breath holding, carbon dioxide inhalation, or acetazolamide injection can be used for measuring the cerebrovascular reserve capacity. Only a subgroup of patients with carotid artery stenosis who were studied with ASL showed compromised cerebrovascular reserve capacity of the affected hemisphere[11]; possibly the ones benefiting the most from surgery. Although further follow-up studies are needed, it can be inferred from reactivity studies using transcranial Doppler (TCD) that this group has the highest risk of a recurrent stroke.[15]

In addition to ASL measurements of global CBF, the possibility of assessing the area of the perfusion territories with ASL may be important in patients with carotid artery stenosis or other cerebrovascular diseases. Patients often present with double-sided stenoses and it is not always clear which side is the symptomatic one, so knowledge of collateral flow could be useful in this decision. In a previous study of subacute patients who had strokes,[16] classifying according to anatomic location of the infarct alone would result in misclassification of the feeding territory in approximately 10% of patients. This error could have implications for patients with multiple stenosed extracranial arteries for whom optimal benefit of operation is expected if the symptomatic vessel is operated on. Intuitively, unless plaque imaging shows otherwise, it would be most beneficial to intervene on the side feeding the smallest area , although further studies are needed to confirm this.

As mentioned earlier, ASL is also capable of measuring the arrival time of the blood at the brain tissue. The arterial transit time parameter includes information on the collateral flow, which may result in a delayed arrival of the arterial blood at the brain tissue level. In patients with more severe obstruction and, for instance, leptomeningeal collateral flow, the ATT is very long. In this regard, the travel time may be an indicator of the quality of the collateral perfusion in patients with extracranial or intracranial stenoses or occlusions. Several studies in patients with carotid artery stenosis or carotid occlusion showed a delayed arrival time in a subgroup of patients in the hemisphere ipsilateral to the carotid lesion. With careful interpretation of ASL images at a single delay time, the delayed arrival of the arterial blood can be appreciated with label still present in the arterial vasculature feeding this specific brain region.[17,18] Especially in patients with a carotid artery occlusion, the arrival times might be delayed to such an extent that the typical time delay between labeling and imaging (1600–2000 milliseconds) is not enough to allow the protons in the labeled water to reach the brain tissue. In patients with carotid artery stenosis, the arrival time is often within normal limits or only increased by a few hundred milliseconds, which still allows the bolus to clear from the feeding arteries at typical postlabeling delays of 1800 milliseconds.

For patients with atherosclerotic carotid artery occlusion, MR imaging examinations are often performed to show the eventual presence of infarcts. Because bypass surgery has not shown a clear benefit for these patients,[19] surgery is nowadays less of an option and the focus is on keeping the remaining vessels open. Identification of the subgroup with a severe stenosis in one of the nonoccluded feeding arteries, such as the contralateral ICA or vertebrobasilar arteries, is important so that the possibilities of endarterectomy or stenting can be considered before further disease progression or a fatal event.[19] Timely intervention on a severe stenosis in one of these nonoccluded arteries

may benefit the patient by augmentation of the collateral flow toward the diseased hemisphere, and this assessment can be done with ASL. Territorial ASL shows the presence and extent of collateral contributions from the external carotid artery, contralateral ICA, and vertebrobasilar arteries, and CVR can be assessed with preacetazolamide and postacetazolamide challenge. In this way, patients with well-developed collateral perfusion and reserve capacity (eg, in chronic ICA stenosis) can be distinguished from the more critical group of patients with inadequate collateral flow and compromised reactivity after a vasodilatory challenge. An example of such a high-risk patient who could benefit from revascularization is shown in **Fig. 1**. The patient has a right internal carotid occlusion and presents with both hypoperfusion and reduced vascular reserve capacity.

In patients with vertebrobasilar stenosis or occlusions, collateral flow at the level of the circle of Willis may compensate flow delivery to the posterior brain areas via the posterior communicating arteries. However, a recent study in patients with vertebrobasilar artery disease[20] using ASL showed lower CBF in the posterior circulation in patients compared with a group of healthy controls. The presence of decreased perfusion or reactivity could therefore indicate the subgroup of patients with vertebrobasilar atherosclerotic lesions that would benefit most from revascularization such as stent placement. Furthermore, in patients with both vertebrobasilar and carotid atherosclerotic lesions, information about the perfusion territories would show which artery is feeding the ischemic area. For instance, in an area such as the thalamus, which can be fed from both the carotid and the vertebrobasilar arteries,[21] it may not be clear which artery is responsible for the presence of an infarct when multiple stenosis of extracranial arteries are present.

Patients with chronic intracranial atherosclerotic lesions may also be at high risk of a recurrent stroke, and ASL can be useful in the depiction of areas with severely decreased perfusion. Furthermore, territorial ASL may show the extent of collateral contributions to specific brain regions. For instance, with an atherosclerotic lesion in the middle cerebral artery, it can visualize possible contributions from the vertebrobasilar arteries via posterior-anterior leptomeningeal collaterals. In these cases, ASL arrival time parameters combined with a vascular challenge can be used to assess the quality of the collateral perfusion (eg, whether autoregulation has been exhausted and how fast the bolus arrives compared with normal tissue). Currently, treatments strategies of both medical and interventional (stent) origin are being evaluated for patients with chronic intracranial arterial lesions.[22,23] Although only a limited number of ASL studies have been performed in these patients groups, ASL may be performed in the future to select patients best suited for different treatments according to perfusion, vascular reserve, and the extent of collateral perfusion.

STROKE

In patients with an acute or subacute infarct, perfusion measurements may show the brain tissue region with a critically decreased blood supply. In addition to CBF, arterial arrival time parameters may also provide important information on tissue fate and patient outcome.[7] When used within an MR imaging protocol, MR imaging perfusion sequences can provide valuable information on cerebral hemodynamics in addition to the sensitive information on the presence and location of cerebral infarct, usually provided by diffusion-weighted MR imaging and anatomic sequences (eg, T2-weighted fluid-attenuated inversion recovery [FLAIR]). In principle, ASL can provide both the information on CBF and arterial timing parameters. However, the number of existing ASL studies in patients with an acute or subacute stroke is limited. Since the first proof-of-principle studies of CBF measurements by ASL in patients who had strokes in 1997 by Siewert and colleagues[24] and 2000 by Chalela and colleagues,[25] only a few studies have been published in this.[16,26,27] The underrepresentation of ASL studies in acute and subacute patients who had strokes is striking because ischemic stroke has a high incidence and a high impact both in terms of death and long-term disability. There are several explanations for the few ASL stroke studies performed thus far. First, most hospitals still prefer CT as the primary imaging modality in the work-up of patients who have strokes to exclude hemorrhage, which limits the number of hospitals where the benefits of new advanced MR imaging methods such as ASL can be tested against the existing perfusion methods. Second, the most advanced ASL methods have only recently been provided commercially on MR imaging machines. For a lot of hospitals and research groups interested in stroke MR imaging research, the ASL methods were not easily available in the past. Also, in the future, the presence of commercially available ASL methods should be coupled with easy methods of postprocessing of the ASL perfusion information for it to be usable in the diagnostic decision making in acute and subacute patients who have had strokes. Because treatment decisions have to be made fast and 24 hours a day by radiologists with varying experience and exposure to modern techniques, the ASL

perfusion information should be readily available and easily interpretable. Readers should be aware of the possible artifacts such as a delayed arrival of the arterial label, which are discussed in more detail later. In addition, a potential problem in the past was the long MR imaging scan time added for ASL to be usable. Typically, ASL sequences in the past lasted 5 minutes or more, which is too long for an acute stroke MR imaging protocol, which should ideally be kept to a scan time of less than 10 minutes. Furthermore, longer MR sequences are often troublesome in acute and subacute patients who have had strokes because patient motion may decrease the image quality and interpretability. With recent advances such as the wide availability of 3 T MR imaging and the development of new ASL sequences, this measurement time could be reduced to 1 to 3 minutes, which makes standard use in acute stroke MR imaging protocols more feasible.[27,28] In addition to higher field strength, other advances such as the introduction of pseudocontinuous ASL[5] and background suppression[8] have helped to increase the SNR and, in so doing, have allowed shorter scan times. An additional development in ASL sequences that has proved to be beneficial in patients who have had strokes is the measurement of the bolus at multiple inversion times with so-called Look-Locker readouts, which allow sampling of the complete arrival curve of the magnetic label arriving at the brain tissue. This measurement is especially important in acute and subacute patients who have had strokes, who often present with large brain regions with a prolonged delay in the arrival of the arterial blood with an occlusion of intracranial arterial branches and presence of collateral perfusion. As mentioned earlier, ASL at multiple delay times may correct for potential underestimation of CBF compared with ASL at a single delay time. For instance, a typical single delay time of 1800 milliseconds may be too early in a brain tissue area behind an intracranial occlusion and the label may not have arrived, or have been exchanged with the brain tissue water, at the moment of imaging. In an individual stroke patient, the delay in arrival is usually unknown. The advantage with ASL acquired at a series of delay times is that no optimization is needed for a specific delay time of the arterial blood. Furthermore, with the sampling of the arrival curve of the label at the brain tissue, both CBF and arterial timing parameters can be measured. These arterial timing parameters may have prognostic importance, as shown previously with contrast perfusion methods. A severe delay in the arrival time of the label may indicate the presence of slow collateral perfusion to a specific brain region, which may be associated with an increased risk of brain tissue infarction. However, ASL methods that use a single delay time may be used in acute and subacute patients who have had strokes, but the results should be interpreted with a knowledge of the typical artifacts with too-early image acquisition.[17] Typically, ASL may underestimate the CBF in brain tissue areas with delayed perfusion when a too-short delay time for image acquisition is used.[29,30] In the future, this may be overcome when pseudo-continuous ASL methods with long labeling durations are combined with longer delay times for image acquisition (>2000 milliseconds). At present, shorter delay times are often used for image acquisition because of the fast decay of the label. The label decays first with the T_1 relaxation time of the arterial blood, and second, once exchanged with the brain water compartment with the T_1 of brain tissue. Consequently, the delay time is a trade-off between the amount of ASL signal (better at earlier delay times) and the long delay times needed to allow the label to perfuse the brain tissue. This trade-off becomes especially obvious in acute and subacute patients who have had strokes in whom the low perfusion in certain brain regions would necessitate more signal (shorter delay times), whereas the delayed perfusion would require longer delay times. Focal hyperintensities are often present together with low perfusion in brain regions, which has been reported in many ASL studies in patients who have had strokes.[25,31] The ASL signal in the arterial collaterals feeding such brain regions is high because the concentrated arterial label is present within these arteries. When such a collateral artery is present in an imaging voxel, the signal change between the label and control ASL images is high because the collateral artery contains pure label. In contrast, in brain tissue perfusion ASL signal, the arterial label mixes with the brain tissue water and the signal is much lower. This pure arterial label in the collaterals often shows up in patients who have had strokes as focal bright areas in ASL images within or around the area of an acute or subacute infarct on the diffusion-weighted images. With knowledge of this common artifact, the reader of ASL images in acute and subacute patients who have had strokes should report the obvious delayed arrival of the label with label still present in the arterial tree, and not as a local hyperperfusion. This information may have prognostic importance. In terms of ASL quantification, label within the vasculature may be troublesome because most CBF quantification models do not take into account the presence of label within the arteries. These quantification models assume that the arterial water protons have been fully exchanged with the brain tissue water. In the voxels with pure label within the arteries, the CBF is typically overestimated. In contrast, in the brain tissue areas around these collateral arteries, where the label did not arrive, an underestimation in the CBF will be present. The effect of such overestimation and underestimation on radiological diagnosis, and ultimately on patient treatment and outcomes, remains to be determined. In daily patient care, the qualitative judgment of images by radiologists is more common than absolute quantification. Clinical T2-weighted FLAIR images are also interpreted qualitatively and T2-FLAIR images are still the cornerstone of MR imaging of the brain. However, training in image interpretation will be important when a new MR imaging method such as ASL is introduced to daily radiological practice. In addition to low perfusion, ASL may also detect hyperperfused brain regions, which are common phenomena after revascularization of occluded arteries in acute patients who have had strokes.[25]

As mentioned earlier ASL also allows the measurement of the perfusion territories of the different brain feeding arteries. In acute and subacute patients who have had strokes, perfusion territory imaging with ASL may show the presence and extent of the collateral perfusion of the brain regions surrounding the areas of the brain tissue infarction. In subacute patients who have had strokes, perfusion territory ASL provides information on the extent of collateral perfusion that is comparable with conventional intra-arterial digital subtraction angiography (iaDSA).[32] Furthermore, in patients who have had strokes, the expected artery feeding a specific infarcted brain tissue region may be different when perfusion territory information is added.[16] The presence and extent of collateral perfusion may have prognostic information in acute and subacute patients who have had strokes, and the artery feeding an area of infarction may influence treatment, for instance on the operation of a stenosis in the extracranial vasculature (discussed earlier). A limitation of ASL perfusion measurements in acute and subacute patients who have had strokes may be the measurements of decreased perfusion in the white matter. With a lower perfusion signal and longer arrival times, the ASL perfusion signal is at the border of the detection limit of current ASL methods. An area with an infarct or reduced perfusion in the white matter is therefore difficult to detect. Although no studies have been performed in this area, it can be expected that, even with the currently most advanced 3 T MR imaging methods, ASL is not able to distinguish normal white matter perfusion from white matter hypoperfusion on a single-subject basis. Although ASL

CBF images should be interpreted with caution, recent clinical studies in acute patients who have had strokes show that ASL CBF measurements may provide an alternative for gadolinium-based perfusion measurements, especially with kidney failure or unknown kidney function.[33] In addition to acute stroke, several recent studies showed the application of ASL CBF measurements in chronic phases of stroke.[34–36]

MOYAMOYA DISEASE

Moyamoya disease is a chronic and progressive stenoocclusive vasculopathy affecting the terminal ICAs, and, at a more severe stage, the proximal main arterial branches of the circle of Willis. Imaging of cerebral hemodynamics in patients with moyamoya disease has been used to quantify the severity of the cerebral hemodynamic impairment at the brain tissue level. In a recent review of hemodynamic measurements in moyamoya, ASL was discussed as one of the potential methods to study perfusion in patients with moyamoya.[37] The clear advantage of MR imaging perfusion measurements compared with PET, SPECT, xenon-enhanced CT, and dynamic perfusion CT is that MR imaging can show with high sensitivity anatomic changes at the brain tissue level, such as new small areas of ischemia. MR cross-sectional imaging of ischemic lesions can be easily combined with the cross-sectional ASL images of cerebral perfusion to show the most critically hypoperfused brain tissue regions. New ischemic lesions in patients with moyamoya may, together with severely disturbed cerebral hemodynamics, indicate the need for interventions such as extracranial to intracranial bypass surgery. The side of the intracranial connection of a superficial temporal artery to middle cerebral artery bypass may be determined based on the middle

cerebral perfusion territory with the most severe hemodynamic impairment. In a head-to-head comparison study, ASL showed similar areas of hemodynamic compromise in a series of patients with moyamoya compared with SPECT before and after an acetazolamide challenge.[38] The ASL-based cerebrovascular reactivity measurements may indicate brain regions with preserved perfusion in a resting situation but an inability to increase the perfusion on a vascular challenge (Fig. 3). In addition, in a previous study in patients with moyamoya and after bypass surgery, ASL perfusion territory measurements showed the perfusion territory supplied by the bypass.[39] The extent of the blood supply measured with perfusion territory ASL of the bypass correlated well with the conventional iaDSA measurements of the bypass.[39] Because of the noninvasive nature of ASL and the short extra scan time of only a few minutes added to a standard MR imaging protocol, we think that ASL will have an important role in the MR imaging follow-up of patients with moyamoya disease.

AVM

In patients with AVM, ASL perfusion territory measurements may be used to show the arterial feeders of the AVM. In addition to showing the different feeders, ASL has the potential to show the relative contribution from each separate feeder. Furthermore, ASL may show the amount of arteriovenous shunting of an AVM,[40] characterized by a high intensity of the labeled signal in the veins draining from the AVM. In addition to the arteriovenous shunting, ASL may show hyperperfused and hypoperfused brain regions surrounding the AVM. In the white matter close to AVMs, increased perfusion has been correlated with the amount of shunting and, in the thalamus,

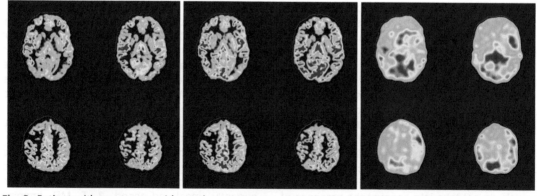

Fig. 3. Patient with moyamoya with no clear asymmetry seen on ASL perfusion images at rest (*left*). After an acetazolamide challenge, a decrease in perfusion of the right middle cerebral artery territory, especially the right-sided basal ganglia, can be appreciated (*middle*). The reactivity images show a clear impairment of the cerebrovascular reactivity of the right hemisphere (*right*).

a decreased perfusion has been reported, which could be the result of a steal effect of the AVM.[40] In addition, ASL can be used in the posttreatment evaluation of AVMs. A recent study used ASL for the evaluation of AVMs after γ knife treatment with both ASL-based evaluation of the AVM nidus and nearby vascular territories.[41]

VASCULAR DEMENTIA

In several other cerebrovascular diseases, ASL may show its value when used in combination with existing MR imaging protocols of the brain anatomy. For instance, in patients with vascular dementia, clinically characterized by the presence of several infarcts in addition to cognitive deficits, ASL perfusion and, potentially, ASL reactivity measurements may show brain tissue areas at risk for future infarcts. Furthermore, in patients with vascular dementia, ASL may help to establish the diagnosis with demonstration of a decreased perfusion at rest or after a vasodilatory challenge. As shown in **Fig. 4**, the perfusion deficits in patients with vascular dementia may be different from those of other types of dementia such as Alzheimer disease and frontotemporal dementia. In general,

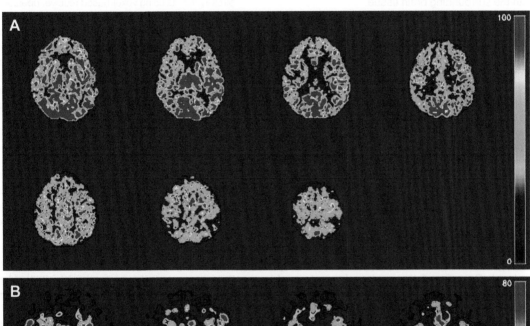
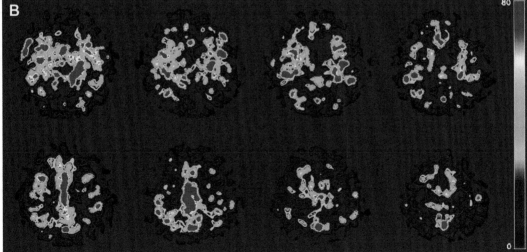

Fig. 4. ASL perfusion images of 2 patients matched for Mini Mental Status Examination scores. (A) Patient with Alzheimer disease; (B) patient with vascular dementia. Note the difference in scales. Although both patients presented with similar degrees of disability, the second patient had little perfusion throughout his brain, possibly because of delayed arrival time through the presence of multiple stenoses. The patient presented in (A) shows typical reduction of perfusion related to reduced metabolism in the frontal and parietal areas. (*Data from* Du AT, Jahng GH, Hayasaka S, et al. Hypoperfusion in frontotemporal dementia and Alzheimer disease by arterial spin labeling MRI. Neurology 2006;67(7):1215–20.)

ASL measurements of perfusion may show altered regional perfusion in patients with age-related changes of the brain tissue such as leukoaraiosis[42] or gray matter atrophy.[43] Quantitative ASL may be especially important in these more generalized diseases. Qualitative interpretation of ASL images may be insufficient in these cases, whereas simple diagnosis of most other cerebrovascular diseases might be possible without quantitative information. Quantification of ASL in dementias and aging will have to deal with the effect of brain atrophy that might potentially result in decrease perfusion caused by partial volume effects of the gray matter with the surrounding brain tissue.

SUMMARY

With the increased availability of advanced ASL methods on the clinical MR imaging scanners of both university and general hospitals, ASL will make a clinical breakthrough in the next few years. An obvious area in which ASL can add important hemodynamic information is in the MR imaging protocols used in patients with acute or chronic cerebrovascular disease. Thus far, most MR imaging protocols in cerebrovascular disease use information on tissue viability (FLAIR, diffusion-weighted imaging) and MR angiography to show the presence of stenosis and occlusions. ASL measurements of cerebral perfusion may show hemodynamically compromised brain regions that appear normal on the standard MR imaging protocol. Because of the noninvasive nature of ASL, the measurements can be easily repeated, such as after a vasodilatory challenge. In patients with cerebrovascular disease, such a measure of cerebrovascular reactivity may add important information on the presence and extent of hemodynamic compromise. In addition, perfusion territory ASL provides noninvasive information on the perfusion territories and the presence of collateral perfusion in patients with extracranial and intracranial arterial stenosis or occlusions.

REFERENCES

1. Kety SS, Schmidt CF. The determination of cerebral blood flow in man by the use of nitrous oxide in low concentrations. Am J Physiol (Legacy Content) 1945;143(1):53–66.
2. Thomsen HS. Nephrogenic systemic fibrosis: history and epidemiology. Radiol Clin North Am 2009;47(5): 827–31, vi.
3. Williams DS, Detre JA, Leigh JS, et al. Magnetic resonance imaging of perfusion using spin inversion of arterial water. Proc Natl Acad Sci U S A 1992; 89(1):212–6.
4. Golay X, Petersen ET. Arterial spin labeling: benefits and pitfalls of high magnetic field. Neuroimaging Clin N Am 2006;16(2):259–68, x.
5. Dai W, Garcia D, de BC, et al. Continuous flow-driven inversion for arterial spin labeling using pulsed radio frequency and gradient fields. Magn Reson Med 2008;60(6):1488–97.
6. Petersen ET, Zimine I, Ho YC, et al. Non-invasive measurement of perfusion: a critical review of arterial spin labelling techniques. Br J Radiol 2006; 79(944):688–701.
7. Christensen S, Mouridsen K, Wu O, et al. Comparison of 10 perfusion MRI parameters in 97 sub-6-hour stroke patients using voxel-based receiver operating characteristics analysis. Stroke 2009;40(6):2055–61.
8. Ye FQ, Frank JA, Weinberger DR, et al. Noise reduction in 3D perfusion imaging by attenuating the static signal in arterial spin tagging (ASSIST). Magn Reson Med 2000;44(1):92–100.
9. Hendrikse J, van der GJ, Lu H, et al. Flow territory mapping of the cerebral arteries with regional perfusion MRI. Stroke 2004;35(4):882–7.
10. Van Laar PJ, van der GJ, Hendrikse J. Brain perfusion territory imaging: methods and clinical applications of selective arterial spin-labeling MR imaging. Radiology 2008;246(2):354–64.
11. Bokkers RP, van Osch MJ, van der Worp HB, et al. Symptomatic carotid artery stenosis: impairment of cerebral autoregulation measured at the brain tissue level with arterial spin-labeling MR imaging. Radiology 2010;256(1):201–8.
12. Wang DJ, Chen Y, Fernandez-Seara MA, et al. Potentials and challenges for arterial spin labeling in pharmacological magnetic resonance imaging. J Pharmacol Exp Ther 2011;337(2):359–66.
13. Rothwell PM, Mehta Z, Howard SC, et al. Treating individuals 3: from subgroups to individuals: general principles and the example of carotid endarterectomy. Lancet 2005;365(9455):256–65.
14. Caplan LR, Hennerici M. Impaired clearance of emboli (washout) is an important link between hypoperfusion, embolism, and ischemic stroke. Arch Neurol 1998;55(11):1475–82.
15. Silvestrini M, Vernieri F, Pasqualetti P, et al. Impaired cerebral vasoreactivity and risk of stroke in patients with asymptomatic carotid artery stenosis. JAMA 2000;283(16):2122–7.
16. Hendrikse J, Petersen ET, Cheze A, et al. Relation between cerebral perfusion territories and location of cerebral infarcts. Stroke 2009;40(5):1617–22.
17. Zaharchuk G, Bammer R, Straka M, et al. Arterial spin-label imaging in patients with normal bolus perfusion-weighted MR imaging findings: pilot identification of the borderzone sign. Radiology 2009; 252(3):797–807.
18. Zaharchuk G, Do HM, Marks MP, et al. Arterial spin-labeling MRI can identify the presence and intensity

of collateral perfusion in patients with moyamoya disease. Stroke 2011;42(9):2485–91.

19. Garrett MC, Komotar RJ, Merkow MB, et al. The extracranial-intracranial bypass trial: implications for future investigations. Neurosurg Focus 2008;24(2):E4.

20. MacIntosh BJ, Marquardt L, Schulz UG, et al. Pulsed arterial spin labeling perfusion MRI correlates with clinical severity in patients with vertebrobasilar artery stenoses. In Proceedings of the 18th Annual Meeting of ISMRM. Stockholm (Sweden), May 1–7, 2010. p. 512.

21. Hendrikse J, Petersen ET, Chng SM, et al. Distribution of cerebral blood flow in the nucleus caudatus, nucleus lentiformis, and thalamus: a study of territorial arterial spin-labeling MR imaging. Radiology 2010;254(3):867–75.

22. Brott TG, Hobson RW, Howard G, et al. Stenting versus endarterectomy for treatment of carotid-artery stenosis. N Engl J Med 2010;363(1):11–23.

23. Bonati LH, Dobson J, Algra A, et al. Short-term outcome after stenting versus endarterectomy for symptomatic carotid stenosis: a preplanned meta-analysis of individual patient data. Lancet 2010; 376(9746):1062–73.

24. Siewert B, Schlaug G, Edelman RR, et al. Comparison of EPISTAR and T2*-weighted gadolinium-enhanced perfusion imaging in patients with acute cerebral ischemia. Neurology 1997;48(3):673–9.

25. Chalela JA, Alsop DC, Gonzalez-Atavales JB, et al. Magnetic resonance perfusion imaging in acute ischemic stroke using continuous arterial spin labeling. Stroke 2000;31(3):680–7.

26. Altrichter S, Kulcsar Z, Sekoranja L, et al. Arterial spin labeling demonstrates early recanalization after stroke. J Neuroradiol 2009;36(2):109–11.

27. Deibler AR, Pollock JM, Kraft RA, et al. Arterial spin-labeling in routine clinical practice, part 2: hypoperfusion patterns. AJNR Am J Neuroradiol 2008;29(7): 1235–41.

28. Zaharchuk G. Arterial spin label imaging of acute ischemic stroke and transient ischemic attack. Neuroimaging Clin N Am 2011;21(2):285–301.

29. Wolf RL, Alsop DC, McGarvey ML, et al. Susceptibility contrast and arterial spin labeled perfusion MRI in cerebrovascular disease. J Neuroimaging 2003;13(1):17–27.

30. Hendrikse J, van Osch MJ, Rutgers DR, et al. Internal carotid artery occlusion assessed at pulsed arterial spin-labeling perfusion MR imaging at multiple delay times. Radiology 2004;233(3):899–904.

31. Viallon M, Altrichter S, Pereira VM, et al. Combined use of pulsed arterial spin-labeling and susceptibility-weighted imaging in stroke at 3T. Eur Neurol 2010;64(5):286–96.

32. Chng SM, Petersen ET, Zimine I, et al. Territorial arterial spin labeling in the assessment of collateral circulation: comparison with digital subtraction angiography. Stroke 2008;39(12):3248–54.

33. Bokkers RP, Warach S, Hernandez D, et al. Whole-brain arterial spin labeling perfusion MR imaging in patients with acute stroke. In Proceedings of the 19th Annual Meeting of ISMRM. Montreal (Canada), May 7–13, 2011. p. 464.

34. Firbank MJ, He J, Blamire AM, et al. Cerebral blood flow by arterial spin labeling in poststroke dementia. Neurology 2011;76(17):1478–84.

35. Richardson JD, Baker JM, Morgan PS, et al. Cerebral perfusion in chronic stroke: implications for lesion-symptom mapping and functional MRI. Behav Neurol 2011;24(2):117–22.

36. Brumm KP, Perthen JE, Liu TT, et al. An arterial spin labeling investigation of cerebral blood flow deficits in chronic stroke survivors. Neuroimage 2010;51(3): 995–1005.

37. Lee M, Zaharchuk G, Guzman R, et al. Quantitative hemodynamic studies in moyamoya disease: a review. Neurosurg Focus 2009;26(4):E5.

38. Noguchi T, Kawashima M, Irie H, et al. Arterial spin-labeling MR imaging in moyamoya disease compared with SPECT imaging. Eur J Radiol 2011;80(3):e557–62.

39. Kitajima M, Hirai T, Shigematsu Y, et al. Assessment of cerebral perfusion from bypass arteries using magnetic resonance regional perfusion imaging in patients with moyamoya disease. Jpn J Radiol 2010;28(10):746–53.

40. Wolf RL, Wang J, Detre JA, et al. Arteriovenous shunt visualization in arteriovenous malformations with arterial spin-labeling MR imaging. AJNR Am J Neuroradiol 2008;29(4):681–7.

41. Pollock JM, Whitlow CT, Simonds J, et al. Response of arteriovenous malformations to gamma knife therapy evaluated with pulsed arterial spin-labeling MRI perfusion. AJR Am J Roentgenol 2011;196(1):15–22.

42. Kawamura J, Terayama Y, Takashima S, et al. Leuko-araiosis and cerebral perfusion in normal aging. Exp Aging Res 1993;19(3):225–40.

43. Chen JJ, Wieckowska M, Meyer E, et al. Cerebral blood flow measurement using fMRI and PET: a cross-validation study. Int J Biomed Imaging 2008. DOI:10.1155/2008/516359.

High-Field Atherosclerotic Plaque Magnetic Resonance Imaging

Chun Yuan, PhD[a],*, Jinnan Wang, PhD[a,b],
Niranjan Balu, PhD[a]

KEYWORDS

- Carotid plaque imaging • High-field MR imaging
- Atherosclerotic plaque composition

Key Points

- Increased SNR (signal-to-noise ratio) at 3 T has allowed new three-dimensional (3D) isotropic sequences with large coverage to be developed with improved slice resolution compared with 1.5 T.
- Criteria for identification of plaque components at 1.5 T are also applicable at 3 T with minor differences for intraplaque hemorrhage (IPH) and calcification.
- Signal from IPH is reduced on time of flight (TOF) compared with 1.5 T because of longer T1 relaxation times at 3 T. Dedicated sequences such as magnetization prepared rapid gradient echo (MPRAGE) can improve both sensitivity and specificity for hemorrhage detection.
- Calcifications are larger at 3 T because of increased susceptibility effects.
- High-field plaque imaging is possible in multiple arterial beds such as carotids, peripheral arteries, and aorta. Intracranial vessel wall imaging is also improved at 3 T. Challenges such as motion, field inhomogeneities, susceptibility, and specific absorption rate (SAR) are yet to be overcome for routine coronary plaque magnetic resonance (MR) imaging.

Atherosclerotic plaque imaging is a branch of cardiovascular imaging whose main goal is to identify vulnerable plaque that poses an increased risk of causing cardiovascular events. Plaque imaging has been extensively validated at 1.5 T and has proved its usefulness in several natural history studies, treatment efficacy studies, and multicenter clinical trials. Since its inception, plaque imaging techniques have also improved significantly. However, the main imaging goals remain to achieve high-resolution images that are able to identify key plaque components such as LRNC, IPH, and calcium; to measure plaque burden; and to detect defects of the luminal surface, such as disruption and fibrous cap conditions. Some of these imaging goals can be further improved by scanning at higher field strengths. This article addresses the opportunities, challenges, and current status of high-field atherosclerotic plaque imaging.

Grant support: This work is partly supported by grant NIH HL56874, NIH HL076378.
Disclaimer: All techniques and devices discussed in this article are investigational, and not yet approved for clinical decision making or diagnoses.
[a] Department of Radiology, University of Washington, Seattle, WA 98109, USA
[b] Clinical Sites Research Program, Philips Research North America, Briarcliff Manor, NY 10510, USA
* Corresponding author. 815 Mercer Street, Room 124, VIL, Seattle, WA 98109.
E-mail address: cyuan@u.washington.edu

HIGH-FIELD PLAQUE MR IMAGING

Plaque MR imaging requires a high SNR for acquisition for several reasons: (1) because of the small size of its imaging target, atherosclerotic plaque MR imaging needs to be acquired at high spatial resolution to faithfully characterize the morphology of the plaque; (2) to visualize the plaque on vessel wall, the bright luminal signal needs to be suppressed; (3) to accomplish large coverage scans in a clinical feasible time also demands a higher SNR to avoid compromised image quality.

Three areas of technological improvements can improve the SNR and contrast between vessel wall, lumen, and the outer wall: scanner field strength, surface radiofrequency (RF) coils and vessel wall imaging sequences. Each of these areas is addressed later along with their respective challenges arising from high-field imaging. Following this, advances in knowledge of the atherosclerotic disease process using these new technologies are described. Throughout this article, 3 T is considered as high-field; 7 T and greater are considered ultrahigh-field.

HIGH-FIELD MR SCANNERS

Compared with lower field strengths, higher field strength promises higher overall SNR. Theoretic analysis predicts that the SNR of the MR imaging system will increase by 100% if the main magnetic field is doubled (eg, from 1.5 T to 3 T). This increased SNR is the primary motivation for moving plaque MR imaging to high-fields. Although the SNR improvement in vivo can vary for different applications,[1–4] this overall improvement makes high-field MR imaging a preferable platform for plaque imaging compared with 1.5 T. The SNR gain can be traded for shortened imaging time, higher spatial resolution, or a combination of the two depending on the imaging needs. Nevertheless, increased magnetic field strengths also represent

new challenges, such as prolonged T1 relaxation time,[2] increased field inhomogeneity, and susceptibility.[4]

Whole-body MR scanners at 1.5 T and 3 T are now well established for vessel wall imaging. 3 T provides an improved contrast/noise ratio of 1.4 to 2.4 times compared with 1.5 T black blood (BB) MR imaging.[2,3] Wide-bore magnets are also desirable, because large patients are generally prone to atherosclerosis.

Fat suppression is necessary in vessel wall imaging to delineate the outer wall. Thus, field inhomogeneity can be challenging at higher field strengths for achieving good fat suppression. Good first-order shimming routines are often adequate for vessel wall imaging. In a few cases, higher order shimming may be necessary. Newer MR systems are equipped with RF shimming capabilities and may prove useful for vessel wall MR imaging.

RF Coils

Body coil transmission is used for vessel wall imaging and is useful for uniform excitation and the large coverage needed for special blood suppression techniques. However, body coil reception does not provide high enough SNR for visualizing the vessel wall. Surface coils pick up signal from a small area, but with increased sensitivity. Because the carotid arteries are superficial, they can be imaged with surface coils to increase SNR. Surface coils with 4, 6, and 8 coil elements have been developed for use at 3 T. Dedicated 4-element phased array coils enable high-resolution imaging at 1.5 T[5] and 3 T.[6] Increasing the number of coil elements provides larger coverage. An 8-element carotid coil not only provided a 1.7-fold SNR increase compared with a 4-element design but also provided increased coverage along the length of the carotid artery. Currently, carotid phased array coils with 4, 6, and 8 coil elements are available commercially on the major scanner platforms. **Fig. 1** shows the design of the 8-element coil and its commercial equivalent. Each coil element is usually read out through a separate RF channel. The noise picked up by the receive chain can be further reduced by digitizing the signal from the coil elements. Newer MR systems digitize the received signal directly at the coil, thereby reducing noise picked up in each of the channels. Such systems can further improve the performance of these coils but require additional components on the coil to digitize the received signal. Improvements in both coil design and the RF receive chain allow plaque imaging with higher SNR and therefore enable higher

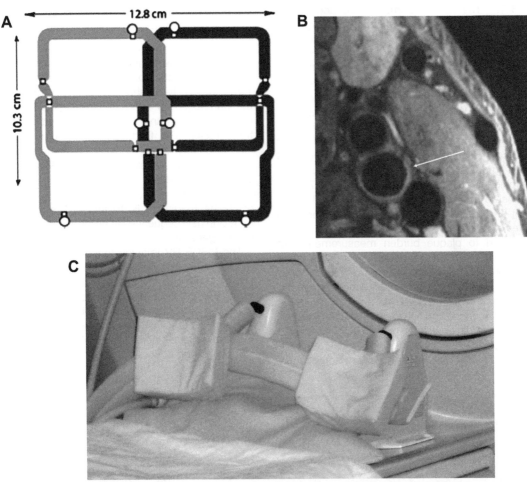

Fig. 1. Eight-element carotid phased array coil for use at 3 T. (*A*) The 4 elements on 1 side. (*B*) High-resolution (0.27 mm² in-plane resolution) T1-weighted MR imaging with excellent delineation of the thin carotid walls (*arrow*). (*C*) Commercial version of the 8-element coil with integrated head rest. (*Adapted from* Balu N, Yarnykh VL, Scholnick J, et al. Improvements in carotid plaque imaging using a new eight-element phased array coil at 3T. J Magn Reson Imaging 2009;30(5):1210, 1213; with permission.)

spatial resolution to be attained. Such improvements will benefit vessel wall imaging in vascular beds such as coronary and intracranial vasculature where high spatial resolution (<0.5 mm in plane) is required.

3D BB Imaging Sequences

Compared with its two-dimensional (2D) counterparts, 3D imaging sequences present several advantages for atherosclerotic plaque imaging. Benefiting from the extra phase encoding direction, a 3D imaging sequence provides significant SNR enhancement because the imaging volume expands in the third dimension. This extra SNR advantage can be used to achieve isotropic resolution, because previous studies have shown that isotropic voxels can potentially reduce registration and segmentation errors,[7] as well as provide more reproducible quantitative measurements[8] for vessel wall imaging.

Despite these benefits, achieving high-resolution 3D isotropic resolution in vivo is challenging. Depending on the field strength, achieving isotropic resolutions may require long scan times. As a result, many of the 3D implementations[9,10] on 1.5 T have adopted anisotropic voxel size to accommodate clinical needs.

The improved SNR offered by high magnetic field strength provides a potential solution to this issue. Recently a 3D turbo spin echo (TSE) with variable flip angle refocusing RF pulses (SPACE) technique was used to achieve high-resolution isotropic (0.72 × 0.72 × 0.72 mm³) large coverage (380 × 374 × 100 mm³) peripheral artery imaging at 3 T.[11] The whole volume can be acquired in 11.32 minutes. A similarly configured 2D sequence would need 20 minutes to cover the same volume at a lower slice direction resolution of 3 mm.

Motion-sensitized driven equilibrium (MSDE)[12] is a new imaging technique that can effectively suppress blood signal by dephasing moving spins in the blood. When combined with proper acquisition schemes, high temporal efficiency can be achieved. In only 2 minutes, the carotid artery tree can be imaged using a 3D MSDE prepared rapid gradient echo (3D-MERGE) sequence[13] with high spatial resolution ($0.7 \times 0.7 \times 0.7$ mm^3) and large coverage (250 mm foot to head direction) (Fig. 2). More importantly, recent research reveals that the 3D-MERGE sequence is not restricted to plaque burden measurement, but can also be used to detect high-risk plaque components if the parameters are properly optimized. Two separate studies have shown the usefulness of 3D-MERGE to detecting LRNC[14] and IPH.[15] These findings suggest that the optimization toward plaque imaging with higher temporal efficiency does not rule out its potential for simultaneous high-risk plaque component detection.

CHALLENGES AND OPPORTUNITIES OF HIGH-FIELD PLAQUE MR IMAGING
Increased Field Inhomogeneity

The magnetic field inhomogeneity describes the level of field fluctuation in the image field of view. Two types of field inhomogeneities are present: the inhomogeneity of the main magnetic field (B0 inhomogeneity), and the inhomogeneity of the transmission RF field (B1 inhomogeneity). In high-field MR systems, both fields are more susceptible to variations than at lower field strengths, especially for complicated anatomic regions like the neck, which is a common target of plaque imaging. It is therefore more important to design new sequences to compensate for these inhomogeneities.

The MSDE BB imaging technique can provide robust blood suppression even in challenging anatomic regions.[12] It relies on dephasing among moving particles to achieve BB effect. Because it does not put any direct requirement on flow velocity like other BB techniques do, MSDE can suppress blood more effectively in regions of complex blood flow.

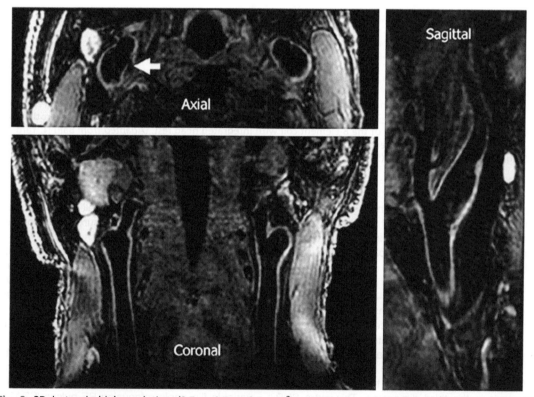

Fig. 2. 3D isotropic high-resolution ($0.7 \times 0.7 \times 0.7$ mm^3) carotid artery image acquired with 3D-MERGE sequence. Arrow on axial reformat shows a small piece of calcification. Vessel wall boundaries are clearly visible on all reformats. (*Reprinted from* Balu N, Yarnykh VL, Chu B, et al. Carotid plaque assessment using fast 3D isotropic resolution black-blood MRI. Magn Reson Med 2011;65(3):631; with permission.)

A practical problem with MSDE at high-field is its sensitivity to B1 inhomogeneity. As shown in **Fig. 3**, when the B1 value drifts away from the nominal value (ie, relative B1 drifts away from 1), significant signal reduction can be observed on the MSDE sequence. At high-fields, SNR can vary across the field of view because of this B1 sensitivity.

To address this issue, an improved MSDE (iMSDE) sequence was proposed.[16] In the iMSDE sequence, the original 90-180-90 RF chain was replaced by the MLEV-4 pulse train (**Fig. 4**), which is known to be more robust to B1 inhomogeneity. Almost no noticeable signal decrease could be observed on the iMSDE pulses in **Fig. 3** even when significant inhomogeneity is present (toward the periphery of the image).

By further incorporating an improved gradient design to compensate for eddy currents, the iM-SDE sequence significantly improved image quality when applied to carotid artery plaque imaging applications (**Fig. 5**). The vessel boundaries on the MSDE image are indistinct because of the lower SNR, whereas the artery can be clearly delineated on the iMSDE image.

Long T1 Effect

Prolonged T1 relaxation time is another well-known effect observed in high-field MR imaging. As reported before,[17] significantly higher T1 relaxation times in different tissues were measured at 3 T than at 1.5 T. This increased T1 relaxation should be factored into sequence pulse sequence

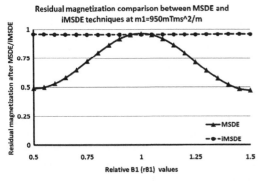

Fig. 3. Comparison of simulated signals as functions of relative B1 inhomogeneity between MSDE and improved MSDE (iMSDE) sequences. The iMSDE sequence provides consistently higher signal intensity compared with the MSDE sequence, and the signal improvement becomes more pronounced when rB1 value drifts further away from unit. (*Adapted from* Wang J, Yarnykh VL, Yuan C. Enhanced image quality in black-blood MRI using the improved motion-sensitized driven-equilibrium (iMSDE) sequence. J Magn Reson Imaging 2010;31(5):1260; with permission.)

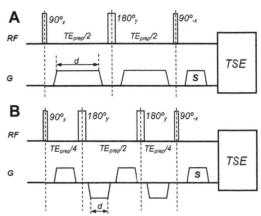

Fig. 4. Pulse sequence diagram of MSDE (*A*) and the iMSDE (*B*) preparations. The adoption of the MLEV-4 pulse in the iMSDE sequence significantly reduced the sequence's sensitivity to the B1 inhomogeneity. (*Adapted from* Wang J, Yarnykh VL, Yuan C. Enhanced image quality in black-blood MRI using the improved motion-sensitized driven-equilibrium (iMSDE) sequence. J Magn Reson Imaging 2010;31(5):1258; with permission.)

parameter optimization to achieve the desired contrast at high-fields.[18]

Longer T1 also helps to improve the efficiency of tissue saturation in MR images because it takes a longer time for the tissue to recover. TOF is a commonly used technique that can generate time-efficient MR angiography data on major arteries without the administration of contrast agents.[19] TOF images visualize flowing blood signals by saturating the static tissue with repetitive RF pulses. On higher magnetic field strengths, static tissues tend to be saturated more effectively, leaving the background signal more uniformly suppressed[4] compared with the more prominent signal variation on 1.5 T images.[20] This efficient background saturation provides higher luminal contrast and better lumen boundary delineation on 3 T scanners, making them a more favorable imaging platform for TOF angiography.

In addition to T1 lengthening, T1 value separation among tissues has also been found to increase,[17] allowing tissues to be more easily separated at higher magnetic strengths. In atherosclerotic plaque imaging, differentiating tissue components based on their respective T1/T2 values is an important approach in detecting high-risk plaque components. Compared with the T2 values, the prolonged T1 relaxation time provides a unique way to better detect high-risk components on T1-weighted images. One example is the detection of IPH tissue, which usually presents a high signal on T1-weighted images. The increased T1 weighting on 3 T

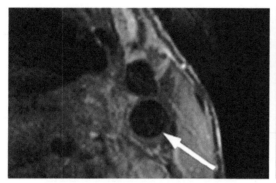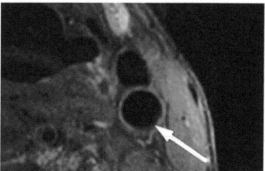

Fig. 5. Significantly improved carotid artery vessel wall delineation (*arrow*) on the iMSDE image (*right*) compared with that on the MSDE image (*left*). (*Adapted from* Wang J, Yarnykh VL, Yuan C. Enhanced image quality in black-blood MRI using the improved motion-sensitized driven-equilibrium (iMSDE) sequence. J Magn Reson Imaging 2010;31(5):1262; with permission.)

systems makes it more reliable to detect IPH in vivo. Compared with the multicontrast approach of combining several T1-weighted sequences for IPH identification on 1.5 T,[20] it is possible to use a single T1-weighted sequence to achieve the same goal at 3 T.[21–23]

At 3 T, magnetization prepared rapid acquisition gradient echo (MPRAGE) sequence has been shown to provide higher sensitivity and specificity in IPH detection compared with the traditional approaches.[24] A recently proposed slab-selective phase-sensitive inversion recovery (SPI) sequence[23] provides even higher tissue contrast between IPH and vessel wall, as well as between vessel wall and lumen, compared with MPRAGE. With its improved IPH contrast, the SPI sequence has the potential to further improve IPH detection accuracy in patients with atherosclerosis.

Increased Susceptibility

Susceptibility effect describes the degree of magnetization of an object in response to the external magnetic field. On MR images, a stronger susceptibility effect usually causes a stronger local magnetic field disturbance, leading to a more pronounced signal void in the vicinity. In high-field MR imaging, stronger susceptibility artifacts are expected compared with lower field strengths.[4] This effect makes plaque components such as calcification more easily identifiable.

A benefit of the increased susceptibility on 3 T is the use of susceptibility-weighted imaging (SWI) to separate lumen and wall signals, thus achieving vessel wall imaging without suppressing blood signal.[25] Because no flow velocity requirement is posed by this technique, the SWI image can theoretically achieve satisfactory lumen/wall separation even in challenging circumstances,

making it a potential alternative for plaque size measurements.

SAR

Although higher field strength provides several benefits for atherosclerotic plaque imaging, it can also cause faster energy accumulation in the human body, reaching the SAR limit more quickly. The major impact on imaging protocol design caused by SAR increase is reduced time efficiency: a higher energy deposition during a certain amount of time forces a delay of the next RF pulse to lower the time-averaged energy deposition, thus making the overall time efficiency decrease significantly.

A potential solution is the use of parallel transmission,[26] which, instead of using only 1 RF transmission source, uses 2 or more sources to achieve more homogeneous energy deposition across the field of view. This technique is able to shorten spatially selective RF pulses in 2 or 3 dimensions, therefore minimizing the overall SAR value.[26]

In vivo 3 T plaque MR imaging
A 3 T MRI protocol for comprehensive assessment of plaque morphology and composition is described in **Table 1**. Criteria for identification of plaque components at 1.5 T[20,27,28] have been validated against histology. These criteria are generally applicable at 3 T with some differences caused by the higher field strength characteristics described earlier. This article discusses studies that focused on differences between 1.5 T and 3 T plaque imaging and how MR imaging of each of the major plaque components is benefited at 3 T.

Comparison with 1.5 T
3 T MR scanners are widely available. Advantages of 3 T compared with 1.5 T have been described

Table 1
Table with recommended MR sequences and protocols. Recommended protocol for high-field plaque MR imaging

Parameters	Scan Type				
	1	2	3	4	5
	3D MERGE	T2 Weighted	TOF	SPI	Pre/Post-contrast T1 Weighted
Sequence	TFE	TSE	FFE	PSIR	TSE
Image mode	3D	2D	3D	3D	2D
Scan plane	Coronal	Axial	Axial	Axial	Axial
TR (ms)	10	4000	20	13	800
TE (ms)	4.8	50	4	3	10
Flip Angle (°)	6	NA	20	15	NA
FOV (cm)	25×16×3.5	14×14	14×14×3.2	14×14×3.2	14×14
Resolution (mm)	0.7×0.7×0.7	0.55×0.55	0.55×0.55×2	0.55×0.55×2	0.55×0.55
Slice thickness (mm)	NA	2	NA	NA	2
Blood suppression	MSDE	MDIR/MSDE	Sat-band for venous flow	NA	QIR/MSDE
Fat suppression	Yes	Yes	No	Yes	Yes

Please refer to the text for detailed description of each sequence.

Abbreviations: FOV, field of view; MDIR, multi-slice double inversion recovery; MERGE, MSDE prepared rapid gradient echo; MSDE, motion sensitized driven equilibrium; PSIR, phase sensitive inversion recovery; QIR, quadruple inversion recovery; SPI, slab-selective phase-sensitive inversion recovery; TE, echo time; TFE, turbo field echo; TR, recovery time; TSE, turbo spin echo.

for MR imaging in several clinical applications.[29] An SNR improvement of 2 times is expected at 3 T compared with 1.5 T. Several investigations have reported improvements close to this theoretical SNR increase. Cury and colleagues[30] reported an increase of 1.8, 1.7, and 1.6 times on proton density weighted, T2-weighted, and T1-weighted vessel wall imaging. Similarly Yarnykh and colleagues[2] found 1.7, 1.8, and 1.5 times improvement on the same contrast weightings. Other studies[1,3] found greater than 2 times improvement but with slightly different sequence parameters and phased array coil configurations at the 2 different field strengths. Blood suppression was equally effective at both field strengths, leading to increased contrast/noise ratio and therefore better delineation of the carotid vessel wall at 3 T. The delineation of the outer wall may also be improved at 3 T because of greater effectiveness of spectral fat saturation methods at higher field strengths. Cury and colleagues[30] reported better fat suppression at 3 T leading to better vessel wall visualization, likely because of increased separation of fat and water peaks at 3 T and thereby improved performance of spectral fat saturation. Together, these studies show the potential benefits of higher field strength for vessel

wall imaging. The improved SNR can be translated into faster scanning by reducing the number of averages required. The increased SNR at 3 T allows reducing the number of averages from 2 (**Fig. 6**).[2] Alternately the resolution can be improved at the expense of SNR. Currently a combination of these approaches is preferred so that in-plane resolution of 0.5 mm is routinely possible at 3 T with short scan times.

Once MR images are available, they must be processed and measured for quantitative plaque burden assessment. Reproducibility of plaque burden assessment at 3 T was similar to 1.5 T. Quantitative measurement of plaque burden showed a coefficient of variation (CV) of 4.2% for wall volume and 3.02% for percent wall volume at 3 T.[31] These CVs were comparable with CVs of 5.8% for wall volume and 3.2% for percent wall volume at 1.5 T using similar MR imaging protocols and measurement methods.[32] The SNR improvement compared with 1.5 T does not necessarily translate into improved reproducibility, likely because of measurement errors secondary to patient positioning[7] as well as different imaging parameters between field strengths.

Methods of plaque composition measurement developed at 1.5 T are also applicable at 3 T,

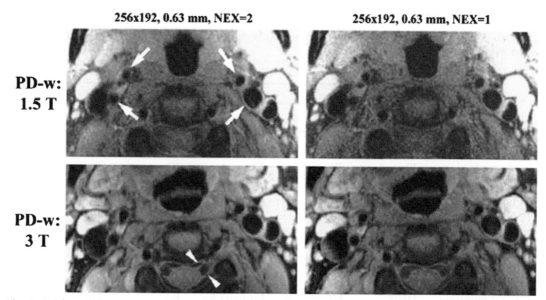

Fig. 6. Axial carotid MR imaging sequences obtained at 1.5 T and 3 T using the same sequence parameters. Note the improved SNR at 3 T with the number of excitations (NEX) = 1 with improved vessel wall delineation (*arrow*) and appearance of small structures as nerve roots (*arrowheads*). With NEX = 2 at 1.5 T, some of the SNR loss can be offset but comes at the expense of increased scan time. (*Adapted from* Yarnykh VL, Terashima M, Hayes CE, et al. Multicontrast black-blood MRI of carotid arteries: comparison between 1.5 and 3 tesla magnetic field strengths. J Magn Reson Imaging 2006;23(5):693; with permission.)

with some differences. Underhill and colleagues[4] showed that there was good agreement between the 2 field strengths for calcification (k = 0.72) and LRNC (k = 0.73). The agreement for hemorrhage was slightly less (k = 0.66) with more hemorrhage being detected at 1.5 T than at 3 T (14.7% vs 7.8%). This finding is attributable to the lengthening of T1 relaxation at high-fields reducing the signal from hemorrhage when using similar imaging parameters between the 2 field strengths (**Fig. 7**). Increased susceptibility at 3 T may also be a contributing factor to reduced sensitivity for hemorrhage at 3 T. Because of the increased susceptibility, calcifications measured larger at 3 T (see **Fig. 7**). To overcome these problems, new sequences have been developed at 3 T. MPRAGE or SPI sequences are added for highly sensitive detection of hemorrhage.[22,23] Ultrashort echo time (UTE) sequences are being explored for accurate quantification of calcification.[33,34] Automated methods of plaque composition measurement developed for 1.5 T have also been shown to be applicable at 3 T (**Fig. 8**). Intraclass correlation coefficient (ICC) for area measurements of lipid core, hemorrhage, fibrous tissue, and calcification ranged from 0.89 to 0.98.[35]

Assessment of disease

Advanced atherosclerotic plaque is composed of several plaque components such as an LRNC with overlying fibrous cap, IPH, calcification, and

loose matrix interspersed among fibrous tissue frameworks. These major components of the plaque can be identified by MR imaging. The qualitative and quantitative measurement of these plaque components have been extensively validated and reported at 1.5 T.[28,36,37] Studies that have benefited from the technical improvements or higher SNR at 3 T are discussed later.

IPH

The association between IPH of carotid atherosclerotic plaque and ischemic brain symptoms has been identified by many studies.[38–41] IPH is visible on T1-weighted images as a hyperintense signal caused by the short T1 relaxation time of methemoglobin, a breakdown product of hemoglobin. Although methemoglobin could be identified using TOF at 1.5 T, it could not be reliably identified at 3 T using TOF (see **Fig. 6**).[42] In a comparison study between 1.5 T and 3 T field strengths[4] using TOF, 32/218 sections showed IPH at 1.5 T, whereas only 17/218 sections showed IPH at 3 T. No IPH that was not detected at 1.5 T was detected at 3 T. In addition, the measured size of IPH was less at 3 T, although the difference was not statistically significant. Use of a highly T1-weighted scan such as MPRAGE[22,43] at 3 T can improve the sensitivity and specificity for IPH (**Fig. 9**).[24] When small IPH (<2.81 mm²; 3-pixel diameter) or calcified IPH was excluded, sensitivity and specificity were

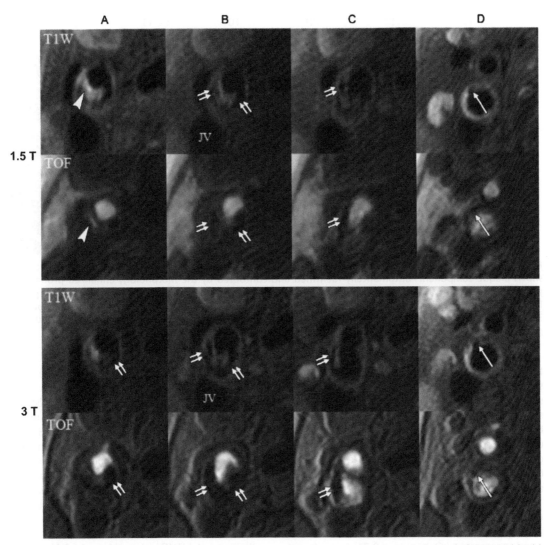

Fig. 7. Serial matched sections of the same subject scanned at 1.5 T and 3 T. Note that calcifications (*double arrows*) appear larger at 3 T (columns A–C). A smaller calcification in the internal carotid (*arrow*, column D) is more easily detected at 3 T because of the higher SNR. IPH (*arrowhead*, column A) is visible at 1.5 T but is not seen at 3 T using TOF. (*From* Underhill HR, Yarnykh VL, Hatsukami TS, et al. Carotid plaque morphology and composition: initial comparison between 1.5- and 3.0-T magnetic field strengths. Radiology 2008;248(2):556; with permission.)

80%, 97% for MPRAGE; 70%, 92% for T1-weighted fast spin echo; and 56%, 96% TOF with histology as gold standard.[24] The sensitivity further increased for larger IPH. Improvements of the MPRAGE technique with suppression of luminal signal (SPI[23]) can further improve the sensitivity of MPRAGE for IPH detection. Such inversion recovery techniques perform better at 3 T for short T1 species with increased SNR because of the higher field strength. An alternative method is the use of precontrast mask image in contrast-enhanced MR angiography studies to identify IPH.[44] Because this sequence is also highly T1 weighted, IPH can be identified as a hyperintense signal. However, sensitivity may be reduced because of a lack of fat suppression with the precontrast mask technique.

IPH has been shown to accelerate plaque growth and is associated with cerebrovascular events and postsurgical brain infarcts. Patients with IPH had an increase in percent change in wall volume (6.8% vs −0.15%) and LRNC volume (28.4% vs −5.2%) over 18 months compared with controls with similar levels of plaque at baseline.[45] They were also more likely to have new IPH (43% vs 0%). In a follow-up study, baseline IPH was strongly associated with subsequent symptoms over 3 years (hazard ratio [HR] 5.2).[41] Although

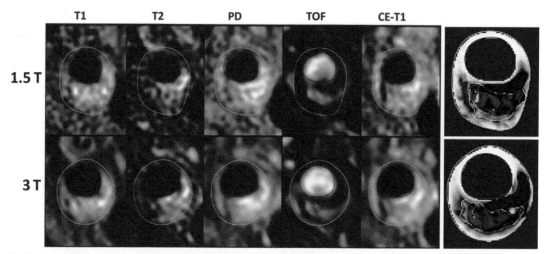

Fig. 8. Carotid boundaries were manually drawn for the same subject scanned at 1.5 T and 3 T. The last column shows plaque components automatically identified and contoured by the morphology-enhanced probabilistic plaque segmentation (MEPPS) algorithm within the carotid boundaries. (LRNC, yellow; loose matrix, purple; IPH, red). (*Adapted from* Kerwin WS, Liu F, Yarnykh V, et al. Signal features of the atherosclerotic plaque at 3.0 Tesla versus 1.5 Tesla: impact on automatic classification. J Magn Reson Imaging 2008;28(4):990; with permission.)

these 1.5 T studies used TOF and T1-weighted spin echo images to identify IPH, studies at 3 T using MPRAGE for IPH detection have reported similar findings. An HR of 9.8 was reported for MPRAGE-detectable IPH baseline over a follow-up period of 28 months.[39] In an asymptomatic group of 91 subjects with 16% to 79% stenosis by ultrasound, 6 events occurred (HR 3.6), with all occurring on the side with IPH.[40]

LRNC
Identification of LRNC at 3 T is similar to 1.5 T. Good agreement (Cohen $\kappa = 0.71$) was found for identification of LRNC between the 2 field strengths.[4] There was no difference in LRNC volume measurements between the 2 field strengths. At 3 T, sequences such as 3D-MERGE

can also contribute to the identification of LRNC.[15] Higher SNR at 3 T allows use of diffusion-weighted imaging (DWI) for identification of LRNC.[46] Although these new 3 T techniques are still being developed, spin echo–based BB MR imaging has been used to follow small changes in LRNC over time. Zhao and colleagues[47] serially imaged subjects with coronary artery disease or carotid disease who were treated with atorvastatin in the Carotid Plaque Composition (CPC) study at 1-year intervals for 3 years. LRNC area reduced from 8.4% to 5.2% over 3 years. During the observation period, LRNC reduced from 14.2 % to 7.4% when slices with normal wall were excluded, with 3.2%, 3.0%, and 0.91% reduction rates in the first, second, and third years, respectively.[48] The corresponding wall volume also decreased by 3.8%

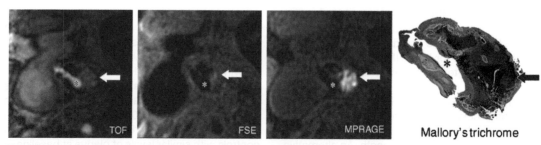

Fig. 9. IPH in a moderately calcified plaque on 3 T1-weighted sequences: TOF, T1-weighted fast spin echo, and MPRAGE. IPH is hyperintense on all 3 sequences but most prominent by MPRAGE, which also corresponds with extent of IPH on histology (*arrow*). Lumen is denoted by an asterisk. (*Adapted from* Ota H, Yarnykh VL, Ferguson MS, et al. Carotid intraplaque hemorrhage imaging at 3.0-T MR imaging: comparison of the diagnostic performance of three T1-weighted sequences. Radiology 2010;254(2):557; with permission.)

over 3 years, with 0.3%, 3.6%, and 0.1% reduction rates in the first, second, and third years, respectively.

Other plaque components

Calcifications at 3 T could be identified to the same extent as 1.5 T (Cohen κ 0.72) but the size measurements were increased because of higher susceptibility at 3 T.[4] Therefore, spin echo sequences are preferable to gradient echo sequences for calcium measurement at 3 T. Newer UTE techniques may improve size measurement of calcium at higher field strengths.[34] Fibrous cap identification and measurement may be improved at 3 T because of higher SNR and improved coil designs but is yet to be shown. Loose matrix tissues can be identified with similar sensitivity and specificity on both field strengths but their contribution to plaque vulnerability is currently unknown.

Ultrahigh-Field Imaging

Along with the gradual adoption of 3 T systems as the mainstay of plaque imaging, MR systems with ultrahigh-field strength, such as 7 T or even higher, are now available. To take advantage of the even higher SNR offered by such systems, several studies have been conducted to explore the feasibility of plaque imaging on these ultrahigh-field systems.

A crucial step in conducting plaque imaging on high-field scanners is development of proper transmit-receive coils because 7 T scanners are not equipped with transmission body coils. As reported by different groups, both 8-channel[49] and 16-channel[50] bilateral carotid coils have been developed for 7 T systems with excellent delineation of the carotid artery. The 16-channel coil is also equipped with a 6-channel transmit coil array to achieve more homogeneous and energy-efficient B1 transmission.[50] As a result, the energy-intense TSE sequence has also been successfully implemented on the 7 T system for high-resolution carotid artery wall imaging.

Another challenge of 7 T imaging is the availability of a dedicated BB imaging technique. Although several BB techniques have been developed for 1.5 T/3 T systems, they cannot be used at 7 T because they all require a global transmission coil for blood nulling. When the body transmission coil is unavailable, as is the case on most 7 T systems, blood suppression is nullified by the strong inflow effect. To overcome this limitation, a local excitation BB imaging (LOBBI) sequence was proposed.[51] The essence of this sequence is to suppress blood signal by destroying its phase coherence similarly to MSDE but after blood is excited by the excitation RF pulse. By doing so, the time gap between blood suppression and data acquisition is shortened, thus minimizing the inflow effect. As shown in a flow phantom experiment (Fig. 10), LOBBI is the only technique that can suppress blood signal successfully with a local transmission coil.

Besides the development in novel coil and pulse sequences, the high SNR at 7 T has found application in new target vessels not commonly imaged at lower field strengths. Recent work using a 7 T

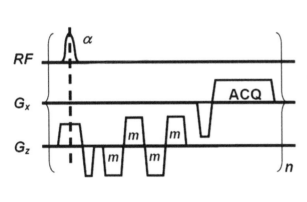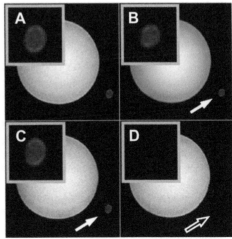

Fig. 10. Pulse sequence diagram of the local excitation black blood imaging (LOBBI) sequence (*left panel*) and a comparison of flow suppression capabilities among different BB techniques (*right panel*). Right panel shows baseline image (*A*), double inversion recovery (DIR) (*B*), MSDE (*C*), and LOBBI (*D*) images. Flow is successfully suppressed on only the LOBBI image. Solid arrows: unsuppressed flow signal on DIR (*B*) and MSDE (*C*) images. Open arrow: suppressed flow signal on LOBBI (*D*) images.

scanner showed the feasibility of intracranial artery vessel wall MR imaging in vivo.[52] Excellent delineation of the circle of Willis vessel wall imaging was achieved at an isotropic 0.8-mm resolution. This isotropic resolution allows for the free reformation of the targeted vessels, which is necessary for tortuous targets like intracranial arteries.

Summary

Although the main focus of atherosclerotic plaque MR imaging has been the carotid artery because of ease of imaging and availability of endarterectomy specimens for validation, many of the techniques presented in this article have already been translated to other vascular beds like peripheral arteries and/or intracranial arteries at 3 T. There are ongoing efforts to translate similar techniques into coronary artery wall imaging. Like other cardiac MR applications, clinical application of coronary wall imaging at 3 T requires further technical development to overcome the challenges of the increased magnetic field inhomogeneities and the large motion of coronary arteries with the cardiac cycle.

In summary, the increased SNR at high-fields benefits atherosclerotic plaque imaging despite increased undesired issues like increased field inhomogeneities. In particular, 3D isotropic imaging of atherosclerotic plaque only becomes clinically feasible with the extra SNR available with high-field MR scanners. The higher SNR, reduced scan time, increased through-plane resolution, and new scan techniques promise faster translation of plaque imaging to the clinics and new applications such as coronary vessel wall imaging in the near future.

REFERENCES

1. Anumula S, Song HK, Wright AC, et al. High-resolution black-blood MRI of the carotid vessel wall using phased-array coils at 1.5 and 3 Tesla. Acad Radiol 2005;12(12):1521–6.

2. Yarnykh VL, Terashima M, Hayes CE, et al. Multicontrast black-blood MRI of carotid arteries: comparison between 1.5 and 3 tesla magnetic field strengths. J Magn Reson Imaging 2006;23(5):691–8.

3. Koktzoglou I, Chung YC, Mani V, et al. Multislice dark-blood carotid artery wall imaging: a 1.5 T and 3.0 T comparison. J Magn Reson Imaging 2006;23(5):699–705.

4. Underhill HR, Yarnykh VL, Hatsukami TS, et al. Carotid plaque morphology and composition: initial comparison between 1.5- and 3.0-T magnetic field strengths. Radiology 2008;248(2):550–60.

5. Hayes CE, Mathis CM, Yuan C. Surface coil phased arrays for high-resolution imaging of the carotid arteries. J Magn Reson Imaging 1996; 6(1):109–12.

6. Balu N, Yarnykh VL, Scholnick J, et al. Improvements in carotid plaque imaging using a new eight-element phased array coil at 3T. J Magn Reson Imaging 2009;30(5):1209–14.

7. Balu N, Kerwin WS, Chu B, et al. Serial MRI of carotid plaque burden: influence of subject repositioning on measurement precision. Magn Reson Med 2007;57(3):592–9.

8. Antiga L, Wasserman BA, Steinman DA. On the overestimation of early wall thickening at the carotid bulb by black blood MRI, with implications for coronary and vulnerable plaque imaging. Magn Reson Med 2008;60(5):1020–8.

9. Luk-Pat GT, Gold GE, Olcott EW, et al. High-resolution three-dimensional in vivo imaging of atherosclerotic plaque. Magn Reson Med 1999;42(4):762–71.

10. Balu N, Chu B, Hatsukami TS, et al. Comparison between 2D and 3D high-resolution black-blood techniques for carotid artery wall imaging in clinically significant atherosclerosis. J Magn Reson Imaging 2008;27(4):918–24.

11. Zhang Z, Fan Z, Carroll TJ, et al. Three-dimensional T2-weighted MRI of the human femoral arterial vessel wall at 3.0 Tesla. Invest Radiol 2009;44(9):619–26.

12. Wang J, Yarnykh VL, Hatsukami T, et al. Improved suppression of plaque-mimicking artifacts in black-blood carotid atherosclerosis imaging using a multi-slice motion-sensitized driven-equilibrium (MSDE) turbo spin-echo (TSE) sequence. Magn Reson Med 2007;58(5):973–81.

13. Balu N, Yarnykh VL, Chu B, et al. Carotid plaque assessment using fast 3D isotropic resolution black-blood MRI. Magn Reson Med 2011;65(3):627–37.

14. Zhao X, Balu N, Liu W, et al. Characterization of carotid atherosclerotic plaque compositions by single magnetic resonance imaging sequence: a comparison study with multicontrast plaque imaging at 3T. Paper presented at: ISMRM Annual Meeting. Montreal (QC), May 6–13, 2011.

15. Balu N, Yarnykh V, Kerwin WS, et al. Interpretation of tissue contrast in a rapid black-blood gradient echo sequence with motion-sensitized driven equilibrium (MSDE) preparation (3D MERGE) for 3D isotropic high-resolution imaging of the vessel wall and its application for hemorrhage detection. Paper presented at: ISMRM Annual Meeting. Montreal (QC), May 6–13, 2011.

16. Wang J, Yarnykh VL, Yuan C. Enhanced image quality in black-blood MRI using the improved motion-sensitized driven-equilibrium (iMSDE) sequence. J Magn Reson Imaging 2010;31(5):1256–63.

17. Stanisz GJ, Odrobina EE, Pun J, et al. T1, T2 relaxation and magnetization transfer in tissue at 3T. Magn Reson Med 2005;54(3):507–12.

18. Yarnykh VL, Yuan C. Multislice double inversion-recovery black-blood imaging with simultaneous slice reinversion. J Magn Reson Imaging 2003; 17(4):478–83.

19. Yarnykh V, Yuan C. Unit 1.4: high-resolution multicontrast MRI of the carotid artery wall for evaluation of atherosclerotic plaques. In: Haacke EM, Lin W, editors. Current protocols in magnetic resonance imaging. New York: Wiley; 2004. p. A1.4.1–18.

20. Chu B, Kampschulte A, Ferguson MS, et al. Hemorrhage in the atherosclerotic carotid plaque: a high-resolution MRI study. Stroke 2004;35(5):1079–84.

21. Leung G, Moody AR. MR imaging depicts oxidative stress induced by methemoglobin. Radiology 2010; 257(2):470–6.

22. Zhu DC, Ferguson MS, DeMarco JK. An optimized 3D inversion recovery prepared fast spoiled gradient recalled sequence for carotid plaque hemorrhage imaging at 3.0 T. Magn Reson Imaging 2008;26(10):1360–6.

23. Wang J, Ferguson MS, Balu N, et al. Improved carotid intraplaque hemorrhage imaging using a slab-selective phase-sensitive inversion-recovery (SPI) sequence. Magn Reson Med 2010;64(5): 1332–40.

24. Ota H, Yarnykh VL, Ferguson MS, et al. Carotid intraplaque hemorrhage imaging at 3.0-T MR imaging: comparison of the diagnostic performance of three T1-weighted sequences. Radiology 2010;254(2): 551–63.

25. Yang Q, Liu J, Barnes SR, et al. Imaging the vessel wall in major peripheral arteries using susceptibility-weighted imaging. J Magn Reson Imaging 2009; 30(2):357–65.

26. Katscher U, Bornert P. Parallel RF transmission in MRI. NMR Biomed 2006;19(3):393–400.

27. Cai JM, Hatsukami TS, Ferguson MS, et al. In vivo quantitative measurement of intact fibrous cap and lipid-rich necrotic core size in atherosclerotic carotid plaque - comparison of high-resolution, contrast-enhanced magnetic resonance imaging and histology. Circulation 2005;112(22):3437–44.

28. Saam T, Ferguson MS, Yarnykh VL, et al. Quantitative evaluation of carotid plaque composition by in vivo MRI. Arterioscler Thromb Vasc Biol 2005; 25(1):234–9.

29. Willinek WA, Schild HH. Clinical advantages of 3.0 T MRI over 1.5 T. Eur J Radiol 2008;65(1):2–14.

30. Cury RC, Houser SL, Furie KL, et al. Vulnerable plaque detection by 3.0 tesla magnetic resonance imaging. Invest Radiol 2006;41(2):112–5.

31. Li F, Yarnykh V, Hatsukami T, et al. Scan-rescan reproducibility of carotid atherosclerotic plaque morphology and tissue composition measurements

using multicontrast MRI at 3T. J Magn Reson Imaging 2010;31(1):168–76.

32. Saam T, Kerwin WS, Chu B, et al. Sample size calculation for clinical trials using magnetic resonance imaging for the quantitative assessment of carotid atherosclerosis. J Cardiovasc Magn Reson 2005; 7(5):799–808.

33. Herzka Jr DA, Nezafat R, Chan R, et al. Imaging of ex vivo human carotid plaques correlates with CT. Paper presented at: Proceedings 16th ISMRM Scientific Meeting and Exhibition. Toronto, May 3–9, 2008.

34. Du J, Corbeil J, Znamirowski R, et al. Direct imaging and quantification of carotid plaque calcification. Magn Reson Med 2011;65(4):1013–20.

35. Kerwin WS, Liu F, Yarnykh V, et al. Signal features of the atherosclerotic plaque at 3.0 Tesla versus 1.5 Tesla: impact on automatic classification. J Magn Reson Imaging 2008;28(4):987–95.

36. Kampschulte A, Ferguson MS, Kerwin WS, et al. Differentiation of intraplaque versus juxtaluminal hemorrhage/thrombus in advanced human carotid atherosclerotic lesions by in vivo magnetic resonance imaging. Circulation 2004;110(20):3239–44.

37. Cai JM, Hatsukami TS, Ferguson MS, et al. Classification of human carotid atherosclerotic lesions with in vivo multicontrast magnetic resonance imaging. Circulation 2002;106(11):1368–73.

38. Altaf N, Beech A, Goode S, et al. Carotid intraplaque hemorrhage detected by magnetic resonance imaging predicts embolization during carotid endarterectomy. J Vasc Surg 2007;46(1):31–6.

39. Altaf N, MacSweeney ST, Gladman J, et al. Carotid intraplaque hemorrhage predicts recurrent symptoms in patients with high-grade carotid stenosis. Stroke 2007;38(5):1633–5.

40. Singh N, Moody A, Gladstone D, et al. Moderate carotid artery stenosis: MR imaging-depicted intraplaque hemorrhage predicts risk of cerebrovascular ischemic events in asymptomatic men. Radiology 2009;252(2):502–8.

41. Takaya N, Yuan C, Chu B, et al. Association between carotid plaque characteristics and subsequent ischemic cerebrovascular events: a prospective assessment with MRI–initial results. Stroke 2006; 37(3):818–23.

42. Underhill HR, Hatsukami TS, Fayad ZA, et al. MRI of carotid atherosclerosis: clinical implications and future directions. Nat Rev Cardiol 2010;7(3):165–73.

43. Bitar R, Moody A, Leung G, et al. In vivo 3D high-spatial-resolution MR imaging of intraplaque hemorrhage. Radiology 2008;249(1):259–67.

44. Qiao Y, Etesami M, Malhotra S, et al. Identification of intraplaque hemorrhage on MR angiography images: a comparison of contrast-enhanced mask and time-of-flight techniques. AJNR Am J Neuroradiol 2011;32(3):454–9.

45. Takaya N, Yuan C, Chu B, et al. Presence of intraplaque hemorrhage stimulates progression of carotid atherosclerotic plaques - a high-resolution magnetic resonance imaging study. Circulation 2005;111(21): 2768–75.

46. Kim S, Jeong E, Shi X, et al. Diffusion-weighted imaging of human carotid artery using 2D single-shot interleaved multislice inner volume diffusion-weighted echo planar imaging (2D ss-IMIV-DWFPI) at 3T: diffusion measurement in atherosclerotic plaque. J Magn Reson Imaging 2009;30(5):1068–77.

47. Zhao X, Dong L, Hatsukami T. Magnetic resonance imaging of plaque lipid depletion during lipid therapy: a prospective assessment of efficacy and time-course. Paper presented at: American College of Cardiology (ACC) 57th Annual Scientific Session. Chicago (IL), March 29 to April 1, 2008.

48. Dong L, Neradilek B, BC. Effects of intensive lipid therapy on atherosclerotic plaque burden and time-course: a prospective, randomized, double blinded study with magnetic resonance Imaging (MRI). Paper presented at: American College of Cardiology (ACC) 57th Annual Scientific Session. Chicago (IL), March 29 to April 1, 2008.

49. Breyer T, Kraff O, Maderwald S, et al. Carotid plaque imaging with an eight-channel transmit/receive RF array at 7 Tesla: first results in patients with atherosclerosis. Paper presented at: ISMRM Annual Meeting; Stockholm (Sweden), May 1–7, 2010.

50. Koning W, Langenhuizen E, Raaijmakers AJ, et al. 6 channel radiative transmit array with a 16 channel surface receiver array for improved carotid vessel wall imaging at 7T. Paper presented at: ISMRM Annual Meeting. Montreal (QC), May 6–13, 2011.

51. Wang J, Balu N, Wilson GJ, et al. Local excitation black blood imaging (LOBBI) for local transmission coil at high field MRI (7T and above). Paper presented at: ISMRM Annual Meeting. Montreal (QC), May 6–13, 2011.

52. Zwanenburg JJ, van der Kolk AG, Hendrikse J, et al. Intracranial vessel wall imaging at 7 Tesla. Paper presented at: ISMRM Annual Meeting. Montreal (QC), May 6–13, 2011.

Head and Neck High-Field Imaging: Oncology Applications

Wessam Bou-Assaly, MD[a],*, Ashok Srinivasan, MBBS, MD, DNB[b], Suresh K. Mukherji, MD[c]

KEYWORDS

- 3 T MR imaging • High-field imaging
- Head and neck cancer • Perfusion • Diffusion

Key Points

- Be familiar with the role of 3 T and high-field magnetic resonance (MR) imaging in head and neck cancer
- Be familiar with different MR imaging techniques and sequences in evaluating head and neck cancer
- Establish an MR imaging protocol in head and neck imaging

In recent decades, head and neck imaging has benefited from the use of 1.5 T magnetic resonance (MR) imaging, providing faster sequences, better soft tissue evaluation, and 3-axis imaging, with less radiation and iodine-based contrast injection. In 2000, the US Food and Drug Administration approved human MR imaging at high-field strength up to 4 T in clinical practice. 3 T MR imaging has become widely available, with the hope of significant advance in the evaluation of the head and neck region. This article reviews the benefits, disadvantages, and challenges of high-field imaging of the head and neck region, mainly focusing on the imaging of head and neck cancer.

CLINICAL RECOMMENDATIONS

MR imaging of head and neck cancer is usually requested in a pretreatment setting for evaluation of local extension of a known primary malignancy, especially into adjacent deep soft tissue planes, difficult to assess by computed tomography (CT) alone, such as intracranial extension of nasopharyngeal malignancy but also to exclude cartilaginous or bony invasion, such as into the thyroid cartilage, which can be difficult to appreciate on neck CT. The use of new techniques such as diffusion and perfusion sequences can play an initial role in differentiating benign from malignant primary lesions, by virtue of assessing the apparent diffusion coefficient (ADC) values and the contrast dynamics over the lesion. Regional lymph nodes can also be assessed by MR imaging to exclude their involvement by secondary metastases using diffusion and perfusion sequences, adding crucial information for the cancer staging.

MR imaging can also be used in a posttreatment setting to monitor a treated primary malignancy, and also to predict the response of a lesion to established treatment. Diffusion and perfusion

[a] Department of Radiology, Neuroradiology Division, University of Michigan, Ann Arbor VA Hospital, 2215 Fuller Court, Ann Arbor, MI 48103, USA
[b] Department of Radiology, Neuroradiology Division, University of Michigan, A. Alfred Taubman Health Care Center, 1500 East Medical Center Drive, Room B1 132D, Ann Arbor, MI 48109-5302, USA
[c] Department of Radiology, University of Michigan Health System, 1500 East Medical Center, Ann Arbor, MI 48109-0030, USA
* Corresponding author.
E-mail address: Wessam@med.umich.edu

Neuroimag Clin N Am 22 (2012) 285–296
doi:10.1016/j.nic.2012.02.013
1052-5149/12/$ – see front matter Published by Elsevier Inc.

sequences as well as conventional MR imaging techniques play an important role in following up treated malignancy to exclude residual or recurrent disease and may play a role in predicting the response of the tumor to treatment.

In our institution, different protocols are preset for different primary sites in the head and neck region. The usual protocols include axial T1 fast spin echo (FSE), axial T2 with fat saturation, diffusion sequence, coronal T2 with fat saturation, coronal T1 FSE, and axial, sagittal, and coronal T1 postgadolinium administration with fat-saturated and possible perfusion sequence.

TECHNICAL CONSIDERATIONS OF HIGH-FIELD IMAGING
Higher Signal-to-noise Ratio

The clear advantage of imaging with 3 T is the increase in signal-to-noise ratio (SNR), caused by the increase number of antiparallel spins at higher field.[1,2] The signal increases in proportion to the field strength B0 and theoretically doubles from 1.5 to 3 T. This increase in SNR can be used for an increase in spatial resolution or for performing faster imaging. Both changes are beneficial when evaluating the head and neck region, where higher resolution images are needed because of the size and closeness of the anatomic and pathologic structures, and also faster images are particularly important for patients with local neoplasm, because they usually have difficulty swallowing and holding still while slowly breathing.

TISSUE CONTRAST ISSUE: EFFECT ON T1 AND T2

Relaxation times are functions of the applied magnetic field. With increasing field strength, spin lattice or longitudinal relaxation time T1 increases by 20% to 40%, whereas the spin-spin or transverse relaxation time T2 slightly decreases.[1,3]

T1 prolongation has a beneficial effect on the postgadolinium-based images, because longer baseline T1 relaxation times are followed by a stronger effect of T1 shortening after contrast material injection, resulting in better postcontrast enhancement.[1,2] The same T1 effect, which is also beneficial in producing superior time-of-flight MR angiography studies, not specifically relevant in neck cancer imaging, leads to reduced contrast resolution on traditional spin echo acquisition.[3] This effect can be corrected by modifying the repetition time (TR) but may result in prolonged acquisition time, which is unsatisfactory for head and neck imaging.[2] Other methods of imaging, such as spoiled gradient recalled (SPGR) or magnetization-prepared technique (eg, inversion recovery or magnetization transfer three-dimensional SPGR) imaging, are not significantly affected by this effect.[3]

The T2 benefit of 3 T is immediately observed in the T2-weighted images using rapid acquisition with relaxation enhancement (RARE; also known as fast spin echo or turbo spin echo), with high matrix size (eg, 512 × 512) and thinner slices, providing high-quality and high-resolution images (**Fig. 1**).[2] These sequences use a radiofrequency (RF) excitation followed by a train of refocusing pulses that suppresses field inhomogeneities and susceptibility effect, which are increased with 3 T MR imaging and are particular to the head and neck region as a result of air, bone, fat, and sharp structural changes.

INCREASE OF CHEMICAL SHIFT AND SUSCEPTIBILITY ARTIFACT

Increase of chemical shift and susceptibility artifact are major challenges with high-field imaging. Chemical shift and susceptibility artifact increase proportionally with the field strength.

Although susceptibility effect could be exploited in brain imaging to improve the sensitivity of FSE imaging to the presence of hemorrhage and mineralization, these are particularly troublesome in head and neck imaging as a result of intimate presence of air, bone, and fat with acute structural changes.[1–3]

Protocol manipulations that manage susceptibility artifact include using shorter echo times (TEs), reducing voxel size, and increasing bandwidth used in 1.5 T.[3]

Susceptibility can be an advantage for dynamic susceptibility-weighted perfusion MR imaging to determine functional parameters like blood flow in head and neck malignancy, but it is also affected by signal loss in areas prone to susceptibility artifact, such as the skull base.[1,3] Minimizing TE can ameliorate these effects.

Chemical shift also increases with higher magnet field, and can be a significant limiting factor in routine anatomic imaging. With appropriate protocols, the high SNR of 3 T and multichannel coils is leveraged by the routine use of higher bandwidth for SE and FSE imaging, reducing the chemical shift effect.[3]

Chemical shift has a beneficial effect, providing a boost in metabolite peak separation for spectroscopy, which has no current definite role in head and neck imaging, and also makes fat suppression more robust in 3 T than at lower field strength.[1]

HIGHER ENERGY DEPOSITION

Energy deposition is also a challenge with high-field imaging and needs to be monitored by measuring the specific absorption rate (SAR). SAR refers to the rate at which energy from RF pulse is deposited in the body and increases by a factor of 4 from 1.5 to 3 T.[1,2] Regulation for RF-induced tissue heating is similar for 3 and 1.5 T and must not exceed 8 W/kg of tissue for any 5-minute period or 4 W/kg for a whole body averaged over 15 minutes.[1,3] Because RF deposition

quadruples from 1.5 to 3 T, the SAR limitations are reached earlier, limiting especially fast pulse sequences with high-power deposition such as fast echo imaging. RARE sequence is particularly affected by SAR because of multiple refocusing pulses. In some cases, it may be necessary to increase the TR or decrease the number of slices.[2]

Manipulations that are traditionally used to limit SAR include reducing acquisition flip angle of refocusing pulse, which could affect the image contrast but has been tolerated well thus far without a noticeable deleterious effect on image contrast.[1–3]

Parallel imaging (PI), such as sensitivity encoding (SENSE), is another powerful method to reduce RF, by reducing the number of phase-encoding steps performed in a given scan. The trade-off in SNR (a PI factor of 2 reduces SNR by 40%) is balanced by the higher signal in 3 T, and facilitated by improved higher SNR high-density 8-channel to 16-channel surface coils.[2,3]

In high-field imaging, increased susceptibility and SAR limitation are challenging. SENSE reduces RF deposition by reducing phase-encoding readouts at a given TE or it allows reduction of echo train length (eg, echo-planar imaging [EPI]), yielding shorter effective TE. This situation results in substantial reduction in image distortion and improves image quality. Shorter TE implies less motion artifact and reduction in blurring in image.

Diffusion Imaging

The greater signal intensity (SI) provided by 3 T is particularly enticing for diffusion-weighted imaging (DWI). 3 T imaging with dedicated 16-channel head and neck coils results in substantial improved SI to noise with better-quality DWI and ADC maps compared with conventional 1.5 T imaging.[3,4]

Recommended sequences										
Slice Orientation	Sagittal T1	DWI (Head)	AX FLAIR (Head)	AX T1	AX T2 F/S	AX FFE With/ Without	AX T1	AX T1 F/S	DWI (Neck)	AX T1 (Head)
FOV	240	230	230	220	220	260	220	220	240	240
RFOV	100	100	80	100	100	100	100	100	100	100
Matrix	272/435	128/256	320/512	256/512	256/400	256/256	256/512	256/512	128/256	256/512
Slice thickness/ gap	5/1.5 mm	4/1 mm	5/1 mm	4/1 mm	4/1 mm	4/default	4/1 mm	4/1 mm	4/1 mm	5/1 mm

Abbreviations: AX, axial; DWI, diffusion-weighted imaging; FFE, fast field echo; FLAIR, fluid-attenuated inversion recovery; FOV, field of view; F/S, fat-saturated; RFOV, rectangular field of view.

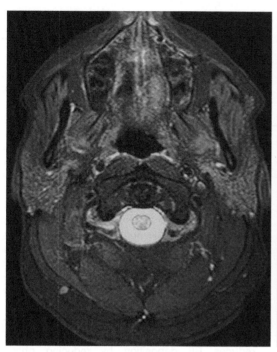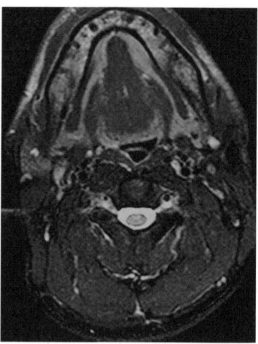

Fig. 1. Axial T2-weighted images on 3 T scanner demonstrate higher resolution with better discrimination of mucosal line, fat plans, lymphoid tissue, muscles, and salivary glands.

DWI is usually acquired by using EPI techniques, which are prone to susceptibility artifact that increases at higher field strength. PI techniques routinely applied in 3 T magnets that are also equipped with optimized surface coils and broadband reconstruction hardware effectively reduce the susceptibility artifact and ameliorate signal loss.[3] Using multishot DWI techniques (eg, PROPELLER [periodically rotated overlapping parallel lines with enhanced reconstruction]), which are less sensitive to susceptibility, have increased usefulness at 3 T.[3]

ONCOLOGIC APPLICATIONS OF HIGH-FIELD IMAGING IN HEAD AND NECK CANCER
Evaluation of a Primary Neck Lesion

Imaging can play a crucial role in determining benignancy in neck diseases, avoiding unnecessary biopsies. However, with conventional MR imaging, there can be overlap of imaging features of benignancy and malignancy, resulting in a diagnostic dilemma, necessitating the search for more advanced techniques. Interest in DWI has been invoked in the last few years because of its potential in characterizing neck pathologies.

ADC values obtained over the lesion in question from diffusion-weighted images were proposed to be helpful in distinguishing benign and malignant neck neoplasms. Reductions in both the extracellular matrix and the diffusion space of water protons in the extracellular and intracellular dimensions (as a result of an increased nuclear/cytoplasm ratio and hypercellularity) have been described as potential reasons for the decreased ADC values within malignant lesions compared with nonmalignant tissue.[4–6]

Although the diffusion characteristics of more obscure lesions are not well known, those of squamous cell cancer, the most common head and neck malignancy, have been extensively studied. At 1.5 T strength, an ADC value of 1.22×10^{-3} mm^2/s was suggested as a threshold less than which a lesion is likely malignant.[5]

3 T imaging with dedicated 16-channel head and neck coils, which results in substantially improved SI to noise, has the potential to produce better-quality DWI and ADC maps compared with conventional field strengths. An ADC value of 1.3×10^{-3} mm^2/s was suggested as a possible threshold for distinguishing benign from malignant lesions in head and neck, with lesions with ADC greater than that being likely benign (**Fig. 2**).[4]

Using the mean ADC value over a lesion may be problematic if the lesion is heterogeneous: some benign diseases may be hypercellular with decreased ADC, and malignant diseases can develop necrotic areas with increased ADC, causing overlap in mean ADC values between these categories. Recent studies suggested

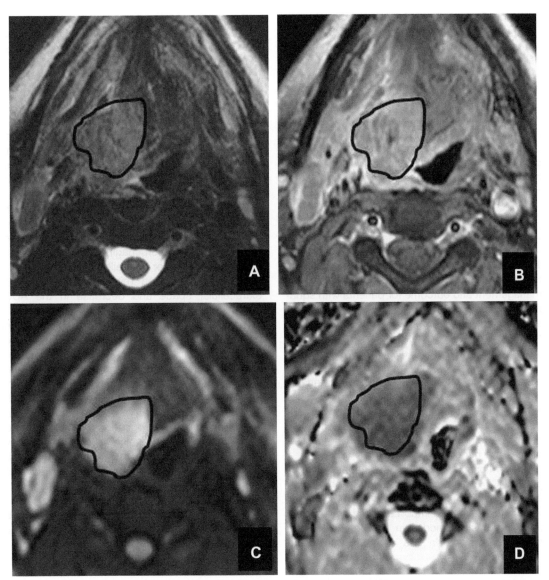

Fig. 2. Axial T2 (*A*), T1 postgadolinium (*B*), B800 diffusion (*C*) and ADC map sequences (*D*). A right tonsillar squamous cell carcinoma demonstrates intermediate to high T2 signal with homogenous postgadolinium enhancement and diffusion restriction on the B800 DWI and a low ADC value of $0.847 \times 10^{-3} mm^2/s$.

separating the ADC within a lesion into multiple clusters (low and high [2-cluster model] or low, intermediate, and high [3-cluster model]) and then evaluating the differences in ADC values generated from the individual clusters between the benign and malignant diseases.[7] By dividing a tumor or lesion into multiple clusters, the heterogeneous components of a lesion were better separated and the true difference in ADC values between benign and malignant lesions was attributed to the fact that malignant lesions have a greater proportion of low ADC voxels.[7] For example, a tumor with 50% of its voxels less than a certain ADC value may have a higher probability of being malignant compared with another lesion with 20% of its voxels less than the same threshold.

ADC has also been shown to be different between malignant diseases like squamous cell carcinoma and lymphoma, because of differences in cellularity between malignant neoplasms of different pathologic types.[8]

Perfusion MR imaging was also suggested as an imaging technique to distinguish benign from malignant head and neck cancer.[9] Tumor angiogenesis with new vessel growth and increased angiogenic activity is mediated by factors released from malignant tumor, which can be images by perfusion. Dynamic contrast-enhanced perfusion-weighted MR imaging yields different quantitative parameters that reflect the angiogenesis, mainly using dynamic susceptibility contrast perfusion-weighted MR imaging (DSC-MR imaging) and dynamic contrast-enhanced MR imaging (DCE-MR imaging). In the study of Abdel Razek and colleagues,[22] the difference in the DSC between malignant and benign head and neck tumors at dynamic susceptibility contrast perfusion MR imaging was statistically significant, explained by highly vascularity with increased capillary perfusion of malignant tumors compared with benign tumors.

Discriminating Benign from Metastatic Cervical Lymph Nodes

The status of the cervical lymph nodes is one of the most important factors influencing therapeutic management and outcome for patients with squamous cell carcinoma of the head and neck. Cross-sectional imaging techniques, such as computed tomography (CT), ultrasonography, and MR imaging provide limited evaluation for cervical lymph node involvement by malignancy. Lymph node size is the most frequently used criteria to discriminate metastatic from benign reactive lymph nodes in the neck. Furthermore, in ultrasonography and CT, internal architecture evaluation can be beneficial for detecting malignant involvement of the node.

Conventional MR imaging does not significantly exceed CT to detect metastatic lymph nodes. Internal architectural abnormality on MR images was suggested as an important hallmark suggestive of metastatic nodes in patients with head and neck cancer. In this context, Curtin and colleagues[10] reported that internal abnormality of the node as judged by the presence of a low signal intensity area on T1-weighted images or an area of high or heterogeneous SI on T2-weighted images improved the diagnostic ability in detecting metastatic nodes in the neck, compared with the diagnostic ability using the size criterion alone. These changes were not sufficient to confidently differentiate benign from malignant nodes and additional specific techniques such as diffusion, perfusion, and magnetic transfer techniques were proposed as additional tools in discriminating metastatic lymph nodes.

Cancer metastasis to a regional cervical lymph nodes is associated with alteration in water diffusivity and microcirculation of the node, a principle on which the diffusion imaging is based. Tumors have larger number of cells, cellular polymorphism, and increased mitosis, which diminish extracellular space and decrease in the ADC (**Figs. 3** and **4**).

Many studies evaluated the role of diffusion imaging and ADC value in discriminating metastatic from benign lymph nodes.[11–16] Although most published data suggested a decreased ADC value in metastatic lymph nodes, only the study of Sumi and colleagues[11] concluded that metastatic lymph nodes had a higher ADC value than normal nodes. These investigators proposed an ADC threshold of 0.4×10^{-3} mm^2/s, which yielded a specificity of 97% and positive predictive value of 93%, with a lower sensitivity of 52% and negative predictive value of 71%. Vandecaveye and colleagues[12] showed lower ADC values in metastatic lymph nodes than benign, with ADC for benign nodes at 1.9×10^{-3} mm^2/s $\pm$ 0.22 versus 0.85×10^{-3} mm^2/s $\pm$ 0.27 for malignant lymph nodes (see **Fig. 4**).

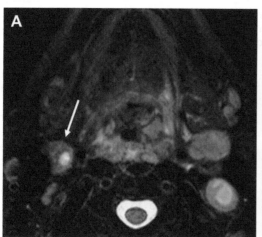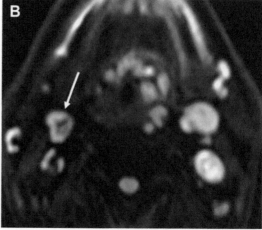

Fig. 3. Axial T2 (A) and axial diffusion B1000 (B) map. Metastatic lymph nodes demonstrate central cystic or necrotic areas seen as area of decreased diffusion signal (raised ADC) (*white arrow*).

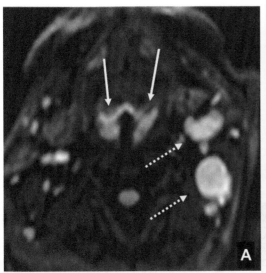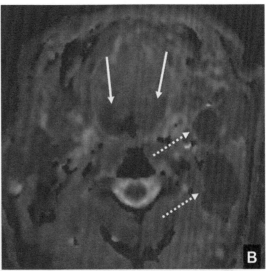

Fig. 4. Axial B1000 (*A*) and ADC map (*B*). Bilateral palatine tonsils squamous carcinomas (*solid arrows*) are associated with left level II enlarged lymph nodes (*dashed arrows*). The primary lesions as well as involved lymph nodes demonstrate diffusion restriction on the B1000 with decreased ADC value of around 0.72×10^{-3} mm^2/s.

False-negative findings for most of the enlarged lymph nodes were associated with intranodal necrosis. Other studies[13–16] also concluded that decreased ADC associated with metastatic lymph nodes compared with benign ones and suggested a threshold of 1.03×10^{-3} mm^2/s less than which a lymph node was most likely to be malignant. Their disagreement with Sumi and colleagues' data was attributed, between other causes, to lower b-values and the large number of necrotic lymph nodes in that study.

Vandecaveye[12] also noted that quantitative DWI enabled the detection of subcentimeter nodal metastases, providing additional information to that generated with anatomic imaging, with higher negative predictive value for the exclusion of metastatic disease. Accurate disease localization is critical for sparing organs at risk and to direct escalated doses of radiation.[17]

The ADC was also suggested to differentiate lymphomatous nodes from squamous carcinoma metastatic nodes, with values of lymphomatous nodes lower than those of metastatic nodes from squamous carcinoma. Also, ADC values of poorly differentiated carcinoma were lower than those of highly or moderately differentiated carcinoma, which was attributed to increased nuclear/cytoplasm ratio and hypercellularity in poorly differentiated cancer.[14,16]

Perfusion MR imaging was also suggested as a method that allows imaging of the physiology of the microcirculation, which is altered in tumors compared with normal tissues (**Fig. 5**).[18,19]

This methodology has been applied to the study of tumors of the brain, breast, uterine cervix, bone, bladder, and prostate as well as primary tumors of head and neck cancer.

Fischbein and colleagues[18] performed high-resolution surface coil anatomic imaging and dynamic contrast-enhanced MR imaging on a group of patients with squamous cell carcinoma of the head and neck who were undergoing clinically indicated neck dissection. These investigators found that time to peak enhancement was longer and that both peak enhancement and maximum slope of washin of contrast agent were lower in tumor-involved compared with nontumor-involved lymph nodes. The washout phase was also less rapid for tumor-involved nodes compared with nontumor-involved nodes. This finding was explained by the facts that normal lymphoid tissue has higher blood flow than squamous cell carcinoma and also by the fact that tumoral tissue has lower transfer of contrast agent to tissue, which is a function of blood flow, blood volume, and vessel permeability, thus lower time to peak and lower maximum upslope. Another potential issue is the enhanced interstitial fluid pressure in tumors, a situation that is believed to represent a major obstacle to delivery of therapeutic agents.[20,21] Abdel Razek and colleagues[22] also studied perfusion imaging in cervical lymph nodes, with a focus on T1-weighted dynamic contrast-enhanced perfusion, T2*-weighted dynamic susceptibility, and arterial spin labeling technique.

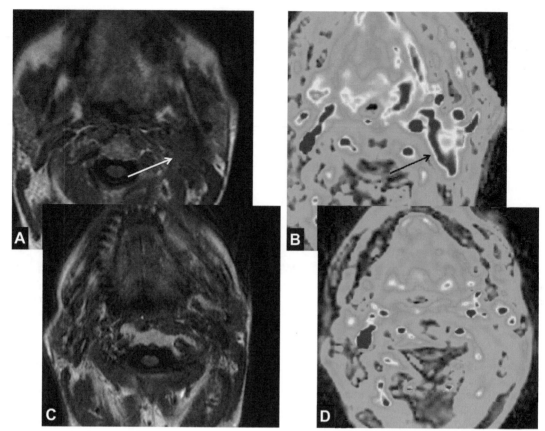

Fig. 5. Axial T1 postcontrast before and after treatment (*A* and *C*) and perfusion sequence images, before (*B*) and after treatment (*D*), demonstrate increased perfusion (*black arrow*) over a left level II soft tissue lesion (*white arrow*) that significantly decreases after treatment.

Prediction and Monitoring of Head and Neck Cancer Treatment

Treatment monitoring

Radiation therapy and concurrent chemotherapy became a leading modality for organ-preserving treatment of head and neck cancer. New developments in radiation treatment, such as combining multifractionated high-dose radiation with chemotherapy, have led to substantial gain in locoregional control and improvement in overall survival.[23–25] Treatment failure in the head and neck after chemoradiotherapy is mainly related to locoregional tumor recurrence, thus, to increase the chances of a salvage procedure to be curative, posttreatment surveillance should aim at detecting locoregional recurrent or persistent disease at an early stage.[26]

Conventional imaging with CT has a relatively high accuracy for detecting recurrent malignancy after radiotherapy (RT); however, as a result of radiation-induced tissue distortion, false-positive and false-negative results occur. Conventional MR imaging does not significantly exceed CT in detecting residual/recurrent disease and fluorodeoxyglucose (FDG) positron emission tomography (PET) CT provides additional information, but cannot resolve the problem, mainly because of inflammatory changes, as well as the low spatial resolution of this technique.[27,28]

Diffusion-weighted (DW)-MR imaging is able to characterize tissue and generate image contrast based on differences in tissue water mobility. Many studies showed a correlation between SI on DW-MR imaging and the ADC value, with tumor cellularity in experimental models. This correlation has been clinically validated in radiation treatment follow-up of brain tumors.[23,29,30] The radiotherapeutically induced nontumoral tissue changes such as edema, inflammation, fibrosis, and necrosis are expected to show low cellularity, in strong contrast with recurrent or persistent tumor. These different microstructures are expected to produce different signal intensities and ADC values on DW-MR imaging.[23]

DW-MR imaging allows accurate ADC-based differentiation of tumoral tissue from postradiotherapeutic alterations and tissue necrosis in the early (<4 months) and late (>4 months) post-RT period, characterizing persistent involved lymph nodes, as small as 6 mm, and persistent primary soft tissue mass.[23,31,32] Tumoral tissue showed significantly higher SI on DWI and a decreased ADC value, compared with postradiotherapeutic tissue changes and necrosis (Fig. 6).

Evaluation of the soft tissue by SI alone yielded low to moderate sensitivity and low specificity, influenced by T2 relaxation and T2 shine-through in areas with high interstitial water content, such as inflammatory or necrotic tissue. The use of the ADC values resulted in a high sensitivity and specificity, with nearly no overlap between tumoral and nontumoral tissue. The presence of malignancy correlated significantly with low ADC values, believed to be caused by the restriction of proton movement in the extracellular extravascular space, secondary to tumor hypercellularity.[5,29,33,34]

However, the presence of necrosis, inflammatory soft tissue changes, or submucosal fibrosis showed high ADC values, correlating with an increased interstitial space and low cell density. Irradiated normal tissue is expected to have high interstitial water content, secondary to the inflammatory or necrotic changes, resulting in substantially increased water mobility when compared with tumoral tissue. Vandecaveye and colleagues[23] also noted the added value of DW-MR imaging for the detection of subcentimetric nodal disease and lower false-positive rate than FDG PET CT for lesions at the primary site and persistent nodal disease.

Predicting tumor response to treatment

MR imaging was also suggested to have a predicting role of the response of the tumor to treatment. Accurate and timely detection of treatment response or presence of nonresponsive tumor can be critical in disease management because

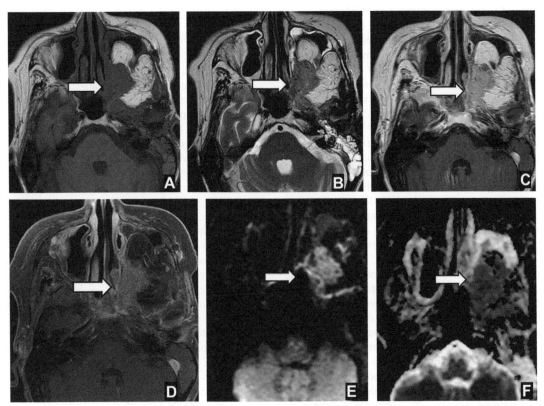

Fig. 6. 60-year-old patient with T4N2M0 squamous cell carcinoma of hard palate treated with resection and chemoradiation, now presenting with neck mass. Axial T1 precontrast (A), axial T2 (B), axial T1 after gadolinium pre (C) and post (D) contrast, axial diffusion sequence at B1000 (E) and ADC map (F). These images demonstrate invasion of the fat graft in the surgical site by a soft tissue mass with low T1 and T2 signal, homogeneous solid postcontrast enhancement and displaying diffusion restriction and low ADC value of around 0.8×10^{-3} mm^2/s (*white arrows*).

the optimal time window for successful surgery or alternative treatment methods may be limited.

DWI has been suggested as the modality of choice for early detection of treatment response in tumors, with the ADC values resulting in lower false-positive results for primary site and persistent nodal disease after radiation therapy compared with spin echo MR imaging or PET.[23,35–37] Clinical studies on the efficacy of ADC for prediction or early detection of treatment response have been reported for brain tumor,[30] breast cancer,[38] and cervical cancer.[39]

Kim and colleagues[35] compared the pretreatment ADC values with treatment outcome and noted that patients who responded favorably to chemoradiation therapy had significantly lower pretreatment ADC than partial responders or nonresponders. The pretreatment ADC values of complete responders ($1.04 \pm 0.19 \times 10^{-3}$ mm^2/s) were significantly lower than those from partial responders ($1.35 \pm 0.30 \times 10^{-3}$ mm^2/s). In complete responders significant increase in ADC was observed within 1 week of treatment, which continued until the end of treatment. Furthermore, a significantly larger increase in ADC values was found in complete responders compared with partial responders by the first week of chemoradiation. The ADC values were measured in the metastatic lymph nodes and not on the primary site, which would be more challenging and also more helpful for daily decision making in clinical routine.

The change in ADC values after the first week of chemoradiation therapy, compared with the pretreatment value, showed the highest test accuracy along with a high sensitivity and specificity of separating complete responders from partial responders, suggesting that ADC can be used as a predictive biomarker for therapeutic response in head and neck cancer and can thus aid in guiding therapeutic options for the patients.

Vandecaveye and colleagues[40] also evaluated the predictive value of the diffusion imaging during chemoradiotherapy for head and neck cancer, by calculating ADC and tumor volume changes between baseline, and 2 and 4 weeks' follow-up and comparing them with recurrence versus complete remission after treatment. These investigators concluded that the ADC changes correlated better with the 2-year tumor outcome after treatment than tumor volume changes and noted that tumoral lesions with complete response to treatment showed significantly higher changes in ADC than tumoral lesions that recurred, relating the ADC increase to the disorganized microstructure in necrosis and the apoptosis in response to cytotoxic and radiation treatment. Absent ADC

increase during chemoradiotherapy corresponded to lesions with a high likelihood of recurrence after treatment, probably correlating with diffusion restriction in the dense microstructure of persistent malignancy.

SUMMARY

High-field MR imaging for head and neck malignancy plays a crucial role in diagnosing, staging, and following the treatment outcome of head and neck cancers, allowing imaging with higher resolution or shorter time, differentiating benign from malignant primary malignancy, detecting regional metastatic lymph nodes, and monitoring and predicting the response of the tumor to established treatment.

REFERENCES

1. Willinek WA, Kuhl CK. 3.0 T neuroimaging: technical considerations and clinical applications. Neuroimaging Clin North Am 2006;16(2):217–28.
2. Aygun N, Zinreich SJ. Head and neck imaging at 3 T. Magn Reson Imaging Clin North Am 2006;14(1):89–95.
3. Tanenbaum LN. Clinical 3T MR imaging: mastering the challenges. Magn Reson Imaging Clin North Am 2006;14(1):1–15.
4. Srinivasan A, Dvorak R, Perni K, et al. Differentiation of benign and malignant pathology in the head and neck using 3T apparent diffusion coefficient values: early experience. AJNR Am J Neuroradiol 2008;29:40–4.
5. Wang J, Takashima S, Takayama F, et al. Head and neck lesions: characterization with diffusion-weighted echo-planar MR imaging. Radiology 2001;220:621–30.
6. Schafer J, Srinivasan A, Mukherji S. Diffusion magnetic resonance imaging in the head and neck. Magn Reson Imaging Clin North Am 2011;19(1):55–67.
7. Srinivasan A, Galbán CJ, Johnson TD, et al. Utility of the k-means clustering algorithm in differentiating apparent diffusion coefficient values of benign and malignant neck pathologies. AJNR Am J Neuroradiol 2010;31(4):736–40.
8. Maeda M, Kato H, Sakuma H, et al. Usefulness of the apparent diffusion coefficient in line scan diffusion-weighted imaging for distinguishing between squamous cell carcinomas and malignant lymphomas of the head and neck. AJNR Am J Neuroradiol 2005;26:1186–92.
9. Razek AA, Elsorogy LG, Soliman NY, et al. Dynamic susceptibility contrast perfusion MR imaging in distinguishing malignant from benign head and neck tumors: a pilot study. Eur J Radiol 2011;77(1):73–9.

10. Curtin HD, Ishwaran H, Mancuso AA, et al. Comparison of CT and MR imaging in staging of neck metastases. Radiology 1998;207(1):123–30.

11. Sumi M, Ichikawa Y, Katayama I, et al. Diffusion-weighted MR imaging of ameloblastomas and keratocystic odontogenic tumors: differentiation by apparent diffusion coefficients of cystic lesions. AJNR Am J Neuroradiol 2008;29(10):1897–901.

12. Vandecaveye V, De Keyzer F, Vander Poor ten V, et al. Head and neck squamous cell carcinoma: value of diffusion-weighted MR imaging for nodal staging. Radiology 2009;251(1):134–46.

13. Perrone A, Guerrisi P, Izzo L, et al. Diffusion-weighted MRI in cervical lymph nodes: differentiation between benign and malignant lesions. Eur J Radiol 2011;77(2):281–6.

14. Holzapfel K, Duetsch S, Fauser C, et al. Value of diffusion-weighted MR imaging in the differentiation between benign and malignant cervical lymph nodes. Eur J Radiol 2009;72(3):381–7.

15. de Bondt RB, Hoeberigs MC, Nelemans PJ, et al. Diagnostic accuracy and additional value of diffusion-weighted imaging for discrimination of malignant cervical lymph nodes in head and neck squamous cell carcinoma. Neuroradiology 2009; 51(3):183–92.

16. Abdel Razek A, Mossad A, Ghonim M. Role of diffusion-weighted MR imaging in assessing malignant versus benign skull-base lesions. Radiol Med 2011;116(1):125–32.

17. Dirix P, Vandecaveye V, De Keyzer F, et al. Diffusion-weighted MRI for nodal staging of head and neck squamous cell carcinoma: impact on radiotherapy planning. Int J Radiat Oncol Biol Phys 2010;76(3): 761–6.

18. Fischbein NJ, Noworolski SM, Henry RG, et al. Assessment of metastatic cervical adenopathy using dynamic contrast-enhanced MR imaging. AJNR Am J Neuroradiol 2003;24(3):301–11.

19. Vaupel P. Tumor blood flow. In: Molls M, Vaupel P, editors. Blood perfusion and microenvironment of human tumors. Berlin: Springer-Verlag; 1998. p. 43.

20. Milosevic MF, Fyles AW, Hill RP. The relationship between elevated interstitial fluid pressure and blood flow in tumors: a bioengineering analysis. Int J Radiat Oncol Biol Phys 1999;43(5):1111–23.

21. Rutz HP. A biophysical basis of enhanced interstitial fluid pressure in tumors. Med Hypotheses 1999; 53(6):526–9.

22. Abdel Razek AA, Gaballa G. Role of perfusion magnetic resonance imaging in cervical lymphadenopathy. J Comput Assist Tomogr 2011;35(1): 21–5.

23. Vandecaveye V, De Keyzer F, Nuyts S, et al. Detection of head and neck squamous cell carcinoma with diffusion weighted MRI after (chemo) radiotherapy: correlation between radiologic and histopathologic findings. Int J Radiat Oncol Biol Phys 2007;67(4): 960–71.

24. Fu KK, Pajak TJ, Trotti A, et al. A phase III randomized study to compare hyper fractionation and two variants of accelerated fractionation to standard fractionation therapy for head and neck squamous cell carcinomas: first report of RTOG 9003. Int J Radiat Oncol Biol Phys 2000;48:7–16.

25. Budach W, Hehr T, Budach V, et al. A meta-analysis of hyperfractionated and accelerated radiotherapy and combined chemotherapy and radiotherapy regimens in unresected locally advanced squamous cell carcinoma of the head and neck. BMC Cancer 2006;6:28.

26. Yom SS, Machtay M, Biel MA, et al. Survival impact of planned restaging and early surgical salvage following definitive chemoradiation for locally advanced squamous cell carcinomas of the oropharynx and hypopharynx. Am J Clin Oncol 2005;28:385–92.

27. Nomayr A, Lell M, Sweeney R, et al. MRI appearance of radiation-induced changes of normal cervical tissues. Eur Radiol 2001;11:1807–17.

28. Fukui MB, Blodgett TM, Snyderman CH, et al. Combined PET-CT in the head and neck: part 2. Diagnostic uses and pitfalls of oncologic imaging. Radiographics 2005;25:913–30.

29. Herneth AM, Guccione S, Bednarski M. Apparent diffusion coefficient: a quantitative parameter for in vivo tumor characterization. Eur J Radiol 2003;45:208–13.

30. Moffat BA, Chenevert TL, Lawrence TS, et al. Functional diffusion map: a noninvasive MRI biomarker for early stratification of clinical brain tumor response. Proc Natl Acad Sci U S A 2005;102: 5524–9.

31. Galbán S, Brisset JC, Rehemtulla A, et al. Diffusion-weighted MRI for assessment of early cancer treatment response. Curr Pharm Biotechnol 2010;11(6): 701–8.

32. Vandecaveye V, de Keyzer F, Vander Poorten V, et al. Evaluation of the larynx for tumour recurrence by diffusion-weighted MRI after radiotherapy: initial experience in four cases. Br J Radiol 2006; 79(944):681–7.

33. Taouli B, Vilgrain V, Dumont E, et al. Evaluation of liver diffusion isotropy and characterization of focal hepatic lesions with two single-shot echo-planar MR imaging sequences: prospective study in 66 patients. Radiology 2003;226:71–81.

34. Hein PA, Kremser C, Judmaier W, et al. Diffusion-weighted magnetic resonance imaging for monitoring diffusion changes in rectal carcinoma during combined, preoperative chemoradiation: preliminary results of a prospective study. Eur J Radiol 2003;45:214–22.

35. Kim S, Loevner L, Quon H, et al. Diffusion-weighted magnetic resonance imaging for predicting and

detecting early response to chemoradiation therapy of squamous cell carcinomas of the head and neck. Clin Cancer Res 2009;15(3):986–94.

36. Chenevert TL, McKeever PE, Ross BD. Monitoring early response of experimental brain tumors to therapy using diffusion magnetic resonance imaging. Clin Cancer Res 1997;3:1457–66.

37. Galons JP, Altbach MI, Paine-Murrieta GD, et al. Early increases in breast tumor xenograft water mobility in response to paclitaxel therapy detected by non-invasive diffusion magnetic resonance imaging. Neoplasia (New York) 1999;1:113–7.

38. Lee KC, Moffat BA, Schott AF, et al. Prospective early response imaging biomarker for neoadjuvant breast cancer chemotherapy. Clin Cancer Res 2007;13:443–50.

39. McVeigh PZ, Syed AM, Milosevic M, et al. Diffusion-weighted MRI in cervical cancer. Eur Radiol 2008; 18:1058–64.

40. Vandecaveye V, Dirix P, De Keyzer F, et al. Predictive value of diffusion-weighted magnetic resonance imaging during chemoradiotherapy for head and neck squamous cell carcinoma. Eur Radiol 2010; 20(7):1703–14.

Pediatric High-Field Magnetic Resonance Imaging

Hisham M. Dahmoush, MBBCh, FRCR,
Arastoo Vossough, PhD, MD, Timothy P.L. Roberts, PhD*

KEYWORDS

- Magnetic resonance imaging • High-field
- Pediatric neuroradiology • 3 Tesla

Key Points

- Most of the added value of using high-field 3 T magnetic resonance imaging derives from being able to take advantage of the spatial and temporal benefits of multichannel coil technology and parallel imaging without unacceptable signal loss.

- Increased spatial resolution is highly desirable or sometimes necessary in pediatrics to delineate small structures and subtle disease especially in younger children, and 3 T high-field imaging can be effectively used toward this goal.

- Using the advantages of high-field 3 T imaging in achieving faster scan times can help reduce the need for sedation or anesthesia, although in practice the signal gain of 3 T high-field imaging is more commonly exploited to increase spatial resolution and image quality than to decrease scan time.

The introduction of 3 T magnetic resonance (MR) imaging systems in clinical practice a decade ago brought about great excitement in neuroradiology. The use of higher magnetic field strengths in daily practice provided the potential for improving image quality and offering exquisite details that would facilitate diagnosis of numerous problematic clinical scenarios. On the other hand, the expected challenges facing the radiological community was based on extensive previous research, in which it had become evident that factors such as altered T1 contrast, increased susceptibility, and safety issues related to specific absorption rate (SAR) would have an impact on how to perform our clinical scans. The same general challenges inherent to 3 T MR imaging are applicable to pediatric imaging as well,[1-3] and in some cases,

especially so. These issues are sometimes further complicated with the inherent difficulties related to MR imaging of young children regardless of magnetic field strength. Modification of certain sequence parameters was mandatory to avoid SAR limits and still provide images of adequate quality. The concomitant advances that occurred in coil technology further mitigated those challenges. In particular, parallel imaging (PI) and multichannel (32) head coils facilitated faster scanning times and improved signal-to-noise ratio (SNR).

This review addresses basic considerations for pediatric neuroimaging at 3 T MR imaging, highlights the many advantages of scanning at higher magnetic fields, and evaluates the impact of 3 T MR imaging on the clinical practice of pediatric neuroradiology, as well as pointing out the

---

Neuroradiology Section, Department of Radiology, Children's Hospital of Philadelphia, Wood 2115, 324 South 34th Street, Philadelphia, PA 19104, USA
* Corresponding author.
E-mail address: robertstim@email.chop.edu

Neuroimag Clin N Am 22 (2012) 297–313
doi:10.1016/j.nic.2012.02.009
1052-5149/12/$ – see front matter © 2012 Elsevier Inc. All rights reserved.

Diagnostic Checklist

- Many medical devices that have been declared safe for use on 1.5 T systems may not be safe using higher field magnets.
- The need for a smaller field of view (FOV) in pediatric imaging results in decreased signal-to-noise ratio (SNR). The increased SNR associated with the use of 3 T magnetic resonance (MR) imaging compensates for the loss of SNR and allows small FOV imaging with adequate image quality.
- The small head of the child should be placed in the center of the FOV when using multielement head coils to decrease image intensity inhomogeneity or shading.
- Specific absorption rate limits have to be taken into consideration when scanning children, particularly small infants who are kept warm in the scanner.
- Susceptibility effects are increased at 3 T. Modification of imaging techniques may be necessary to reduce susceptibility in patients, especially those with metallic implant and devices.
- The smaller FOV and better SNR makes 3 T favored for delineating small parts such as the temporomandibular joints, inner ear structures, and cranial nerves.
- In patients with epilepsy, the higher spatial resolution possible with the improved SNR makes 3 T imaging favored for detecting small malformations and epileptogenic foci.
- The improved contrast-to-noise ratio and SNR provide better details in MR angiography.
- Stronger chemical shifts, increased SNR, and higher order shimming allow for improved spectral quality in MR spectroscopy.
- High-field imaging allows more robust arterial spin labeling perfusion imaging in the assessment of cerebral blood flow without the need for intravenous contrast administration.
- Optimization of 3 T imaging of the pediatric spine (particularly T1-weighted images) is necessary to provide adequate image quality.

difficulties and opportunities faced during day-to-day clinical work.

PRINCIPLES OF HIGH-FIELD 3 T IMAGING AS APPLIED TO PEDIATRICS

Applying a higher magnetic field strength increases longitudinal magnetization and results in improvement of SNR.[4] MR signal increases by a factor of 4 at 3 T compared with 1.5 T, but the noise also increases by a factor of 2.[5] This situation should theoretically double the SNR at 3 T compared with 1.5 T, but, in practice, the SNR increase is mostly less than double.[6–8] A combination of factors including sequence modifications as a result of SAR limits, coil design, B_0 and B_1 inhomogeneity, and certain imaging parameter alterations for maintaining good image contrast result in an SNR that is less than this promised factor of 2.[2,9] For example, if the repetition time (TR) in a spin echo sequence is kept constant despite the longer T1 relaxation times of tissue at 3 T (see subsequent section), there is a T1-weighting reduction in SNR, confounding the increase derived from field strength. Increasing the TR to compensate for the longer T1 increases the acquisition time.[2] The use of higher receiver bandwidth to reduce susceptibility effects also contributes to loss of SNR.

The SNR increase (even if <2 times) can be invested to substantially increase the spatial resolution, yielding better depiction of anatomic structures,[7] and in turn, in principle, increase diagnostic confidence. Thinner slices can be acquired to improve spatial details of subtle abnormalities and small structures.[2] Imaging of small structures is more problematic in children than in adults, especially in neonates and very young children. The better detail in brain lesions becomes relevant in malformations of cortical development, which can be challenging to diagnose and classify (**Fig. 1**). The higher signal can also facilitate high-resolution imaging of small fluid-filled intracranial structures such as the inner ear and internal auditory canal (IAC). The higher resolution provides increased confidence in making diagnoses such as absence or thinning of cranial nerves, for example those within the IAC (**Fig. 2**). The introduction of multichannel head coils has for the most part obviated use of small surface coils. The combination of high magnetic field and multichannel coils allows exquisite imaging of small articulations, which is exemplified in evaluations of the temporomandibular joints (**Fig. 3**).

The SNR increase can alternatively be used to increase the temporal resolution, facilitated by reducing the number of needed averages to obtain

Pediatric brain 3 T MR imaging protocol at the Children's Hospital of Philadelphia (Siemens)

Routine Sequences[a]

T1 MPRAGE–sagittal 0.9-mm isotropic voxels reformatted into orthogonal planes

Axial two-dimensional (2D) turbo spin echo T2–2-mm thickness–384 × 384 matrix

Axial 2D FLAIR–4-mm thickness–320 × 320 matrix

Axial spin echo T1–4-mm thickness–256 × 256 matrix

Pulsed arterial spin labeling perfusion–8-mm thickness–64 × 64 matrix

Coronal or sagittal 2D fast spin echo T2–2-mm thickness–384 × 384 matrix–orientation depending on indication and if performed as part of a contrast brain study, performed immediately after gadolinium contrast injection

Diffusion–30 directions–2.5-mm thickness–128 × 128 matrix–b = 1000

[a] Most are performed with GRAPPA (generalized autocalibrating partially parallel acquisition) 2 parallel acceleration.

Optional Sequences Depending on Indication

Coronal 2D FLAIR–4-mm–320 × 320 matrix

MRA–3D TOF–0.5-m isotropic voxels

MRV–2D TOF–both axial and coronal acquisitions–3-mm thickness–256 × 256 matrix

GRE susceptibility–4-mm thickness–256 × 256 matrix

SWI–2-mm thickness–320 × 320 matrix

CISS–0.5-mm thickness–256 × 256 matrix–small FOV

Repeat T1 MPRAGE after contrast with same parameters as above, reconstructed in orthogonal planes

Repeat SE T1 after contrast with same parameters as above (patients receive both T1 MPRAGE and SE T1 after contrast)

Abbreviation: MRV, magnetic resonance venography.

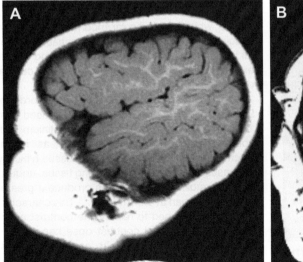 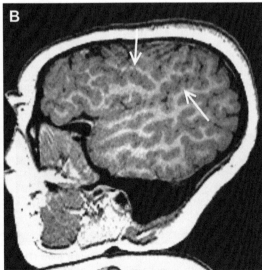

Fig. 1. Malformation of cortical development and polymicrogyria at different field strengths. Sagittal T1-weighted images of the brain at 1.5 T (*A*) are compared with 3 T (*B*). There is perisylvian and frontal polymicrogyria with small irregular gyri with lumpy gray-white junction, which is readily detectable on the higher-resolution and contrast 3 T image (*arrows*), but which is difficult to identify on the 1.5 T T1-weighted image. The polymicrogyria had not been fully appreciated until the 3 T scan.

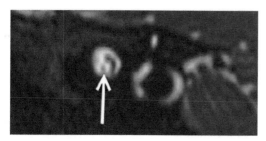

Fig. 2. Cochlear nerve hypoplasia in a young boy with unilateral sensorineural hearing loss. Sagittal oblique reformation high-resolution three-dimensional T2-weighted image through the IAC identifying a cochlear nerve (*arrow*), which is smaller and brighter than the facial nerve, consistent with nerve hypoplasia.

a good-quality image. Theoretically, an SNR advantage of times 2 can be traded for up to a 4-fold increase in temporal resolution. By doing so, the acquisition time can be reduced and the same spatial resolution maintained.[7] This situation is useful in children, who are typically more anxious and distracted, and hence move more frequently than adults during MR imaging examinations. The improved temporal resolution at higher magnetic field strengths coupled with motion-insensitive or motion-compensated sequences (eg, PROPELLER [periodically rotated overlapping parallel lines with enhanced reconstruction] and BLADE) contribute to the reduction of studies requiring pharmaceutical sedation.[10] Sedation has to be performed by trained personnel, requires

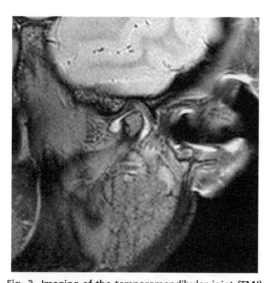

Fig. 3. Imaging of the temporomandibular joint (TMJ) in a patient with juvenile idiopathic arthritis at 3 T. Sagittal oblique proton density of the right TMJ showed the anatomic details in exquisite detail, including the meniscus, joint effusion, and small erosions. This image was obtained with the use of a standard 32-channel head coil and without dedicated surface coils.

MR-compatible equipment for monitoring and rescue (if needed), is time-consuming, and carries potential inherent risks, particularly respiratory depression (albeit an uncommon occurrence).[11,12]

Many of the clinical applications that were made possible by high-field imaging at 3 T are dependent on the ability to either generate images with better spatial resolution or perform quicker studies and maintain adequate spatial resolution. In our experience, and especially for the smaller field of view (FOV) required for pediatric applications, often the former is true and the increased signal is more commonly exploited to acquire higher spatial resolution images.

T1 relaxation times increase with increasing field strength, whereas the absolute differences between tissue T1 values become smaller. Therefore, the overall T1 contrast between tissues tends to decrease at higher magnetic fields (Fig. 4). However, because the SNR is improved at higher magnetic fields, the contrast-to-noise ratio (CNR) is typically higher.[13] The decreased T1-weighted contrast can be overcome by sequence change, for example using inversion recovery fast-segmented gradient sequences such as three-dimensional (3D) magneti-zation-prepared gradient echo (MPRAGE) and 3D fast magnetization-prepared spoiled gradient echo instead of spin echo sequences (see Fig. 4). These sequences offer superb gray-white matter contrast and have the additional advantage of being a 3D acquisition, which can be easily acquired in an isotropic or near isotropic fashion and later reformat-ted into any desired plane. The latter advantage can be helpful in reducing overall scanning times (by eliminating extra sequences showing different planes), which is of particular importance in pediatric imaging. The sharp gray-white differentiation is help-ful in identifying subtle areas or delineating the full extent of malformations, such as those of cortical development.

The T1 of many tissues increases in the order of 20% to 50% as the field strength is increased from 1.5 T to 3 T. The T1 of chelated gadolinium (Gd) contrast agents does not increase as much. Because the T1 of the unenhanced tissue typically increases more than the enhancing tissue, equiva-lent doses of Gd chelate often produce a greater effect at 3 T than at 1.5 T (Fig. 5).[14] This character-istic has been used to reduce the contrast agent dose.[15] The reduced contrast dose has obvious favorable financial and health care implications. Shapiro[16] compared the conspicuity of enhancing lesions on T1 fast spin echo with fast spoiled gra-dient recalled (FSPGR). Although most lesions were well delineated on both sequences, they varied in conspicuity. Furthermore, some lesions were identified on one but not the other sequence.

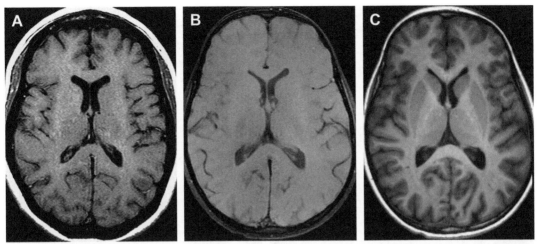

Fig. 4. Differences in T1 contrast between gray and white matter using different magnetic field strengths and pulse sequences. (*A*) T1-weighted spin echo axial MR image without fat suppression or magnetization transfer on a 1.5 T magnet showing modest contrast between gray and white matter. (*B*) T1-weighted spin echo axial MR image with fat suppression on a 3 T magnet showing poor T1 contrast between gray and white matter. (*C*) MPRAGE axial T1 MR image showing superb T1 gray-white matter contrast.

Our experience is mostly in agreement with these data, although we sometimes note better lesion conspicuity on T1 spin echo sequences compared with the higher-resolution T1 MPRAGE sequences, even considering differences in timing between contrast injection and image acquisition (**Fig. 6**). However, the reformation of thin slices while maintaining good image quality made possible by 3D volumetric acquisitions may allow better identification of the internal architecture of enhancing lesions on MPRAGE aiding in diagnosis (**Fig. 7**). Similar to Shapiro, at time of writing, we tend to acquire both sequences after contrast administration, which results in lengthening of the scanning session.

The intrinsic magnetization transfer (MT) effect associated with multislice (with other slices serving as off-resonance excitation) acquisitions can be used in pediatric neuroimaging at higher magnetic field strengths. In our experience, dysplastic lesions such as cortical dysplasia and tubers associated with tuberous sclerosis (TS) often show MT effect, which increases the

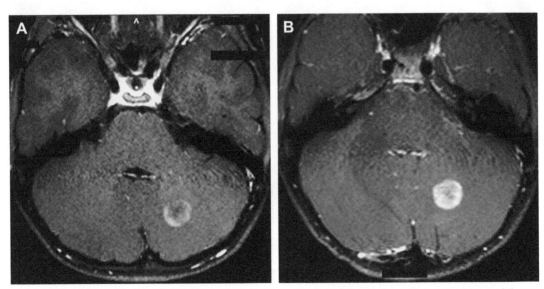

Fig. 5. Left cerebellar enhancing lesion (presumably a glioma) in a patient with neurofibromatosis type I. (*A*) At 1.5 T, peripheral enhancement is noted in the lesion 3.5 minutes after contrast injection. (*B*) At 3 T, more homogeneous and avid enhancement is seen 2.25 minutes after injection. (*From* Zimmerman RA, Bilaniuk LT, Pollock AN, et al. 3.0 T versus 1.5 T pediatric brain imaging. Neuroimaging Clin North Am 2006;16(2):233; with permission.)

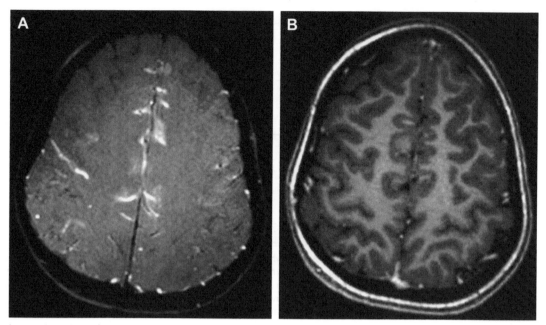

Fig. 6. Disseminated supratentorial leptomeningeal metastases in a patient with brainstem glioma. (*A*) Extensive avid leptomeningeal enhancement within the sulci is well seen on a postcontrast spin echo T1-weighted image. (*B*) However, on the postcontrast T1 MPRAGE sequence, only subtle leptomeningeal enhancement is visualized.

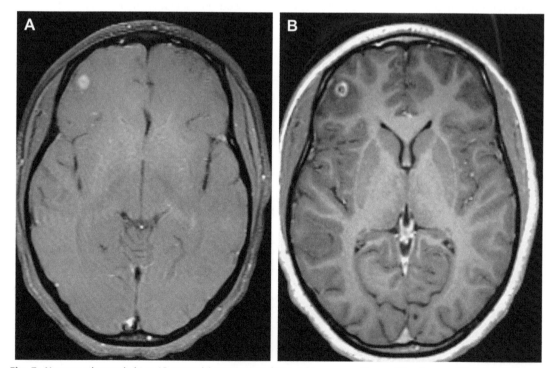

Fig. 7. Neurocysticercosis in a 13-year-old immigrant from Africa presenting with seizures. (*A*) Fairly homogeneous solid enhancement identified in the right frontal lobe on a postcontrast spin echo T1-weighted image. (*B*) Rim-enhancement and a marginal nodule (scolex) are appreciated on thin-section postcontrast MPRAGE T1-weighted image, in keeping with the colloidal vesicular stage of neurocysticercosis.

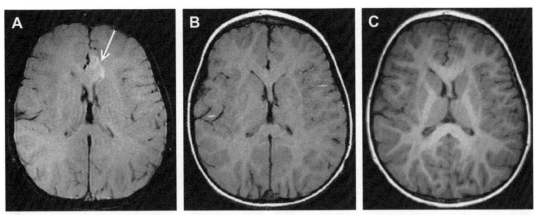

Fig. 8. Left medial frontal focal cortical dysplasia at 3 T. (*A*) Spin echo T1-weighted 3 T image with fat suppression and without magnetization transfer pulse shows high signal intensity in the medial frontal cortex and subcortical white matter (*arrow*), enabling easy detection of the abnormality. (*B*) Spin echo T1-weighted 1.5 T image without fat suppression or magnetization transfer pulse is unremarkable. (*C*) MPRAGE 3 T image showing only subtle blurring of the gray-white matter junction at this location.

detectability and allows for more confident diagnosis of focal cortical dysplasia (**Fig. 8**) and aids in accurate estimation of the lesion burden in TS (**Fig. 9**). However, if a discrete MT pulse is inadvertently applied to the T1-weighted sequences, many normal structures such as the basal ganglia and parts of the cortex may seem to have abnormal high signal, which could lead to false diagnoses (**Fig. 10**).

DIFFUSION IMAGING

The improved SNR at 3 T makes the use of higher b-values, thinner slices, and (without the need for signal averaging) larger number of diffusion-encoding directions practically possible. This situation results in better quality of diffusion imaging.[2] The inherent sensitivity to susceptibility artifacts in echo-planar imaging (EPI) (which is typically used in diffusion imaging) at 3 T poses a problem by causing image distortion and blurring. These detrimental effects can be partially remedied by the implementation of PI. PI reduces magnetic susceptibility effects and decreases the number of phase encoding steps, shortens the echo train length, and consequently diminishes the effective echo time (TE), making diffusion imaging less sensitive to motion, distortion, and blurring.[17] The result is increased lesion conspicuity and consequently better image quality.[17–19] Despite the reduction of SNR intrinsic to PI, its use on a 3 T system still generates more SNR than similar sequences performed without PI on

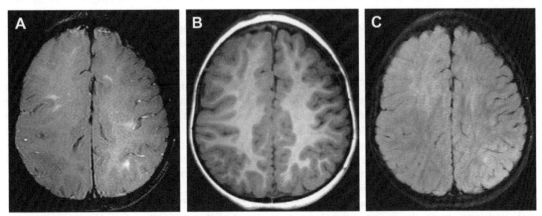

Fig. 9. Parenchymal tubers in TS. (*A*) Spin echo T1-weighted image with fat suppression and without MT shows multiple cortical tubers of high signal with excellent lesion conspicuity, some of which are seen to extend into the white matter toward the ventricles. (*B*) MPRAGE image shows only subtle signal abnormalities in the same regions. (*C*) Fluid-attenuated inversion recovery image shows some of the tubers, but many lesions are inconspicuous.

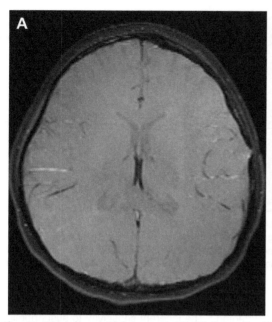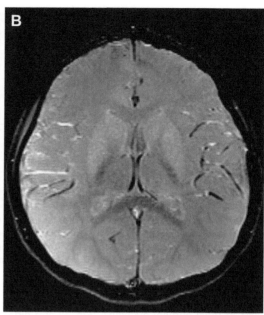

Fig. 10. MT pulse on T1 images at 3 T. (*A*) Spin echo T1 with fat suppression and without MT pulse. Note the expected poor gray-white matter contrast at 3 T. (*B*) Spin echo T1 with fat suppression and MT pulse applied. The normal gray matter structures (particularly the basal ganglia and thalami) show apparent increased signal, which may lead to false diagnoses.

1.5 T magnets. (SNR varies linearly with field and is reduced only by the square root of 2 by using PI with a factor of 2.) In addition, diffusion tensor imaging (DTI) measurements at 3 T are more accurate than 1.5 T,[20] benefiting from reduced distortion and shortened TE (increased SNR, less T2-weighting), DTI quality is improved, and white matter fiber tracking is easier to obtain.[5] This situation helps evaluate the relationship of tumors to the adjacent white matter tracts more accurately, which can play a role in surgical planning. It can also aid in the evaluation of certain brain abnormalities (eg, absence of the decussating fibers of the superior cerebellar peduncles in Joubert syndrome) (**Fig. 11**).[21]

ARTERIAL SPIN LABELING PERFUSION

Arterial spin labeling (ASL) perfusion imaging is based on magnetic tagging of arterial blood water protons, which are used as an endogenous tracer of flow.[22] This technique allows the quantification of cerebral blood flow (CBF). The fact that ASL does not require the rapid injection of intravenous contrast as opposed to Gd (Gd-diethylenetriaminepentacetate)-based dynamic susceptibility contrast perfusion methods is an advantage in younger children, given the potential difficulties associated with obtaining good intravenous access. An additional advantage is that if the patient moves during the acquisition, something that

commonly occurs in pediatric MR imaging, the ASL sequences can be immediately repeated, whereas this is not immediately possible in Gd-based methods (because the presence of previously administered Gd contrast agent contaminates subsequent signal assessments).

ASL imaging greatly benefits from the use of high-field imaging. This benefit is not merely because of the intrinsically increased SNR. The transit time for the flow of blood from the tagged region to the imaging slices is comparable with the T1 of the blood.[23] The longer T1 of blood at higher fields increases the lifetime of tagged blood, allowing for more robust ASL imaging, especially in cases of slower flow or delayed arterial transit.[7] Both prolonged T1 times and intrinsic SNR increase factors contribute to the increased CNR in clinical ASL perfusion at 3 T[24] compared with 1.5 T. Practically, these advantages can be considered as enabling for the technology. The improvements in the quality of ASL perfusion in some children compared with adults can be attributed to combined effects of shorter transit time allowing faster delivery of the tagged blood to the imaging slices, increased blood water signal, higher baseline CBF, and longer T1 relaxation time in the pediatric population.[25,26] However, there are limitations associated with ASL. It provides only CBF information as opposed to other perfusion parameters (such as cerebral blood volume [CBV] or vascular permeability). Furthermore, it is

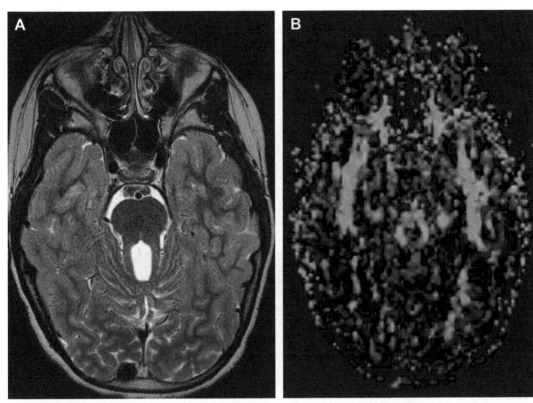

Fig. 11. Patient with clinical manifestations of Joubert syndrome. (A) Axial T2-weighted image showing the classic molar tooth appearance of the brainstem and superior cerebellar peduncles. (B) Axial DTI shows absence of the normal decussation (absent red transverse crossing fibers) of the superior cerebellar peduncles.

sensitive to motion because it relies on image subtraction, which becomes more problematic in children, who are often less cooperative in staying motionless for MR imaging. From a clinical standpoint, this motion problem remains a challenge despite the use of motion correction techniques.

The assessment of brain perfusion in children without the need for contrast injection can play a role in many diseases. Evaluation of brain perfusion in patients with moyamoya disease may potentially identify tissues that are most affected, and the hope is that this may contribute to the process of stratifying patients who may benefit from revascularization surgery. Many vasculopathies that involve the intracranial arteries (eg, sickle cell disease) also have altered perfusion patterns, which can be demonstrated noninvasively (Fig. 12). Strouse and colleagues[27] found an inverse relationship between IQ and CBF in patients with sickle cell disease before detectability of abnormalities with transcranial Doppler or conventional MR imaging. Similar to in adults, ASL may show the tissue at risk after an ischemic stroke. In children who present with symptoms concerning for ischemic stroke but who display no abnormalities on

diffusion-weighted imaging, alterations in cerebral perfusion may suggest alternative diagnoses such as complicated migraine or a vasoconstrictive syndrome. A rough estimate of the vascularity of the tumors can also be obtained. CBV measurements are not easily obtainable with this technique, in this application in particular, in contrast to Gd-based perfusion.

SUSCEPTIBILITY AT HIGH-FIELD

The effective transverse relaxation rate R2* (=1/T2*) describes the susceptibility-induced gradient-echo signal loss and it greatly increases at higher magnetic fields.[6] Although this situation can result in artifacts (signal mismapping or geometric distortions) and lead to challenging imaging situations, it can also be advantageous in the detection of iron, blood products, and mineralization in a variety of pulse sequences and applications (Fig. 13).[18] Artifacts are most frequently encountered in pediatric neuroimaging with orthodontic devices, spinal fusion hardware, programmable ventriculoperitoneal shunts, and at air-tissue interfaces (particularly in the frontal regions and skull base). They are most

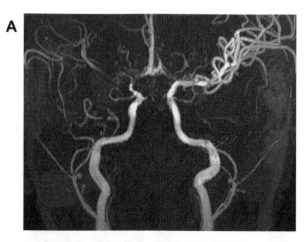

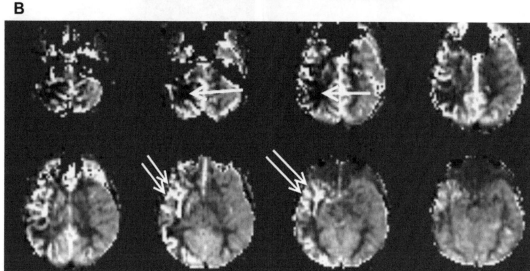

Fig. 12. Perfusion changes in the right cerebral hemisphere (predominantly in the territory of the middle cerebral artery) in a patient with known arteriopathy caused by sickle cell disease. (A) Maximum intensity projection TOF MRA shows severe narrowing/occlusion of the distal right internal carotid artery and the A1 and M1 segments of the anterior and middle cerebral arteries. (B) ASL perfusion CBF map shows superficial high signal intensity (*double arrows*) attributed to tagged blood, which remains within the vasculature because of delayed transit time and underlying low parenchymal signal intensity (*single arrows*).

pronounced on susceptibility-weighted imaging (SWI), gradient echo sequences (GRE), and EPI acquisitions such as functional MR (fMR) imaging, diffusion-weighted imaging, and ASL. Manipulations that can reduce susceptibility artifacts include the use of higher receiver bandwidth, shorter TE, PI to reduce the echo train length, and decreasing the voxel size, although each of these modifications can have its own disadvantages.[7,28,29]

SWI is more sensitive in detection of susceptibility effects than conventional GRE sequences, by incorporating signal loss as well as phase information.[30] SWI has been shown to be extremely sensitive for detection of paramagnetic and diamagnetic substances and to offer additional

information over and above routine imaging sequences for the evaluation of neurodegenerative diseases, trauma, cerebrovascular disorders, intracranial hemorrhage, and calcification and has rapidly expanding applications in other brain diseases (Fig. 14).[31] Because susceptibility effects increase at 3 T, more lesions are appreciated at 3 T compared with 1.5 T on SWI, and just like other sequences, higher-resolution images can be obtained at 3 T. Although the increased detection of lesions is an obvious advantage, the clinical significance and prognostic value of some of these tiny lesions remain uncertain.

Venous blood has higher T2* effect compared with arteries because of the higher concentration

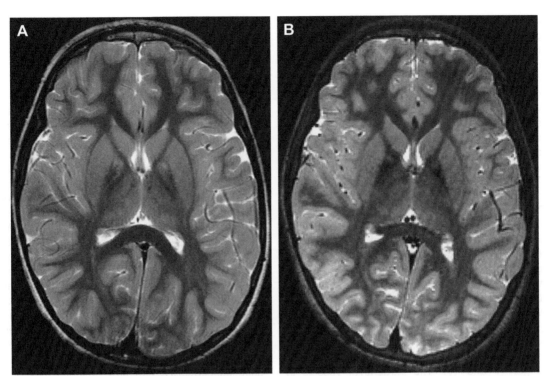

Fig. 13. Panthonate kinase-associated neurodegeneration (PKAN) at 1.5 T and 3 T imaging. (*A*) Axial T2-weighted image on a 1.5 T magnet shows faint bilateral and symmetric T2 prolongation the globi pallid, which are diagnostically nonspecific. (*B*) Axial T2-weighted image on a 3 T magnet identifies T2 shortening in the globi pallidi around the central hyperintensities, giving the classic eye-of-the-tiger appearance of PKAN.

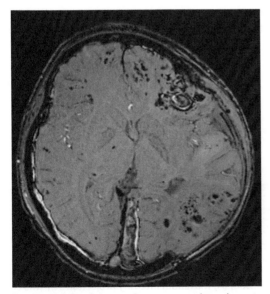

Fig. 14. Subdural hemorrhage, parenchymal contusion, and diffuse axonal injury in a teenager after a motor vehicle accident. SWI shows widespread small parenchymal hemorrhages at the gray-white matter junction, more focal blood products in the left frontal lobe superficially, as well as bilateral convexity and interhemispheric subdural blood.

of deoxyhemoglobin in veins. As a result, arteries and veins can be differentiated by SWI using a long TE. Use of minimum intensity projection enhances visualization of small venous structures.[32] These small vessels can be globally prominent in patients with chronic hypoxemia (congenital heart disease). The regional reduction in number of small veins suggests either local hyperperfusion with decreased deoxyhemoglobin content in the venous structures or focal gyral swelling with consequent compression of the veins. Prominence of medullary veins in noncardiac patients may suggest venous hypertension or medullary vein thrombosis. SWI also has the potential to differentiate hemorrhage from calcification on phase images in many cases.[31] The increased susceptibly enhances the blood oxygen level-dependent contrast at 3 T, resulting in more robust fMR imaging studies.[33]

MR ANGIOGRAPHY

The T1 relaxation time of background tissues increases, whereas the signal from inflowing blood is essentially T1-independent, resulting in increased CNR at 3 T on time-of-flight (TOF) MR angiography (MRA), through improved background suppression (T1-weighting). In addition, there is increased SNR at 3 T. Both these factors result in improvement of vessel-to-background contrast[6,34–36] and overall improvement in image quality. Overall, MRA at 3 T has promising results, with ability to perform imaging with increased spatial resolution, decreased scan time, and for contrast MRA studies, decreased amount of administered intravenous contrast agent.[37] Increased pulsatile flow artifact compared with 1.5 T may potentially degrade the image[35] but this can be overcome by using lower flip angles.[38] The larger vessels of the circle of Willis itself are marginally better visualized at 3 T; however, there is marked increase in SNR and visualization of first-order and second-order branches.[39] This greater ability of 3 T MRA in depicting small vessels also applies to more accurate delineation of areas of stenosis within the larger caliber native vessels. The superior image quality of MRA at 3 T provides more accurate information about the vasculature in pediatric arteriopathies such as sickle cell disease and moyamoya syndrome (Figs. 15 and 16). The intracranial vessels in neonatal and small infants are small and may carry turbulent flow. Therefore, 3 T MRA is particularly suited in evaluation of the intracranial vessels in this population.[40] The high spatial and temporal resolution achievable at 3 T has made high-resolution dynamic enhanced spinal MRA possible in children using 3D GRE. This technique allows diagnosis and initial evaluation of spinal dural arteriovenous fistulae and arteriovenous malformations without the invasiveness of catheter angiography.[41]

PEDIATRIC SPINE IMAGING

Imaging of the spine is particularly challenging at 3 T. The increased (and converging) T1 relaxation times reduce the apparent contrast resolution on T1-weighted images.[42] The increased cerebrospinal fluid (CSF) signal intensity decreases the contrast between the spinal cord and the surrounding CSF.[2] Although this situation can be partially improved by using sequences such as T1 fluid-attenuated inversion recovery (FLAIR), the contrast remains worse compared with 1.5 T.[42] In our experience, the poor T1 contrast is exaggerated in very small children. Furthermore, the appreciation of subtle areas of abnormal enhancement is less than what can be detected on 1.5 T magnets (Fig. 17). Although high-resolution 3 T spine imaging better shows smaller structures such as nerve roots and neural foramina, the larger number of artifacts (chemical shift, susceptibility, and flow artifacts) may obscure details.[2,14,16,42] Flow artifacts are also more pronounced in children because of the high pulsatile CSF flow.

MR SPECTROSCOPY

Many factors contribute to the advantages of performing MR spectroscopy at 3 T. The stronger

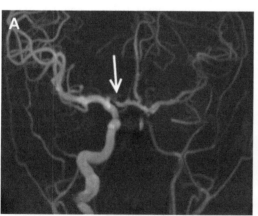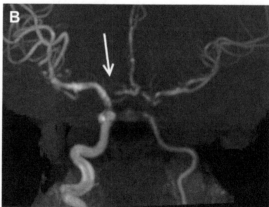

Fig. 15. Sickle cell disease arteriopathy and moyamoyalike vessels. (A) Maximum intensity projection TOF MRA at 3 T shows narrowing of the left internal carotid artery with severe stenosis/occlusion of its most distal segment, severe stenosis of the origin of the A1 segment of the right anterior cerebral artery, and decreased caliber of the M1 segment of the left middle cerebral artery. Also note prominent anterior communicating artery. (B) Maximum intensity projection TOF MRA at 1.5 T performed 2 years earlier shows similar changes; however, it overestimates the degree and extent of occlusion of the left internal carotid artery terminus and A1/M1 segments. MRA performed 2 years before (B) at 3 T showed identical vasculature to (A) (not shown). The collateral vessels on the right are also better seen at 3 T than at 1.5 T (arrow in A).

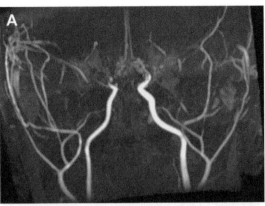

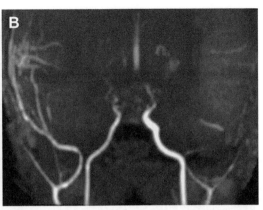

Fig. 16. Moyamoya syndrome with synangiosis surgery. (A) Maximum intensity projection TOF MRA at 3 T shows severe narrowing, leading to occlusion of the distal internal carotid arteries, A1 segments of the anterior cerebral arteries, and M1 segments of the middle cerebral arteries. Collateral vessels are seen around the occluded termination of the internal carotid arteries. Bilateral synangiosis are noted with more pronounced flow-related enhancement on the right. (B) Although these findings are redemonstrated on maximum intensity projection 1.5 T TOF MRA, more distal and smaller vessels are better identified on the 3 T image. Subsequent 3 T MRA 2 years after (B) showed similar vasculature to (A) (not shown).

chemical shift at higher fields increases the spread of individual peaks, resulting in improved spectral resolution and identification of metabolites that were mostly obscured at 1.5 T.[43] The improved SNR increases the signal derived from each metabolite, so the metabolite peaks are easier to differentiate from background noise (Fig. 18). The SNR gain is most pronounced at short TE, whereas long TEs are minimally affected because

T2 relaxation signal loss increases with increasing field. These factors allow the use of smaller voxels, which translates into an improved quantification of metabolites and decrease in the partial volume effect.[44] More recently, the wider availability of higher order shimming on high-field scanners has helped improve field homogeneity, reducing the peak width and increasing the peak height. The shorter echo sampling times can lead to significant

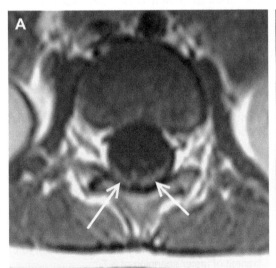

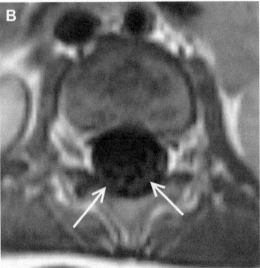

Fig. 17. Disseminated suprasellar pilocytic astrocytoma in a 4-year-old girl. (A) Axial spin echo T1-weighted image at the lower L1 level on a 1.5 T system clearly shows enhancement and thickening along the cauda equina roots (arrows). (B) Axial spin echo T1 FLAIR image at the same level on a 3 T system (A) shows barely discernable enhancement in the nerve roots (arrows). Similar enhancement to (A) was noted on a study performed 3 months before (B) (not shown).

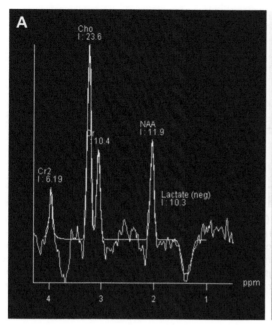
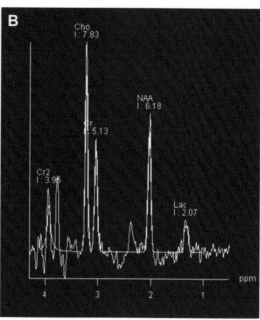

Fig. 18. Cytochrome C oxidase deficiency. (A) MRS with TE 144 milliseconds at 1.5 T shows the inverted lactate doublet at 1.3 ppm (B) MRS with TE 144 at 3 T shows lactate peak at 1.3 ppm, which is not inverted below the baseline. Note the better spectral separation and the decreased baseline noise at 3 T.

reduction in total scan time.[45] Faster scanning times are particularly helpful in the pediatric population.

The clinical use of spectroscopic data is perhaps more relevant in pediatric than adult neuroimaging. Many metabolic diseases typically present in childhood, and many have characteristic spectral peaks on MR spectroscopy, allowing the accurate diagnosis of such disorders.[46] Response to therapy can sometimes be evaluated by monitoring these peaks. Spectroscopic evaluation for lactate can help in appreciating the full extent of perinatal asphyxia[47] or contribute to the diagnosis of certain metabolic disorders[46] in the appropriate clinical setting. MR spectroscopy may help predict the neurologic outcome in premature babies because it allows assessment of the developing brain.[48] Similar to adult practice, spectroscopy can be used to characterize intracranial masses in children and assess the effects of therapy for brain tumors.

The increased chemical shift can sometimes be detrimental because it can cause misregistration, resulting in poor lactate inversion at intermediate TE values. This situation may make it difficult to separate lactate from lipid peaks. For this reason, we typically perform spectroscopy at short TE to detect abnormal metabolite levels that may be helpful in diagnosis of metabolic disorders and also at long TE because the lipid peak is neutralized with longer TE values to help bring out the lactate peak.

SAFETY ISSUES

SAR is a measure of energy deposition within the human body. By doubling the magnetic field strength, the SAR increases by a factor of 4.[8] Therefore, SAR becomes a practical problem with increasing field strength. Certain sequences are associated with higher SAR such as turbo spin echo, FLAIR, and sequences that use either very short TR such as CISS (constructive interference into steady state) and FIESTA (fast imaging employing steady state acquisition) or large flip angles.[8,49] Factors that can reduce SAR, but at the expense of decreased SNR, include PI and using variable flip angles.[50–52] Therefore it is possible to use these techniques and maintain acceptable signal. SAR can be further reduced by using transmit/receive array coils, by decreasing the number of slices, and by having a delay between sequences. Potential increase in body temperature via energy deposition particularly in neonates who are typically kept warm in the scanner is the main challenge related to SAR at 3 T.[2] The introduction of delays between sequences to mitigate this problem can be a hindrance to the benefit of faster scanning at 3 T.

Most medical devices have been tested at 1.5 T for safety and compatibility.[53] Although an increasing number of devices have been tested at 3 T, some devices have not been approved as safe at high-fields. Therefore it is mandatory to keep in mind that the phrase "MR safe" does not necessarily translate into being "3 T MR safe." Vagus nerve stimulators (VNSs), which are commonly used in treatment of medically refractory epilepsy in children, has been declared safe at 1.5 T if the study is performed under certain safety measures.[54] There are promising results regarding the safety of scanning patients with VNSs on 3 T systems using a transmit/receive head coil, but further more extensive testing is perhaps needed[55] before widespread routine use. At our institution, we often opt to scan patients in the immediate postoperative period at 1.5 T to decrease potential safety hazards related to recently used surgical devices or implants, although this may not be necessary in many cases.

SUMMARY

Although often adequate evaluation can be achieved using either 3 T or 1.5 T MR imaging, we tend to favor particular applications for each field strength. We generally prefer 3 T imaging for evaluation of epilepsy, subtle brain malformations, brainstem abnormalities, cranial nerves, IACs, and cerebrovascular evaluation (MRA). We prefer 1.5 T for complete spine evaluation for assessment of drop metastases and in patients with extensive orthodontic or other metal hardware. We use 1.5 T scanners for imaging patients who have foreign bodies not cleared for 3 T imaging. We exclusively use 1.5 T imaging for fetal MR imaging.

The impact of high-field MR on pediatric neuroimaging has modified practice by both neuroimagers and referring physicians. The improved quality of many aspects of MR imaging has driven the demand for these systems from both sides. Nevertheless, the challenges arising from factors such as increased T1 relaxation, increased susceptibility, and safety issues continue to provide obstacles in many high-field MR imaging applications. It is easier to be frustrated with the problems and image quality issues of higher field systems, because expectations are often higher from these expensive systems. However, turning these imaging challenges into opportunities for better patient care requires a more in-depth understanding of the nuances and basic aspects of MR imaging on the part of MR technologists and radiologists.

REFERENCES

1. Zimmerman RA, Bilaniuk LT, Pollock AN, et al. 3.0 T versus 1.5 T pediatric brain imaging. Neuroimaging Clin North Am 2006;16(2):229–39, ix.

2. Dagia C, Ditchfield M. 3T MRI in paediatrics: challenges and clinical applications. Eur J Radiol 2008; 68(2):309–19.

3. Chavhan GB, Babyn PS, Singh M, et al. MR imaging at 3.0 T in children: technical differences, safety issues, and initial experience. Radiographics 2009; 29(5):1451–66.

4. Weishaupt D, Köchli VD, Marincek B. How does MRI work?: an introduction to the physics and function of magnetic resonance imaging. 2nd edition. Berlin: Springer; 2006. p. 170.

5. Lin W, An H, Chen Y, et al. Practical consideration for 3T imaging. Magn Reson Imaging Clin North Am 2003;11(4):615–39, vi.

6. Frayne R, Goodyear BG, Dickhoff P, et al. Magnetic resonance imaging at 3.0 Tesla: challenges and advantages in clinical neurological imaging. Invest Radiol 2003;38(7):385–402.

7. Willinek WA, Kuhl CK. 3.0 T neuroimaging: technical considerations and clinical applications. Neuroimaging Clin North Am 2006;16(2):217–28, ix.

8. Soher BJ, Dale BM, Merkle EM. A review of MR physics: 3T versus 1.5T. Magn Reson Imaging Clin North Am 2007;15(3):277–90, v.

9. Wen H, Denison TJ, Singerman RW, et al. The intrinsic signal-to-noise ratio in human cardiac imaging at 1.5, 3, and 4 T. J Magn Reson 1997; 125(1):65–71.

10. Runge VM, Case RS, Sonnier HL. Advances in clinical 3-tesla neuroimaging. Invest Radiol 2006;41(2): 63–7.

11. Stokowski LA. Ensuring safety for infants undergoing magnetic resonance imaging. Adv Neonatal Care 2005;5(1):14–27 [quiz: 52–4].

12. Edwards AD, Arthurs OJ. Paediatric MRI under sedation: is it necessary? What is the evidence for the alternatives? Pediatr Radiol 2011;41(11): 1353–64.

13. de Graaf RA, Brown PB, McIntyre S, et al. High magnetic field water and metabolite proton T1 and T2 relaxation in rat brain in vivo. Magn Reson Med 2006;56(2):386–94.

14. Bernstein MA, Huston J 3rd, Ward HA. Imaging artifacts at 3.0T. J Magn Reson Imaging 2006;24(4): 735–46.

15. Krautmacher C, Willinek WA, Tschampa HJ, et al. Brain tumors: full- and half-dose contrast-enhanced MR imaging at 3.0 T compared with 1.5 T–initial experience. Radiology 2005;237(3):1014–9.

16. Shapiro MD. MR imaging of the spine at 3T. Magn Reson Imaging Clin North Am 2006;14(1):97–108.

17. Bammer R, Keeling SL, Augustin M, et al. Improved diffusion-weighted single-shot echo-planar imaging (EPI) in stroke using sensitivity encoding (SENSE). Magn Reson Med 2001;46(3):548–54.

18. Willinek WA, Gieseke J, von Falkenhausen M, et al. Sensitivity encoding for fast MR imaging of the brain

in patients with stroke. Radiology 2003;228(3): 669–75.

19. Kuhl CK, Gieseke J, von Falkenhausen M, et al. Sensitivity encoding for diffusion-weighted MR imaging at 3.0 T: intraindividual comparative study. Radiology 2005;234(2):517–26.

20. Alexander AL, Lee JE, Wu YC, et al. Comparison of diffusion tensor imaging measurements at 3.0 T versus 1.5 T with and without parallel imaging. Neuroimaging Clin North Am 2006;16(2):299–309, xi.

21. Poretti A, Boltshauser E, Loenneker T, et al. Diffusion tensor imaging in Joubert syndrome. AJNR Am J Neuroradiol 2007;28(10):1929–33.

22. Gevers S, Majoie CB, van den Tweel XW, et al. Acquisition time and reproducibility of continuous arterial spin-labeling perfusion imaging at 3T. AJNR Am J Neuroradiol 2009;30(5):968–71.

23. Wang J, Alsop DC, Li L, et al. Comparison of quantitative perfusion imaging using arterial spin labeling at 1.5 and 4.0 Tesla. Magn Reson Med 2002;48(2): 242–54.

24. Franke C, van Dorsten FA, Olah L, et al. Arterial spin tagging perfusion imaging of rat brain: dependency on magnetic field strength. Magn Reson Imaging 2000;18(9):1109–13.

25. Wang J, Licht DJ, Jahng GH, et al. Pediatric perfusion imaging using pulsed arterial spin labeling. J Magn Reson Imaging 2003;18(4):404–13.

26. Wolf RL, Detre JA. Clinical neuroimaging using arterial spin-labeled perfusion magnetic resonance imaging. Neurotherapeutics 2007;4(3):346–59.

27. Strouse JJ, Cox CS, Melhem ER, et al. Inverse correlation between cerebral blood flow measured by continuous arterial spin-labeling (CASL) MRI and neurocognitive function in children with sickle cell anemia (SCA). Blood 2006;108(1):379–81.

28. Vargas MI, Delavelle J, Kohler R, et al. Brain and spine MRI artifacts at 3Tesla. J Neuroradiol 2009; 36(2):74–81.

29. Dietrich O, Reiser MF, Schoenberg SO. Artifacts in 3-T MRI: physical background and reduction strategies. Eur J Radiol 2008;65(1):29–35.

30. Chavhan GB, Babyn PS, Thomas B, et al. Principles, techniques, and applications of T2*-based MR imaging and its special applications. Radiographics 2009;29(5):1433–49.

31. Mittal S, Wu Z, Neelavalli J, et al. Susceptibility-weighted imaging: technical aspects and clinical applications, part 2. AJNR Am J Neuroradiol 2009;30(2):232–52.

32. Thomas B, Somasundaram S, Thamburaj K, et al. Clinical applications of susceptibility weighted MR imaging of the brain–a pictorial review. Neuroradiology 2008;50(2):105–16.

33. Gati JS, Menon RS, Ugurbil K, et al. Experimental determination of the BOLD field strength dependence in vessels and tissue. Magn Reson Med 1997;38(2):296–302.

34. Al-Kwifi O, Emery DJ, Wilman AH. Vessel contrast at three Tesla in time-of-flight magnetic resonance angiography of the intracranial and carotid arteries. Magn Reson Imaging 2002;20(2):181–7.

35. Bernstein MA, Huston J 3rd, Lin C, et al. High-resolution intracranial and cervical MRA at 3.0T: technical considerations and initial experience. Magn Reson Med 2001;46(5):955–62.

36. Willinek WA, Born M, Simon B, et al. Time-of-flight MR angiography: comparison of 3.0-T imaging and 1.5-T imaging–initial experience. Radiology 2003; 229(3):913–20.

37. Michaely HJ, Kramer H, Dietrich O, et al. Intraindividual comparison of high-spatial-resolution abdominal MR angiography at 1.5 T and 3.0 T: initial experience. Radiology 2007;244(3):907–13.

38. Tanenbaum LN. Clinical 3T MR imaging: mastering the challenges. Magn Reson Imaging Clin North Am 2006;14(1):1–15.

39. Nowinski WL, Puspitasaari F, Volkau I, et al. Comparison of magnetic resonance angiography scans on 1.5, 3, and 7 Tesla units: a quantitative study of 3-dimensional cerebrovasculature. J Neuroimaging 2011. [Epub ahead of print].

40. Malamateniou C, Adams ME, Srinivasan L, et al. The anatomic variations of the circle of Willis in preterm-at-term and term-born infants: an MR angiography study at 3T. AJNR Am J Neuroradiol 2009;30(10): 1955–62.

41. Vargas MI, Nguyen D, Viallon M, et al. Dynamic MR angiography (MRA) of spinal vascular diseases at 3T. Eur Radiol 2010;20(10):2491–5.

42. Phalke VV, Gujar S, Quint DJ. Comparison of 3.0 T versus 1.5 T MR: imaging of the spine. Neuroimaging Clin North Am 2006;16(2):241–8, ix.

43. Larsson EM, Stahlberg F. 3 Tesla magnetic resonance imaging of the brain. Better morphological and functional images with higher magnetic field strength. Lakartidningen 2005;102(7):460–3 [in Swedish].

44. Gruetter R, Weisdorf SA, Rajanayagan V, et al. Resolution improvements in in vivo 1H NMR spectra with increased magnetic field strength. J Magn Reson 1998;135(1):260–4.

45. Dydak U, Schar M. MR spectroscopy and spectroscopic imaging: comparing 3.0 T versus 1.5 T. Neuroimaging Clin North Am 2006;16(2):269–83, x.

46. Cecil KM. MR spectroscopy of metabolic disorders. Neuroimaging Clin North Am 2006;16(1):87–116, viii.

47. Barkovich AJ, Westmark KD, Bedi HS, et al. Proton spectroscopy and diffusion imaging on the first day of life after perinatal asphyxia: preliminary report. AJNR Am J Neuroradiol 2001;22(9): 1786–94.

48. Vigneron DB. Magnetic resonance spectroscopic imaging of human brain development. Neuroimaging Clin North Am 2006;16(1):75–85, viii.

49. Barth MM, Smith MP, Pedrosa I, et al. Body MR imaging at 3.0 T: understanding the opportunities and challenges. Radiographics 2007;27(5): 1445–62 [discussion: 1462–4].

50. van den Brink JS, Watanabe Y, Kuhl CK, et al. Implications of SENSE MR in routine clinical practice. Eur J Radiol 2003;46(1):3–27.

51. Pruessmann KP, Weiger M, Scheidegger MB, et al. SENSE: sensitivity encoding for fast MRI. Magn Reson Med 1999;42(5):952–62.

52. Hennig J, Scheffler K. Hyperechoes. Magn Reson Med 2001;46(1):6–12.

53. Shellock FG, Crues JV 3rd. MR Safety and the American College of Radiology White Paper. AJR Am J Roentgenol 2002;178(6):1349–52.

54. Benbadis SR, Nyhenhuis J, Tatum WO 4th, et al. MRI of the brain is safe in patients implanted with the vagus nerve stimulator. Seizure 2001;10(7): 512–5.

55. Gorny KR, Bernstein MA, Watson RE Jr. 3 Tesla MRI of patients with a vagus nerve stimulator: initial experience using a T/R head coil under controlled conditions. J Magn Reson Imaging 2010;31(2): 475–81.

Imaging of the Spine at 3 Tesla

Marc Shapiro, MD[a,b,c,*]

KEYWORDS

- 3 Tesla (T) • Spine • MR imaging
- Magnetic field strength (B0) • Signal/noise ratio (SNR)
- Specific absorption rate (SAR) • T1 FLAIR
- Radio frequency (RF) transmission

Key Points

- 3 T imaging of the spine shows improvements compared with 1.5 T.
- Increased signal/noise ratio (SNR) allows for thinner slices and increased in-plane resolution and therefore better spatial resolution.
- There is increased conspicuity of paramagnetic contrast at 3 T.
- At 3 T, increased SNR also improves diffusion imaging, diffusion tensor imaging (DTI), spectroscopy, functional magnetic resonance (MRI) imaging, spinal magnetic resonance (MRA) angiography and arterial spin labeling (ASL).
- Increased susceptibility on T2 weighted (T2WIs) images and increased SNR produces improved blood level oxygen dependence (BOLD) effect at 3 T. The same combination with low dose gadolinium enhances perfusion imaging.
- Increased chemical shift effect at 3 T improves spectroscopy and fat saturation (FS).
- Parallel Imaging (PI) has a synchronous effect with 3 T which permits the use of higher PI factors. This shortens scan times thus ameliorating the increased SAR that is inherent when doubling the B0 from 1.5 T to 3 T.

Since its introduction into the clinical realm in the early 1980s, MR imaging has evolved into the gold standard for evaluating the bone marrow of the spine as well as the soft tissues within and adjacent to the spinal canal. Early MR imaging field strengths ranged from 0.3 to 0.6 Tesla (T). In the mid-1980s, 1.5 T was introduced and, within a few years, achieved widespread acclaim as the optimal field strength for clinical MR imaging despite the presence of a 2 Tesla system in that era.

Nearly a decade has passed since 3 T was first made practical for spine MR imaging with the advent of a compatible 8-channel phased array spine coil. A limited supply of these coils prevented widespread use until late 2004. Most first-generation 3 T systems were not ready for routine clinical use. The only way that early 3 Ts could cope with the increased energy deposited in patients with the doubled magnetic field strength (B0) was by interrupting the scan to allow cooling.

Our first-generation 3 T was a long-bore (215 cm) system that was delivered in early 2003, followed by our first spine coil in May 2003. There were frequent scan interruptions and inadequate computer processing power to rapidly formulate the increased data generated by the thinner slices and increased matrices (in-plane resolution) that

---

[a] NeuroImaging Institute of Winter Park, 2111 Glenwood Drive, Winter Park, FL 32792, USA
[b] Department of Diagnostic Radiology, University of Miami School of Medicine, Miami, FL, USA
[c] Section of Neuroradiology, University of Central Florida, Orlando, FL, USA
* NeuroImaging Institute of Winter Park, 2111 Glenwood Drive, Winter Park, FL 32792.
E-mail address: ShapMD@NeuroimagingWinterPark.com

Neuroimag Clin N Am 22 (2012) 315–341
doi:10.1016/j.nic.2012.03.001
1052-5149/12/$ – see front matter © 2012 Published by Elsevier Inc.

Diagnostic Checklist

- The goal is to improve the image quality and spatial resolution for each and every pulse sequence compared with 1.5 T.

- Use thin slices and increased in-plane resolution in evaluation of cervical and thoracic spines. With T2 sagittal spin-echo sequences, BLADE helps diminish patient motion artifacts when scanning patients; especially young children and patients with movement disorders.

- Use 2 mm sagittal and 2.5 mm slice thickness in the axial plane with T2 turbo spin echo (TSE) with or without FS, or use ultrathin sections with either T2 SPACE (sampling perfection with application optimized contrast by using different flip angle evolution) for subtle foraminal or lateral recess encroachment in patients with radiculopathy, and ultrathin three-dimensional (3D) or even two-dimensional (2D) imaging with the best sequence your manufacturer provides for differentiating cord gray and white matter.

- 3D sequences mitigate flow (pulsation) artifacts that are exacerbated at 3 T.

- T2 SPACE should be obtained only when seeking very high spatial resolution with pulsation dampening. SAR friendly but lacks adequate intramedullary contrast resolution and shouldn't be used tor detecting subtle abnormalities in cord signal.

- T1 fluid-attenuated inversion recovery (FLAIR) should be the only T1 sagittal sequence for any region in the spine. It allows for best differentiation of all interfaces between all of the following; bone, disc with spinal cord, conus and cauda equina and best delineates soft tissue and/or bone with CSF. FS is as robust with T1 FLAIR as with T1 spin echo sequences.

- For T1-weighted images in the axial plane for the thoracic or cervical regions, use T1 volumetric interpolated breath-hold examination (VIBE) or your manufacturer's comparable sequence. Cord–cerebrospinal fluid (CSF) interfaces are obscured with T1 spin echo or conventional spin echo (CSE) in any plane. T1 VIBE and other 3D T1 gradient echo (GRE)-based techniques permit adequate detection of contrast enhancement while providing excellent spatial resolution and superb delineation of cord dimension as well as differentiation between cord-CSF and/or nerve root–CSF. The dampening of pulsation artifacts makes it even better for delineating these soft tissue–CSF interfaces. This author prefers VIBE FS for pre and post contrast axial T1 WIs.

- In the author's experience, STIR and T1 FLAIR with phase contrast are the two best sagittal sequences for evaluating demyelinating disease at 3 T; a new 3-point Dixon technique (IDEAL on GE medical systems MRI systems) that should be available on all fourth-generation and upgraded third-generation 3 T systems. This sequence provides better FS in patients who have pronounced susceptibility artifact from metal after surgery. It also provides excellent FS at the cervicothoracic junction for both soft tissue neck and brachial plexus imaging at 3 T.

- There are multiple techniques (increasing bandwidth, turbo factor and matrices and decreasing, slice thickness and TE; orienting the frequency direction parallel to the long axis of metal may also help) mitigate susceptibility artifact thus improving image quality at any field strength because susceptibility scales with field strength.

- Because susceptibility artifacts occur in the frequency direction, orienting frequency encoding parallel to the long axis of metal will help diminish these artifacts in patients with spine hardware.

- There is a new sequence available on latest generation scanners that decreases both the in-plane and out-of-plane distortion that occurs with metal. It is designated slice encoding for metal artifact compensation (SEMAC).

- Try advanced imaging techniques with late-generation 3 T systems. The author routinely does diffusion and DTI on all patients with multiple sclerosis (MS) spectroscopy and perfusion for tumors. The author tries T2-weighted perfusion technique (CBV) and dynamic contrast enhancement (DCE) with permeability (Ktrans).

- The authors, facility has lost less than 10 patients in 3 years due to claustrophobia or body habitus related to the ultrashort, 70 cm bore size. The short bore length also decreases SAR as with single-voxel spectroscopy when differentiating between an infectious-inflammatory lesion involving the cord and a primary cord tumor. Tractography can help differentiate between a cord glioma and ependymoma because ependymomas usually arise from the ependymal surface of the central canal and should theoretically splay white matter tracts apart, whereas gliomas tend to infiltrate tracts.

- Similar to 3 T of the brain, when performing spinal cord perfusion, only half to one quarter the standard dose of gadolinium given at 1.5 T is necessary for all contrast enhanced spine imaging at 3 T.

- Despite the significantly increased cost associated with new-generation wide-bore and shorter-bore systems, the financial burden is compensated by the imager's ability to scan obese or extremely large, muscular patients whose body habitus may result in MR imaging that is nondiagnostic or equivocal if imaged on an open MRI scanner or perhaps even a 1.5 T, system. Most claustrophobic and very large patients tolerate being scanned in a 70-cm diameter, short-bore 3 T system.

should be obtained using 3 T. As a result, patient scan times were excessively long and susceptible to motion artifact. Patient throughput was impossible and the quality of spine scans was not equal to those imaged on our 1.5 T.

One manufacturer's first 3 T system precluded the user from adjusting receiver bandwidth, inversion times (TI), or turbo factor (TF; TF = ETL), resulting in poor susceptibility compensation and suboptimal contrast for certain pulse sequences including T1 FLAIR, which, in many experienced 3 T users' opinions, is important for optimizing 3 T spine protocols (Table 1).

The problems inherent in first-generation 3 Ts are detailed here not just for historical background; they had a pejorative effect on some neuroradiologists' opinions and publications regarding the value of 3 T (or the lack thereof) for clinical imaging of the brain and spine. Examples of both were published in reputable journals.[1,2] This author's opinion of 3 T for brain and spine imaging was negative until after we switched to a second-generation 3 T system General Electric (GE)'s HD system with a slightly shorter bore (200 cm), improved radio frequency (RF) transmission, and faster, dual processors. These features enabled us to improve quality and decrease imaging times for routine spine and brain scans to 30 minutes or less, which increased throughput to 25 scans/d with spatial resolutions exceeding those of the same scans at 1.5 T. Referring specialists thereafter specifically requested their patients be scanned on the 3 T system.

In January 2009, we obtained a third-generation 3 T scanner (Siemens 32-channel Verio) with a shorter (163 cm) and wider (70 cm) bore, better SAR efficiency, and an anterior neck bridge that increased signal and homogeneity for cervical spine and soft tissue neck scans. The Verio had BLADE (PROPELLER) capability for spine imaging. BLADE is a method of suppressing motion artifact that obtains data with multiple radially oriented blades extending through the center of k space. Its reconstruction algorithm eliminates the overlapping sections with the most motion.[3] We had prior experience with PROPELLER for brain imaging with our prior 3 T HDX system manufactured by General Electric using an axial T2 FLAIR pulse sequence that improved our detection of

white matter lesions.[4] We have routinely used BLADE on sagittal T2 TSE sequences for the cervical and thoracic spine for almost 3 years (Fig. 1). BLADE (PROPELLER) may also be used in the other planes for T2 TSE sequences as well as T1 FLAIR if a longer TE is acceptable.

Others have shown that BLADE is beneficial for improving the quality of sagittal T2 imaging of the cervical spine.[5] In May 2011, we performed our 25,000th spine on 3 T using the 3 different 3 T systems discussed earlier. More than 24,900 of these were scanned on the second-generation or third-generation systems.

The major advantage 3 T has compared with 1.5 T is the doubling SNR. Signal quadruples over 1.5 T because signal is proportional (α) (B0).[2] Noise at 3 T is doubled compared with 1.5 T because N is α B0. Thus, 3 T SNR is double that at 1.5 T. The increased SNR at 3 T can be used to decrease slice thickness, increase matrices (in-plane resolution), or decrease imaging time (eg, decrease number of averages) or any combination of these factors by adjusting these variables accordingly for virtually any pulse sequence. The increased SNR at 3 T enables the reader to routinely visualize some normal structures such as the normal central canal gray matter on sagittal T2 or PD-weighted sequences that are not identified on the same sequences at 1.5 T (Fig. 2).[6]

The enhanced detection of normal structures in the spine by 3 T because of increased SNR was later validated by other investigators who compared 3 T with 1.5 T using a T1 FSE pulse sequence. They also found that 3 T is more sensitive in the detection of abnormal bone marrow because of increased SNR.[7]

A second significant advantage of 3 T is the superior conspicuity of contrast enhancement at 3 T compared with 1.5 T, even though T1 relaxivity of gadolinium is constant between 3 T and 1.5 T.[8] This disparity is related to 2 factors; the increased SNR and prolonged T1 relaxation of background tissues by 20% to 40% and CSF by 26% to 38%.[9] Most radiologists are confident that this is so, and they use only half the standard dose (0.05 mmol/kg) of gadolinium for scans at 3 T compared with the recommended for scans at 1.5 T (Fig. 3).

Table 1
Protocols for 3 T

CSPx Routine

	TR	TE	TI	TA	Matrix	BLADE	IPAT	Turbo Factor	Gated	ST (mm)	BW Roffset (Hz/px)
Sagittal T2 TSE 22 cm	3000	100	n/a	2:50	320 × 320	Yes	Yes 2	21	No	2.0	260
Sagittal T1 FLAIR 22 cm	2000	18	800	3:06	320 × 256	No	Yes 2	6	No	3	217
Axial T2 TSE FS 16 cm	5000	84	n/a	5:02	256 × 192	No	Yes 2	16	No	2.5	279
Axial T2 MEDIC	650	17	n/a	5:33	512 × 384	No	n/a	n/a	No	2.5	399
7 elements											

Abbreviations: BW, bandwidth; n/a, not applicable.

CSP Cord

	TR	TE	TI	TA	Matrix	BLADE	IPAT	Turbo Factor	Gated	ST (mm)	BW (Hz/px)
Sagittal T2 STIR 22 cm	4000	47	220	2:50	320 × 256	No	No	16	No	2.0	252
Sagittal T1 FLAIR 22 cm	2000	18	800	3:06	320 × 256	No	Yes 2	6	No	3	217
Axial T2 FS 16 cm	5000	84	n/a	5:02	256 × 192	No	Yes 2	16	No	2.5	279
Axial T1 VIBE 16 cm	6.37	2.45	n/a	2:54	256 × 248	no	Yes 2	n/a	No	3	360
Sagittal T1 FLAIR FS after 22 cm	000	18	800	3:06	320 × 256	No	Yes 2	6	No	3	217
Axial T1 VIBE after 16 cm	6.37	2.45	n/a	2:54	256 × 248	No	Yes 2	n/a	No	3	360

C and T Spine for Cord DW Imaging

	TR	TE	EPI Factor	TA	Matrix	BLADE	IPAT	Number of Shots	Diffusion Weightings	ST (mm)	BW (Hz/px)
Sagittal multishot echoplanar DW imaging	2000	60	64	2:44	128 × 128	No	2	5	0 400 600	3	1028

TSP Routine

	TR	TE	TI	TA	Matrix	BLADE	IPAT	Turbo Factor	Gated	ST (mm)	BW (Hz/px)
Sagittal T2 TSE 32 cm	2500	89	n/a	4:22	384 × 307	No	Yes 2	16	Yes	2.0	266
Sagittal T1 FLAIR 32 cm	2000	21	800	3:50	320 × 256	No	Yes 2	8	No	3	217
Axial T2 FS 18 cm	3500	88	n/a	3:18	256 × 192	No	No	12	Yes	3	337
11 elements	—	—	—	—	—	—	—	—	—	—	—

TSP Cord

	TR	TE	TI	TA	Matrix	BLADE	IPAT	Turbo Factor	Gated	ST (mm)	BW (Hz/px)
Sagittal T STIR 32 cm	4000	57	220	4:42	384 × 288	No	No	17	Yes	2	250
Sagittal T1 FLAIR 32 cm	2000	21	800	3:50	320 × 256	No	Yes 2	8	No	3	217
Axial T2 FS ran upper and lower 18 cm	2800	75	n/a	3:32	256 × 192	No	No	12	Yes	3	337
Axial T1 VIBE 18 cm	5.38	2.45	n/a	2:49	256 × 248	No	Yes 2	n/a	No	3	360

	TR	TE	TI	TA	Matrix	BLADE	IPAT	Turbo Factor	Gated	ST (mm)	BW (Hz/px)
Sagittal T1 FLAIR FS after 32 cm	2000	21	800	3:50	320 × 256	No	Yes 2	8	No	3	217
Axial T1 VIBE after	5.38	2.45	n/a	2:49	256 × 248	No	Yes 2	n/a	No	3	360

LSP Routine	TR	TE	TI	TA	Matrix	BLADE	IPAT	Turbo Factor	Gated	ST (mm)	BW (Hz/px)
Sagittal T2 TSE 26 cm	4300	85	n/a	2:41	384 × 288	no	Yes 2	16	No	3	266
Sagittal T1 FLAIR 26 cm	1800	19	733	4:32	320 × 256	No	Yes 2	7	No	3	265
Axial T2 FS 18 cm	4300	80	n/a	3:54	256 × 192	No	no	16	No	3	305
Axial T1 18 cm	700	23	n/a	4:37	256 × 192	No	No	4	No	3	300
9 elements	—	—	—	—	—	—	—	—	—	—	—

LSP for Metastases, Primary Tumor, Infection, Inflammation, Substitute STIR 2.5 mm for Sagittal T2 TSE plus T1 FLAIR Sagittal with FS Before and After Gadolinium for these and After Surgery

Light Metal: CSP	TE	BW	TF	ST
T2 sagittal TSE	74	488	24	2.5
T1 sagittal FLAIR	14	488	6	3
T2 axial FS	84	434	21	2.5
T1 FSE	11	362	4	3

Heavy Metal: CSP	TE	BW	TF	ST
T2 sagittal TSE	76	751	36	2.5
T1 sagittal FLAIR	14	401	6	3
T2 axial FS	84	454	24	2.5
T1 axial FSE	11	362	4	3

Light Metal: LSP	TE	BW	TF	ST
T2 sagittal TSE	73	482	24	3
T1 sagittal FLAIR	19	347	6	3
T2 axial FS	69	488	24	3
T1 axial FSE	23	349	4	3

Heavy Metal: LSP	TE	BW	TF	ST
T2 sagittal TSE	73	766	38	3
T1 sagittal FLAIR	19	265	6	3
T2 FS	69	781	36	3
T1 FSE	23	300	4	3

Abbreviations: CSP, cervical spine; px, pixel.

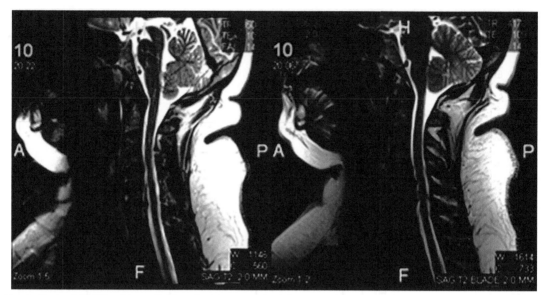

Fig. 1. Sagittal T2 TSE without (*left*) and with BLADE (*right*). BLADE (PROPELLER) decreases patient motion artifact on T2 TSE and T1 FLAIR. It can be used in any orthogonal plane.

For perfusion imaging with dynamic susceptibility contrast (DSC), 1 study showed that only 25% of the standard dose of gadolinium used at 1.5 T produced the same diagnostic results and quality for mean transit time (MTT) performed at 3 T.[10] Dynamic spinal MR angiography is significantly improved at 3 T because of both increased SNR and the increased conspicuity of gadolinium.[11] The increased SNR combined with increased susceptibility also results in improved BOLD signal on fMR imaging, which is performed

in the spinal cord at some institutions for evaluating the extent of damage by various diseases including MS.[12]

Diffusion-weighted (DW) imaging for detection of acute cord infarcts and active MS plaque is also improved by the increased SNR at 3 T if PI and other techniques are used to overcome susceptibility (Fig. 4).

We have also used DW imaging at 3 T to help us to differentiate between an island of red marrow and a metastasis and between normal but

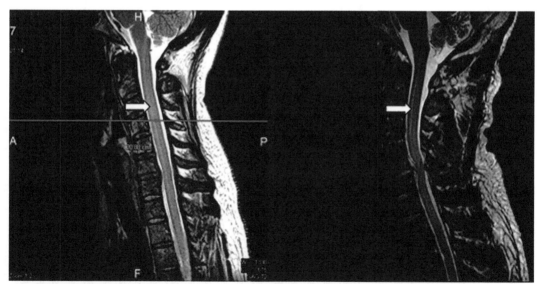

Fig. 2. Sagittal T2 FSE and T2 TSE on 2 patients with disc disorders imaged on 2 different 3 T systems. Both show a normal central canal (*white arrows*) routinely identified at 3 T but not at 1.5 T.

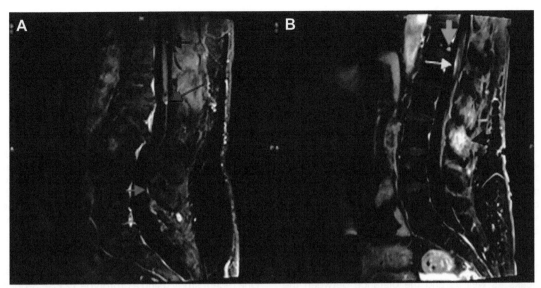

Fig. 3. Sagittal T1 FLAIR with FS after injection of 0.05 mmol/kg, showing the excellent conspicuity of gadolinium with half standard dose at 3 T in 2 different patients. (*A*) Punctate foci of recurrent ependymoma at inferior tip of conus (*red arrow*), on dorsal surface of the spinal cord (*black arrow*), and on filum terminale (*blue arrow*). (*B*) Metastatic breast disease involving vertebral body (*green arrow*), spinous process (*purple arrow*), and anterior cord surface (*yellow arrow*).

prominent enhancing central basivertebral venous complexes in a patient with a known primary cancer (**Fig. 5**).

It has also been our experience that purely blastic metastases (**Fig. 6** images in top row) at 3 T produce neither T2 prolongation nor restricted DW imaging, whereas purely lytic and partially blastic metastases (see **Fig. 6** images in bottom row) have increased signal on DW imaging without reduced apparent diffusion coefficient (ADC) indicating T2 shine through. DW image signal has been reported to improve detection of subtle, metastatic foci.[13] Non-contrast T1 FLAIR or T1 TSE or T1 CSE are the best sequences at 3 T or at 1.5 T for detecting bone marrow metastases (**Fig. 7**). In our experience, diffusion has not been accurate at 3 T or at 1.5 T for differentiating between benign and malignant compression fractures. It is one of several imaging parameters that should be considered when trying to distinguish between the 2 (see **Fig. 6** images in bottom row).

The RESOLVE sequence permits acquisition of multishot diffusion-weighted echo planar scans.[14] This feature is necessary for 3 T because bulk susceptibility artifacts can markedly degrade DW images, rendering them nondiagnostic. Acceptable image quality has been achieved at 3 T by using PI. This technique decreases the impact of the susceptibility differences, which otherwise lead to substantial artifact.[14]

DTI and cord tractography are superior at 3 T to 1.5 T (**Fig. 9**).[15,16]

Spectroscopy of the brain, spinal cord, and other regions of the body are improved by both the increase in both SNR and chemical shift effect.

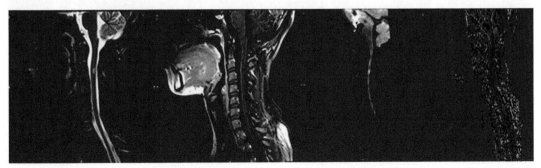

Fig. 4. Restricted diffusion in active MS plaque at C2 to C3 without enhancement. From left to right: sagittal STIR, postcontrast T1 FLAIR FS, DW imaging, and DTI.

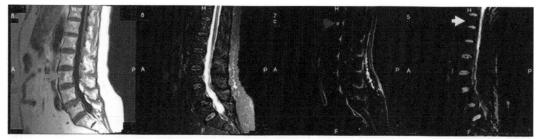

Fig. 5. Sagittal sequences: T1 FLAIR (*far left*), T2 STIR (*second left*), T1 FLAIR FS after gadolinium (*second right*), and DW imaging (B0 = 500) (*far right*) in a patient with primary breast cancer who was told that she had lumbar spine metastases by an outside facility. Heterogeneous bone marrow on T1 FLAIR with a probable island of red marrow in L3 (*blue arrow*). STIR shows no suggestion of metastases. T1 FLAIR FS post shows enhancement in mid-body of T12 (*red arrow*). Possible metastasis versus central basivertebral complex. DW imaging shows the same signal pattern in the T12 location as in other vertebral bodies. It is probably not a metastasis. Subsequent bone scan and positron emission tomography computed tomography (CT) were negative.

The latter increases the individual metabolite peaks as well as and the distance between the different metabolites (**Fig. 10**).[17]

The increased chemical shift effect also improves FS at 3 T.

However, on some patients, at the cervicothoracic junction, FS may still be suboptimal in homogeneity on T2 TSE. A work in progress (WIP) T2 TSE 3-point Dixon technique (IDEAL) for the Verio remedied this issue (**Fig. 11**). This sequence produces fat and H_2O-suppressed images as well as in-phase and out-of-phase combined images. One recent study using a prototype T2 FSE 3-point Dixon (TDSE) sequence for imaging the spine was equal to short tau inversion recovery (STIR) in lesion conspicuity with less motion and less blurring.[18] This technique is now available on the latest generation 3 T systems.

When B0 is doubled, challenges arise in the form of patients' physiologic responses, alterations in their tissues' relaxation properties, and amplification of certain imaging artifacts. Of major

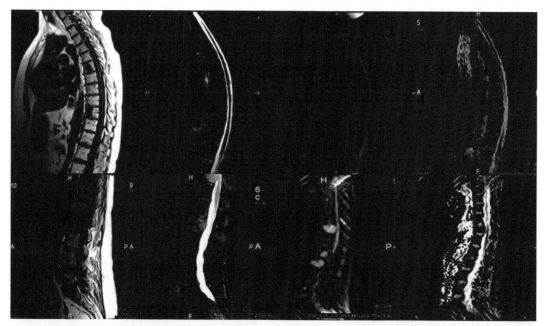

Fig. 6. Purely blastic prostate metastasis T spine are shown in the top row: sagittal T1 FLAIR, STIR, and multishot DW imaging and ADC. There is decreased signal on all. Lytic breast metastases are shown in the bottom row: multiple metastases with dark signal intensity on T1 FLAIR and increased signal on short tau inversion recovery (STIR) and multishot DW imaging; there is expansion on some but it is minimally increased on ADC, indicating increase on DW imaging related to T2 shine through.

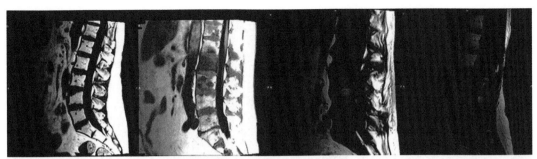

Fig. 7. Bone marrow signal alterations shown at 3 T using T1 FLAIR with smaller metastases (*left*) large and small metastases (*second on left*), total marrow replacement in patient with chronic lymphocytic leukemia (*third left*), and postradiation complete fatty replacement of normal marrow from T12 to L2 (*right*).

significance is the increased energy that is deposited in patient's tissues by the RF pulses during an MR imaging scan, which, when divided by that patient's weight, is designated as the specific absorption rate (SAR). This added power results in increased heating of local tissues that dissipates into the patient's whole body mass. To limit the increase in core body temperature to no more 1° C, The International Electrotechnical Commission (IEC) established safety limits, subsequently adopted by the US Food and Drug Administration (FDA), for power deposition, independent of field strength, of 8 W/kg of a given tissue, not to exceed 5 minutes or 4 W/kg for the entire body averaged over 15 minutes. SAR is proportional (α) to field strength (B0),[2] flip angle (FA),[2] and duty cycle (D) At 3 T, SAR is 4 times greater than at 1.5 T unless the FA and duty cycle are decreased. Recovery time (TR), TF (ETL), and TE are the most important factors that affect the duty cycle. Decreasing the FA at 3 T from 180 to 120° does not change tissue contrast significantly but it substantially lowers SAR.[19] Decreasing TF = ETL does not degrade image quality unless there is susceptibility, and increasing TR allows for tissue cooling between RF pulses, but at the expense of imaging time. Decreasing ETL means fewer 180° RF pulses per TR. GrE sequences with low FAs are the most SAR friendly; CSE is less SAR intensive than TSE (FSE), which requires a longer TE. T2-weighted TSE (FSE) seem well suited for 3 T because they can be used with high matrices and thin sections, but they require a large number of slices for complete coverage of an adult patient's thoracic or lumbar (L) spine and, as a result, these long TE sequences are SAR intensive.

All manufacturers now use tailored RF pulse designs (VERSE, LOW SAR, and TAPS) that manipulate the RF pulse and the resulting B1 inhomogeneity while using gradient modulation that changes trajectory in k space.[20] These designs are particularly useful for T2 TSE sequences with

a 30% to 40% reduction in SAR on these long ETL sequences. Another alternative available on the Verio is 3D T2 TSE, which can provide practical imaging times with a sequence called T2 SPACE. This FSE technique (also designated CUBE by another manufacturer), uses different interecho spacing that is minimized and the FAs for refocusing pulses that can be kept constant or variable. The combination of using minimal interecho spacing and keeping flip angle refocusing pulses with most FAs less than 180° yields a large number of echoes per excitation, which produces a SAR-efficient and fast T2 pulse sequence with high spatial resolution and excellent CSF-cord separation. Because this sequence is spin echo based, it helps diminish susceptibility artifacts. The combination of high T2 signal intensity, high spatial resolution, with low energy deposition and thin sections, makes T2 SPACE ideally suited for delineating fine structures (eg, nerve roots traversing CSF or in the foramina) on 3 T MR imaging of the spine (**Fig. 12**).[21]

However, T2 SPACE is inadequate for the detection of many intramedullary signal alterations caused by most disorders. Another powerful tool for reducing SAR is PI, a technique using phased array coils that are arranged spatially in the phase direction. These coils substitute for a certain percentage of phase encoded steps, which results in faster scan times. An integrated parallel imaging technique (IPAT) (ASSET, SENSE)[22] factor of 2 reduces phase encoding steps by 50% but decreases SNR by 40%. IPAT factors of 3 and 4 use one-third and one-quarter of the usual phase encoding in k space but result in 50% and 60% loss in SNR since the decrease in SNR is proportional to the square root of the acceleration (IPAT) factor.[23] PI has been touted as having a synergistic effect with 3 T because there is more than enough signal to compensate for the loss when increasing IPAT factors (**Fig. 13**).

Improved magnet design with significant reduction in bore length uses shorter body coils that

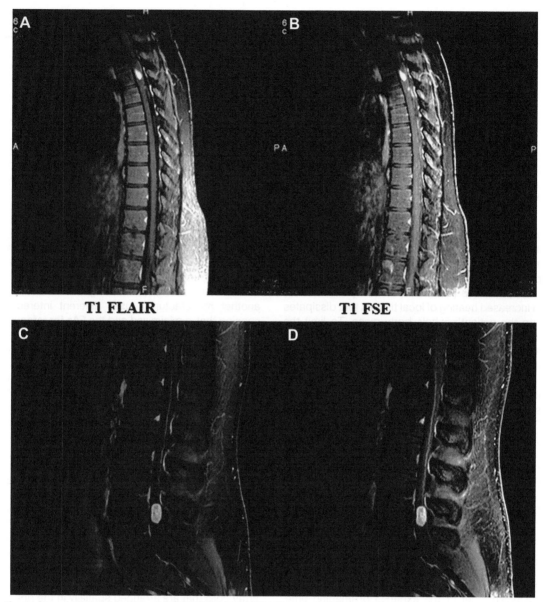

T1 FLAIR   **T1 FSE**

Fig. 8. (*A* and *C*) T1 FLAIR. (*B* and *D*) T1 FSE. T1 FLAIR FS (*A*) versus T1 FSE FS (*B*) for cord glioma and myxopapillary ependymal (*C* and *D*). Contrast enhancement is equal for both sequences in both tumors. True cord dimensions as well as cord, conus medullaris, and cauda equina interfaces with CSF are better delineated on T1 FLAIR because of prolonged T1 relaxation at 3 T on T1 FSE. The CSF nulling effect of the inversion pulse (TI) on T1 FLAIR negates this problem for T1 spines at 3 T.

expose less of a patient's body to the increased RF at 3 T. Ideally, all future coil design will be multichannel transmit-receive to allow for optimal SAR reduction.[19]

Prolonged T1 relaxivity, another factor and a potential obstacle, must be considered when imaging at 3 T. Prolonged T1 relaxation times of body tissues and fluids at higher field strength require longer TRs for T1 CSE or TSE pulse sequences to optimize T1 relaxation times at the higher B0. For spine imaging, the greatest impact is the change in CSF signal on both T1 pulse sequences from a darker signal at 1.5 T to a more intermediate gray signal at 3 T. This change results in decreased conspicuity of normal interfaces between CSF and cord, conus medullaris, cauda equina, and nerve roots as well as interfaces of disc and bone with CSF. If one still chooses to use short TR, short TE spin echo sequences at 3 T, the gray signal intensity of CSF will diminish

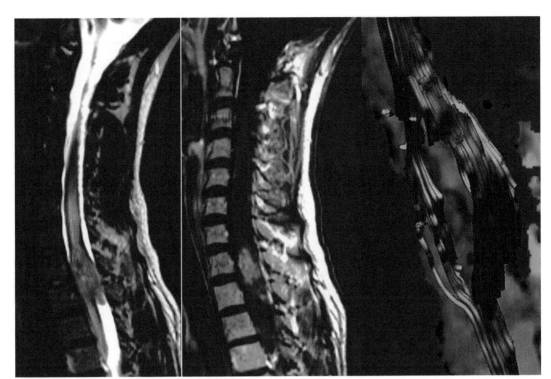

Fig. 9. 3 T sagittal (SAG). T2, T1 postcontrast, and tractography show expansile, intramedullary tumor at T1 to T3 with adjacent edema. Increased SNR at 3 T is helpful for cord tractography, which is beneficial in this case for differentiating between glioma and ependymoma, as is shown by the splaying of tracts typical of ependymoma. (Case *Courtesy of* Meng Law; with permission from Elsevier and Magn Reson Clin NorthAm.)

the reader's ability to detect subarachnoid involvement by infectious, inflammatory, or neoplastic diseases on noncontrast 3 T MR imaging of the spine.[6] This impediment disappears if T1 CSE (FSE) is replaced by T1-weighted FLAIR. This sequence was tried and compared with T1 FSE at 1.5 T with the following results: "T1-weighted fast FLAIR sequence revealed superior contrast at the CSF-cord interface, better conspicuity of lesions of the spinal cord and bone marrow, and reduced hardware-related artifacts as compared with conventional T1-weighted spin echo sequences."[24]

In 2005, our group prospectively scanned 110 (50 lumbar, 50 cervical, 10 thoracic) patients' spines on our second-generation 3 T system with both T1 FLAIR and T1 FSE in the sagittal plane. The parameters that were evaluated were cord, conus and cauda equina interfaces with CSF, as well as interfaces of vertebral body and disc with CSF, differentiation of normal from abnormal bone marrow, and size of

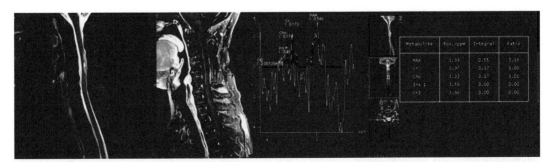

Fig. 10. Cord MS. Sagittal STIR and T1 FLAIR FS post gadolinium, short TE 2D single-voxel spectroscopy improved by the increased chemical shift at 3 T, which improves both the height of individual metabolite peak and separation between metabolite peaks for cord spectroscopy. Diminished *N* acetyl aspartate (NAA) with a normal choline (Ch) peak is consistent with MS plaque.

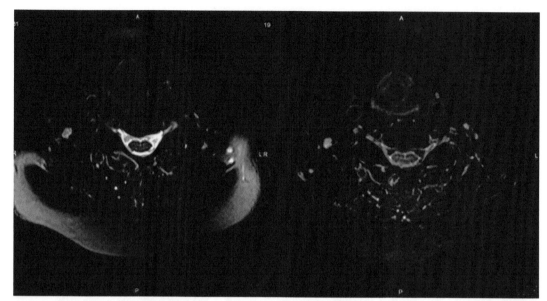

Fig. 11. (*Left*) Axial T2 TSE with chemical FS that is inhomogeneous with incomplete FS of posterior subcutaneous fat. (*Right*) Three-point Dixon provides homogeneous, robust FS in the same patient on the water-suppressed image. This technique is particularly helpful for cervical spines near the cervical-thoracic junction for imaging the brachial plexus and soft tissue neck.

susceptibility artifacts in patients with spine hardware. Similar to the results found at 1.5 T, T1 FLAIR was superior for delineating normal and abnormal soft tissue–CSF interfaces and vertebral body and disc-CSF interfaces. Susceptibility artifacts were smaller on T1 FLAIR because of its longer ETL. The T1 pulse sequences were equal in separating normal from pathologic bone marrow (see **Figs. 6** and **7; Fig. 14**).[25] See neoplastic changes in **Figs. 6** and **7** and radiation changes in **Fig. 7** (extreme right image) and signal alterations caused by fractures in **Fig. 14**A, C.

Recently, other investigators have obtained similar results comparing T1 FLAIR and T1 FSE of the lumbar spine imaging at 3 T.[26]

We subsequently prospectively evaluated 88 enhancing lesions in 100 patients at 3 T whom we scanned with both T1 FLAIR and T1 FSE sequences in the sagittal plane following contrast injection (see **Fig. 14**A, C). All enhancing disorders were detected on both sequences, most with equal conspicuity. When a sequence showed superior contrast enhancement, it was invariably found with the one imaged with a longer time delay after injection in the few patients in whom there was a disparity in contrast conspicuity. Seventy of these patients were scanned with chemical FS added to both sequences (**Fig. 8**). The quality and homogeneity of FS were equal on both pulse sequences (see **Fig. 8**).[27]

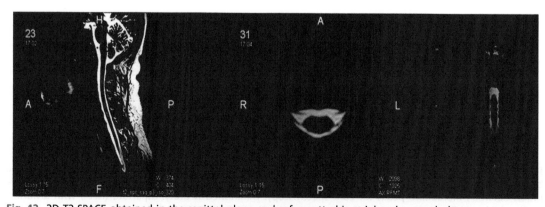

Fig. 12. 3D T2 SPACE obtained in the sagittal plane and reformatted in axial and coronal planes.

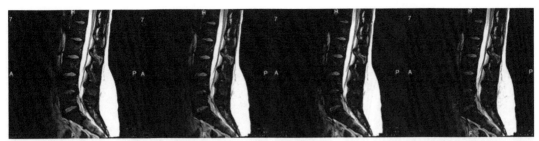

Fig. 13. T2 TSE with IPAT factors increasing from left to right (0, 2, 3, and 4) and SNR decreasing from left to right (100%, 60%, 50%, and 40%), and decreasing acquisition times of 5:15, 2:41, 1:58, and 1:20. Other factors: TR = 4300, TE = 85, FA = 120, matrices = 384 × 288.

The findings discussed earlier were also confirmed on a later study performed at MD Anderson with the conclusion that "T1 FLAIR post contrast imaging in the spine results in significantly improved CSF suppression and increases the conspicuity of bone lesions, disc herniations and epidural metastasis compared to T1FSE."[28] Whenever T1 axial images are required before and after contrast is administered, a variant of a 3D GrE technique, VIBE using non–breath hold adaptation that can be used without or with FS with short TE, small voxel size, high bandwidth, and low FA. This combination of factors minimizes pulsation (ultrashort TE) and susceptibility (high bandwidth) artifacts, is SAR friendly (low FA), and produces excellent 3D T1 data sets with excellent contrast resolution between cord and CSF, which makes this sequence well suited for spine imaging at 3 T. The one exception at our institution is in the lumbar spine, where we prefer our axial T1-weighted sequence to be multislice and multiangled through the disc spaces. On lumbar spines, we obtain axial T2 TSE sequences as a stack perpendicular to the vertebral bodies. In biologic tissues, T2 relaxation values are the same or minimally decreased at 3 T compared with 1.5 T. However, T2* scales directly with field strength. At 3 T, T2-weighted

images, including T2 TSE FSE, are more sensitive to susceptibility effects of blood breakdown products and metals (Figs. 15 and 16).

Susceptibility was the second most commonly encountered artifact (27%) after pulsation artifacts (56%) in a study performed with more than 2000 patients.[29] Susceptibility-weighted (SW) imaging has been reported to further enhance detection of petechial hemorrhage in acute spinal cord injury at 3 T.[30] SW imaging is a technique that uses a long TE GrE sequence that combines phase and magnitude. It is exquisitely sensitive for deoxyhemoglobin, intracellular methemoglobin, hemosiderin, calcium, and venous blood. We use SW imaging routinely as part of all brain protocols.

Some radiologists prefer 1.5 T for imaging patients with spine hardware because of increased susceptibility artifact (signal loss and geometric distortion) at 3 T because susceptibility scales α B0. In this author's opinion, this is not necessary because imaging parameters can be altered to minimize susceptibility artifact. Increasing receiver bandwidth, TF (ETL) and matrices, decreasing slice thickness, field of view (FOV) and TE as well as using PI and orienting frequency encoding direction parallel to the long axis of metal (when possible) all help decrease susceptibility artifact whether

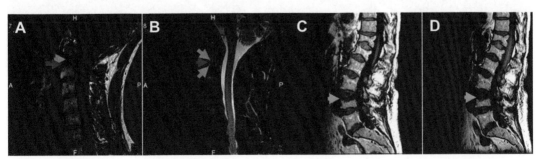

Fig. 14. (A and B) Demonstrates a subacute type 2 odontoid fracture (red arrow). (A) Sagittal T1 FLAIR and (B) sagittal STIR. Adjacent edema (blue arrows) is above and below on STIR but only above on T1 FLAIR. (C) Sagittal T1 FLAIR and (D) sagittal T1FSE. Represent both acute and as well as old osteoporotic compression fractures of the lumbar spine (green arrows). Note that the CSF - conus and vertebaral body-CSF interfaces with T1 FLAIR are better delineated than with T1 FSE on images C and D.

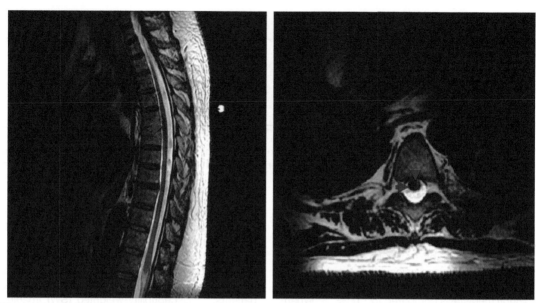

Fig. 15. Sagittal and axial T2 FSE show the effect of shortening of T2* relaxation times at 3 T compared with 1.5 T, which is responsible for the detection of intramedullary hemosiderin (*red arrow*) that was not detectable on a recent 1.5 T scan. Susceptibility is α B0.

scanning at 3 T, 1.5 T, or a lower field strength.[31] Our experience has been that, when susceptibility artifact with spine hardware is sufficiently strong to result in nondiagnostic spine MR imaging at 3 T, even after appropriately maximizing and minimizing all parameters mentioned earlier, it will also be nondiagnostic at 1.5 T.

2D GrE sequences exacerbate susceptibility more at 3 T. 3D GRE with small voxel size and very short TE perform well when imaging patients with metal. The doubling of SNR at 3 T is beneficial when increasing receiver bandwidth by a factor of 2, which results in a 40% decrease in SNR. If PI is also used, signal loss is additive.

Recently, a robust technique that reduces distortion (both in and through plane) by spine hardware known as SEMAC has been used at both 1.5 and 3 T.

The SEMAC technique uses a modified spin echo or STIR sequence that corrects metal artifact distortion using robust encoding of each excited slice against metal-induced field inhomogeneity. In-plane distortion is reduced by extending a view-angle-tilting (VAT) spin echo sequence with additional z-phase encoding. Both techniques are used in a modified spin echo pulse (STIR can be used) sequence that is time consuming but can be accelerated significantly by using PI. This technique

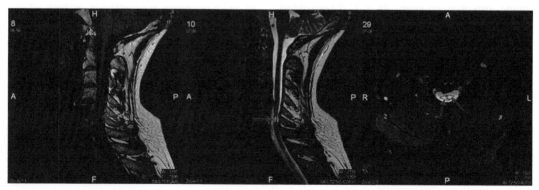

Fig. 16. Posttraumatic cystic myelomalacia involving central gray matter shown on sagittal T1 FLAIR (*left*) and T2 FSE and axial (best for delineating gray matter involvement) in spite of the fusion hardware by adjusting the imaging parameters. Increasing bandwidth, ETL, and matrices; decreasing slice thickness, TE, and field of view (FOV); using PI; and orienting frequency parallel to the long axis of metal all help to decrease susceptibility artifact, particularly when scanning at higher field strengths.

initially required close to 10-minute scan times (**Fig. 17**).[32]

This innovative technique requires no additional hardware and should be available on all manufacturers' 3 T systems in the near future. We have imaged the spines of more than 30 patients with multilevel fusions to date using a Siemens' work in progress (WIP) pulse sequence (WARP), which has enabled us to visualize the spinal canal in 10 patients for whom, without adding this sequence, the MR imaging was nondiagnostic. Recently a 3-point Dixon technique, IDEAL, has been described at 1.5 T to improve T1 FS postcontrast imaging as well as T2-weighted imaging when there is spine hardware present.[33] This technique is available as a WIP on the Verio and will be available as a product soon (**Fig. 18**).

PULSATION OR FLOW ARTIFACTS

Pulsation artifacts were the most common artifact identified on 3 T MR imaging in the 2000-plus patient study discussed earlier.[29] They are exacerbated by increasing B0. They are diminished by using a superior-to-inferior direction phase encoding direction (**Fig. 19**). The use of 1 or crossed saturation pulses anterior to the spine and posterior to the heart and great vessels helps diminish these artifacts. 3D imaging sequences such as VIBE and SPACE for T1 and SPACE for T2 sequences with ultrasmall voxels and extremely thin (0.6 mm) slice thickness help mitigate pulsation artifact. We use cardiac gating when necessary to mitigate heart pulsations for thoracic spine imaging at 3 T.

Chemical Shift Effects

Chemical shift effects scale with field strength, which increases metabolite peak height and separation between peaks. Increased B0 at 3 T also improves RF fat suppression. An increase in chemical shift artifact on 3 T also produces an undesirable increase in fat-H_2O misregistration. By imaging with higher bandwidths (32–125 kHz),

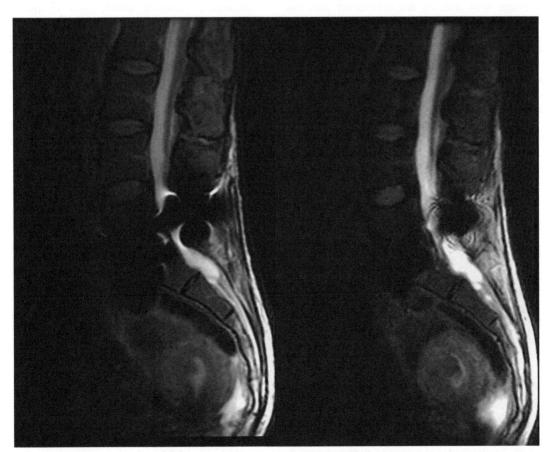

Fig. 17. The SEMAC technique (with VAT) reducing both in-plane and through-plane distortion caused by disc replacement device and posterior and posterior fusion and/or spacer device. (*Courtesy of* Pauline Worters; Brian A. Hargreaves, PhD; Wenmiao Lu, PhD; Weitian Chen, PhD; and Kim Butts Pauly.)

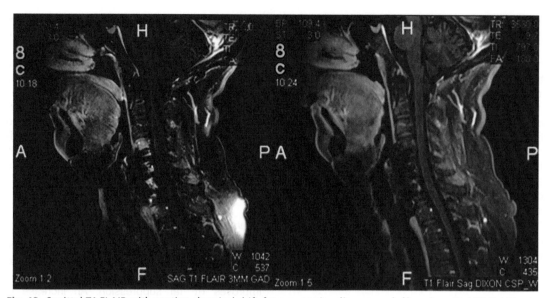

Fig. 18. Sagittal T1 FLAIR with routine chemical shift fat suppression (*image on left*) and sagittal T1 FLAIR using 3 point Dixon technique (*image on right*) both post Gadolinium demonstrate significant improvement in homogeneity of fat suppression both adjacent to anterior fusion and at cervico-thoracic junction.

chemical shift artifacts are diminished with the associated decrease in SNR (**Fig. 20**).

There is a decrease in SNR by approximately 47% but 3 T still has adequate signal. The increased fat-water misregistration at 3 T can also be diminished by decreasing voxel size or using fat suppression techniques when clinically suitable to remedy this issue (**Fig. 21**).

Increased chemical shift artifact on 3 T is remedied by the use of FS.

Increased dielectric effect, also known as standing wave, at 3 T results in marked in homogeneity in tissue signals associated with changes in RF wave pattern (shorter and slower at 3 T) represents a significant issue (signal loss) for body imaging, particularly in patients with ascites. The Siemens Verio has an improved RF transmitter that has diminished the increased standing wave effects on spine imaging. At least 2 manufacturers now (and probably all will in the near future) market

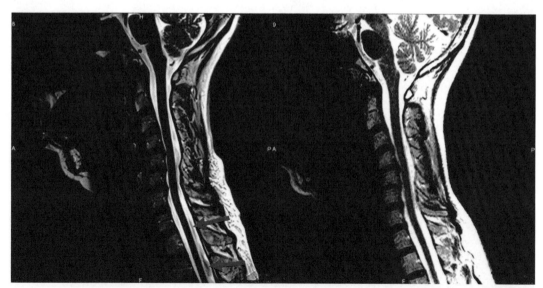

Fig. 19. Sagittal T2 TSE (2.5 mm) 3 T (*left*) and using 3 mm slice thickness at 1.5 T (*right*). Increased pulsation artifact (*red arrows*) at 3 T with phase encoding in superior to inferior (S-I) direction. Note the obvious disparity in SNR between 3 T and 1.5 T.

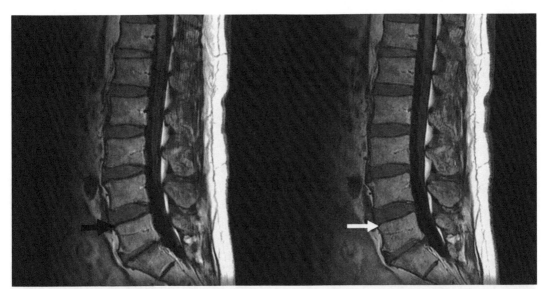

Fig. 20. Effect of increasing receiver bandwidth on chemical shift artifact image on left has chemical shift artifact resulting in spuriously thickened superior end plate (*black arrow in image on left*) with a receiver bandwidth of 16 kHz. The same slice in the same patient with the bandwidth increased to 42 kHz decreases chemical shift artifact (*white arrow*).

3 T systems with digital, multicoil, parallel RF transmitters at increased cost to further negate dielectric effects with higher B0.[34]

Ambient Noise

Sound pressure levels (SPLs) increase with field strength and decrease magnet length. The noise levels of an ultrashort-bore (163 cm) 3 T with high gradient levels is twice that of 1.5 T in excess of 130 dBA. Similar to SAR regulations, the IEC and FDA limit sound levels to 99 dBA. The Verio and other ultrashort-bore, high-performance 3 T systems have acoustically shielded vacuum bore liners and patients are given strong noise-dampening headphones to meet regulations.

THE CLINICAL ROLE OF DIFFERENT PULSE SEQUENCES AVAILABLE AT 3 T FOR EVALUATING SPINAL CORD DISORDERS

As mentioned earlier, 3D T2 SPACE has superb spatial resolution (0.6 mm) and is extremely SAR efficient. However, its intramedullary contrast is inadequate for detection of spinal cord signal alterations (**Fig. 22**).

A recent publication without separating field strengths asserted that double-echo (PD and T2)

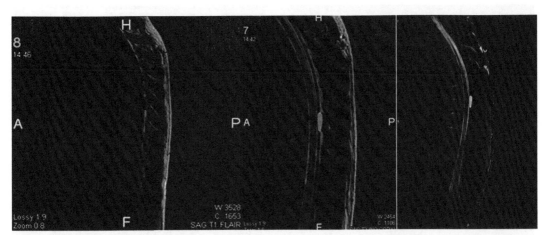

Fig. 21. T1 FLAIR, T2 FSE, and STIR: an arachnoid cyst surrounded by epidural fat with chemical shift artifact seen in the frequency encoding direction (anterior to posterior) posterior to the arachnoid cyst on T2 FSE, which disappears on STIR.

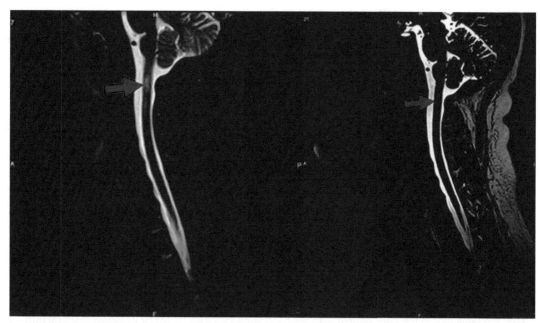

Fig. 22. Cord MS. Sagittal STIR (*left*) and T2 SPACE (*right*) MS plaques are not well seen on T2 SPACE, a sequence designed for submillimeter spatial resolution and separation of cord and CSF but not cord signal alterations.

spin echo is superior to STIR for detecting spinal cord MS because of pulsation and other artifacts with STIR.[35] In the same article, the investigators promulgate that T1 FLAIR with phase sensitivity reconstruction true inversion recovery (IR) is the most sensitive sequence for detecting MS in the spinal cord. 3 T T1 FLAIR with phase-sensitive reconstruction (true IR) was noted as the most sensitive sequence in a study in 2008 that had a limited number of patients in whom approximately 10% more plaques were detected with true IR than STIR. Less than half were identified on PD and T2.[36]

Our experience at 3 T concurs with the finding of Poonawalla and colleagues[36] that STIR at 3 T is more sensitive than PD TSE and T2 TSE (with and without FS). We performed 2 prospective studies (50 and 75 patients), the first comparing sagittal STIR with T2 TSE with FS and subsequently with PD TSE and T2 TSE in the cervical cord.[37–40]

Figs. 23–25 indicate the detection and conspicuity of multiple sclerosis plaques. STIR at 3 T proved to be superior to all 3 sequences separately, and superior to PD and T2 TSE combined. In addition, some imagers at 3 T have had

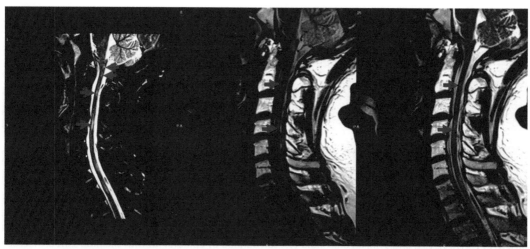

Fig. 23. Sagittal STIR (*left*) at 3 T is superior to proton density TSE (*middle*) and T2 TSE (*right*) separately and combined for the detection of MS plaques (*red arrows*) in the cervical and thoracic cord.

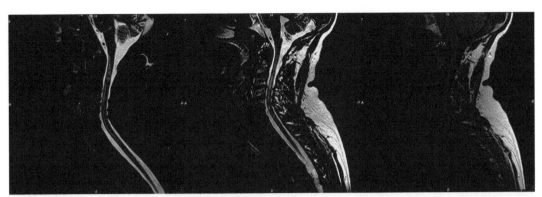

Fig. 24. Patient with longstanding relapsing and remitting MS; 3 T sagittal STIR 2.5 mm performed at our institution (*left*), outside 3 T T2 FSE 3 mm (*middle*), and T2 FLAIR 3 mm (*right*). STIR delineates the true dimensions of several plaques extending from the top of the odontoid to C4 better than T2 FSE. Plaques not identified on T2 FLAIR. As with 1.5 T, T2 FLAIR should not be used to image spinal cord MS plaques at 3 T.

a renewed enthusiasm regarding T2 FLAIR for imaging spinal cord MS. In this author's experience, although T2 FLAIR, especially with BLADE (PROPELLER), is a robust tool for imaging brain MS plaques but, similar to 1.5 T, it should not be used at 3 T for imaging cord demyelination (see **Fig. 24**).

We have examined more than 50 patients with MS to date with known or suspected spinal cord MS with both STIR and T1 FLAIR with phase sensitivity (see **Figs. 24** and **25**). Although this author agrees that true IR is a sensitive sequence for detecting MS plaques in the cord at 3 T, every plaque we detected was also identified on our STIR sequence, which has a smaller FOV, shorter TE, slightly longer inversion time (TI), and smaller TF, higher matrices, and 1 average that varies significantly from the study that favored true IR. We identified a few plaques that were present only in retrospect on the T1 FLAIR with phase sensitivity, only after first identifying them on STIR (**Fig. 26**). Our conclusion regarding these 2 sequences for imaging spinal cord MS at 3 T is that they are complimentary and that they both should be

obtained and not PD TSE and/or T2 TSE (see **Fig. 25**; **Fig. 27**).

As mentioned previously, the increased SNR at 3 T permits the use of thinner sections (2–2.5 mm) with higher in-plane resolution than typically used at 1.5 T in both the cervical and thoracic regions. We frequently image patients with MS or who have had prior 1.5 T scans with STIR. With rare exceptions, the 3 T scan is superior (**Fig. 28**).

CLINICAL USE OF T2-WEIGHTED AXIAL SEQUENCES

As mentioned previously, if one is merely interested in spatial resolution and spinal cord–CSF interfaces, then T2 SPACE is excellent, but the sequence is suboptimal for detecting intrinsic cord disorders. We use either T2 TSE FS or (Merge) multiecho data image combination (MEDIC) for evaluating foramina. This sequence also delineates intramedullary gray-white matter borders in addition to separating cord from CSF with thin sections (**Fig. 29**).

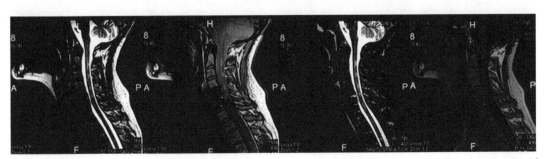

Fig. 25. 3 T comparison of sagittal T2 TSE (*far left*), PD TSE (*second left*), STIR (*second right*), and T1 FLAIR with phase sensitivity reconstruction (*far right*) for the detection of MS plaques. STIR and T1 FLAIR with phase sensitivity best delineate the margins of plaques. Note susceptibility caused the anterior cervical fusion hardware is not an issue for cord evaluation on all sequences.

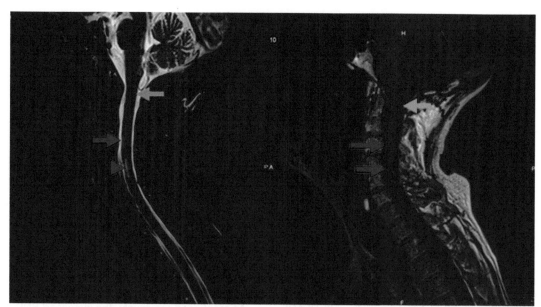

Fig. 26. Patient with relapsing and remitting MS with multiple plaques in medulla and cord. Plaque in dorsal cord posterior to odontoid identified clearly on STIR (*green arrow, image on left*) but only in retrospect on T1 FLAIR with phase sensitivity reconstruction (*image on right*). Slice thickness is 2 mm on both sequences.

The thinner sections and higher in-plane resolution obtained with the increased SNR of 3 T is also advantageous compared with 1.5 T for imaging spondylosis, degenerative and traumatic disc disease, and any associated soft tissue (cord, muscles, and ligaments) signal abnormalities (**Figs. 30–32**).

Congenital Anomalies

The detection and evaluation of congenital abnormalities is particularly improved by the increased SNR, thinner slices, and increased matrices at 3 T. We have imaged newborns referred from neonatal intensive care units at local hospitals

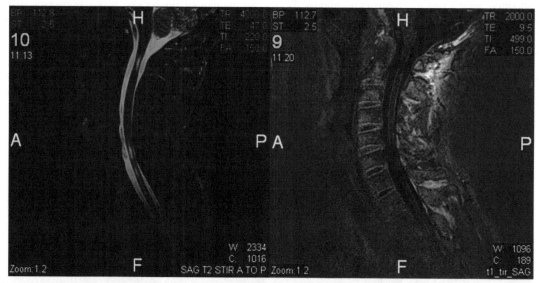

Fig. 27. Patient with multiyear history of MS (relapsing and remitting). Sagittal STIR (*left*) and T1 FLAIR with phase sensitivity reconstruction (*right*) are comparable in sensitivity for cord MS plaques at 3 T. In this author's experience these are the two most sensitive sequences in the detection of spinal cord MS plaques in the sagittal plane. At our institution, we no longer perform PD and T2 TSE sequences in the sagittal plane for our spinal MS protocol. We also obtain sagittal T1 FLAIR pre and post gadolinium as well as axial T2 TSE FS and VIBE pre and post contrast.

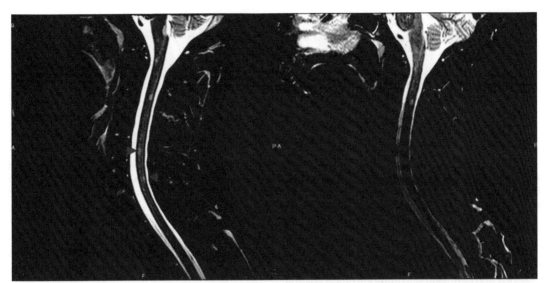

Fig. 28. Sagittal STIR 2.5 mm (*left*) versus STIR 3 mm in same patient imaged at 1.5 T (*right*) 2 months earlier at another facility. Using thinner slice thickness and higher in-plane resolution, the SNR at 3 T is higher with increased conspicuity of MS plaques (*red arrows* pointing to 2 plaques not visualized on image obtained at 1.5 T).

that do not have 3 T for either detection of an anomaly or for a more detailed assessment of a previously recognized abnormality of the brain and/or spine. The same abnormalities are usually better delineated as the child gets older (**Fig. 33**).

TUMORS AND SEPARATING INFLAMMATION FROM INFECTION

Virtually all of the imaging tools that neuroradiologists frequently use to analyze tumors in the brain

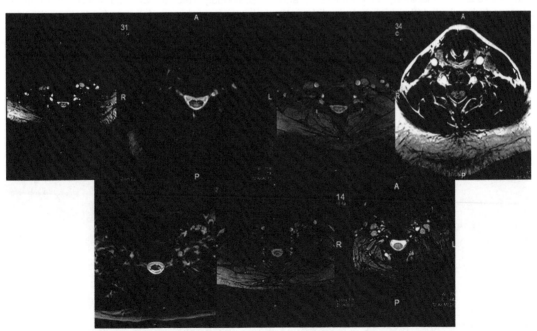

Fig. 29. T2 axials for MS: axials: MEDIC with FS (*upper left*), T2 TSE FS (*top, second to left*) on MEDIC non-FS (*top second to right*), postgadolinium T1 VIBE non-FS (*top right*) all depict central posterior plaque well including VIBE. Bottom row; left is T2 TSE FS and bottom center is MEDIC FS: Both depict plaque left posterior aspect of cord well. The author prefers the T2 TSE FS cord-CSF interface. Bottom right is normal MEDIC depicting central gray matter very well.

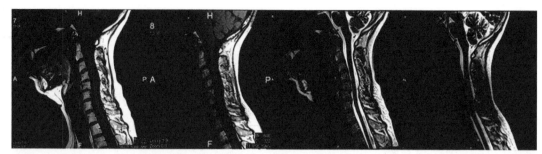

Fig. 30. Mild cervical spondylosis. Sagittal 3 T T1 FLAIR (*left*) and 1.5 T T1 TSE (*second left*) 3 T T2 TSE (*second right*), and 1.5 T T2 TSE. Cord-CSF and disc-vertebral body-CSF interfaces are better at 3 T. SNR is better at 3 T on both T1 and T2 sequences. *Note:* improved visualization of anterior anatomic structures related primarily to anterior bridge with 3 T cervical spine coil and increased SNR.

(routine imaging without and with contrast, diffusion with ADC values, DTI with tractography, spectroscopy and perfusion with cerebral blood volume (CBV) and dynamic contrast enhancement (DCE) permeability (K_{trans}) are currently available at 3 T for evaluating and separating intramedullary, intradural, extramedullary, and extradural neoplasms. The exceptions at the time of this writing are ASL and 3D CSI. At this time, there is only 2D CSI for spectroscopy in the spinal cord. All techniques are more robust at 3 T than 1.5 T because of increased SNR enabling the use of thinner slices with higher in-plane resolution, increased susceptibility, increased conspicuity of gadolinium, and increased chemical shift, which help in differentiating between types of tumor (see **Fig. 9**) and separating tumor from inflammatory-infectious lesions,

particularly with DCE and spectroscopy (see **Figs. 9** and **10; Figs. 34–36**).

Alterations in Magnet Design

Late-generation 3 T scanners with a shorter Z axis (163 cm) are more SAR friendly but infrequently require an additional axial sequence(s) for tall patients with long torsos when scanning their thoracic spines or performing a metastatic spine survey with a large FOV. A bore width of 70 cm enables users to image obese and large, muscular (eg, high-performance athletes) patients who previously had to be examined on open MR imaging systems of lower field strength, which often resulted in suboptimal spatial resolution, particularly in the detection of subtle but clinically

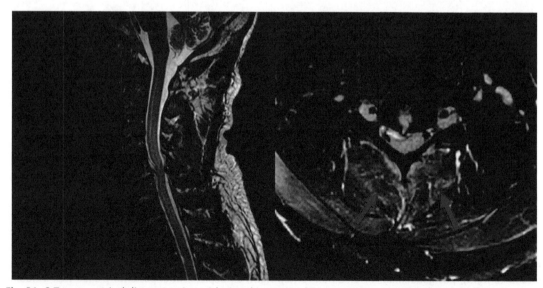

Fig. 31. 3 T acute cervical disc protrusion with signal intensity changes consistent with a fissure in the right paracentral location of the posterior annulus with contusion to posterior paraspinal muscles (*red arrows*). Sagittal T2 TSE (*left*) and axial T2 TSE FS (*right*). *Note:* visualization of normal central canal on sagittal T2 TSE.

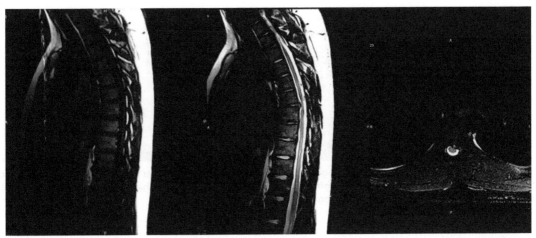

Fig. 32. T SPINE protrusion: sagittal T1 FLAIR (*left*), T2 TSE (*middle*), and axial T2 TSE FS (*right*). Slice thickness of 2 and 2.5 mm with higher in-plane resolution than was used at 1.5 T with 3 to 4 mm produces a more accurate evaluation of the thoracic spinal cord.

significant cord disorders or a mild stress fracture of a single pars interarticularis. The increased bore dimensions also helps diminish the anxiety experienced by claustrophobic patients and makes the scan experience easier for the general population (personal experience). During our 32 months' experience, we have encountered only 2 patients who could not be scanned because of size or claustrophobia. The heaviest patient that we have imaged weighed 223 kg. The scan table accommodates up to 250 kg. We experienced no imaging penalties associated with the larger-diameter bore. All 3 T manufacturers (Siemens; GE; Philips and Toshiba) currently offer MR imaging systems with 70-cm diameter bores. In 2010, 17% of all new MR imaging equipment sold worldwide and 25% sold in the United States were 3 T systems. It is this sector of new MR imaging systems that is still increasing in market share. The dominant factor preventing 3 T from garnering a larger market share is the increased purchase cost in an environment in which an inexorable trend of diminishing reimbursement pervades. The same market forces may prevent advances and proliferation of 7 T MR imaging systems for imaging the brain and spine, although the development of a compatible phased array spine coil has recently been described.[41]

In addition, there has been a single publication to date on imaging the spine at 7 T in 5 volunteers and a single patient with spinal dysraphism using a combination of VIBE, CISS, DESS, and T2 TSE. T2 TSE was useful in only 2 of the 5 volunteers. There were significant issues with susceptibility. VIBE was best for displaying nerve roots and neural foramina.

The investigators stated that "None of the presented sequences, which are all established at

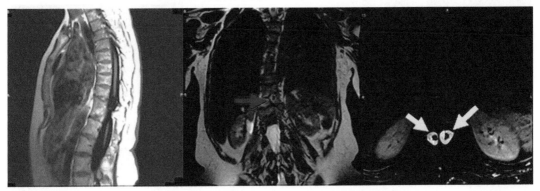

Fig. 33. Sagittal T1 FLAIR (*left*), cororonal T2 FSE (*middle*), and axial T2 FSE FS (*right*) show classic findings of midline cleft (*red arrow*) in thoracic vertebrae as well as diplomyelia (*yellow arrows*) associated with diastematomyelia.

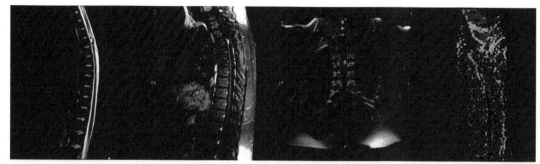

Fig. 34. Spinal cord glioma after biopsy. Sagittal STIR (*left*) and T1 FLAIR FS after gadolinium (*second left*) and coronal T1 FLAIR FS after biopsy (*second right*) and DTI (*far right*) show hemorrhage from biopsy and residual, enhancing, infiltrative tumor as identified on DTI.

lower field strengths, was able to demonstrate all anatomic structures of the lumbar spine owing to the various described limitations. Imaging quality was not competitive with the standard attained at 1.5 or 3 T, with a few exceptions owing to better spatial resolution. A combination of different sequences at 7 T can demonstrate most structures with moderate quality. The custom-built coil used for this investigation is a prototype that allows first insights into spine imaging at 7 T. With optimization of the hardware (RF coil and RF power), improvements in image quality can be expected in the future that may overcome the described limitations."[41]

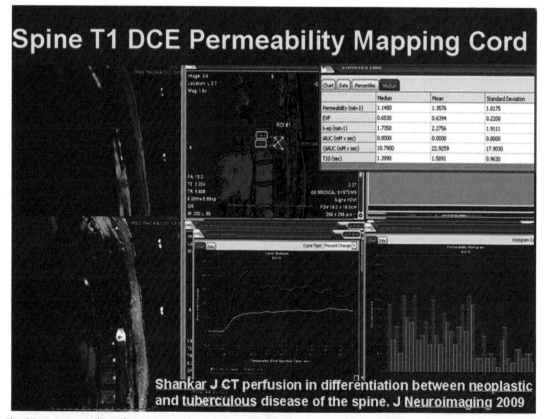

Fig. 35. An expansile, enhancing intramedullary mass that has moderate T2 signal intensity on a 3 T T2 sagittal sequence with extensive adjacent edema. The permeability map (K_{trans}) value suggests tumor; probably an infiltrating glioma. The reference cited on the slide relates to separating spinal tuberculosis involving the cord from tumor by using CT perfusion in 51 patients. (*Courtesy of* Meng Law.)

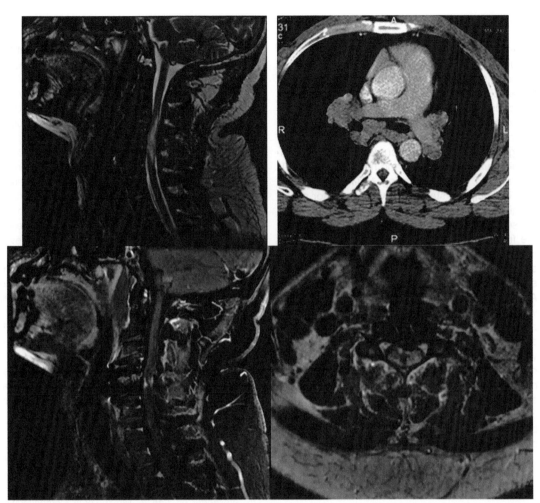

Fig. 36. Patient with a history of previously treated B cell lymphoma limited to the abdomen and pelvis 4 years prior presented with a myelopathy in 2005 when these images were obtained. Spinal cord biopsy was required to make the diagnosis of sarcoidosis. In 2012 with current advanced techniques including dynamic contrast enhancement (perfusion) with permebility (k trans) and MR spectroscopy now available to better differentiate between intramedullary inflammatory lesions and tumors, the biopsy may not be mandatory.[39] Sagittal T2 FSE (*top left*) and contrast-enhanced CT of the chest (*top right*), sagittal T1 FLAIR FS after gadolinium (*bottom left*), and axial T1 FSE after gadolinium (*bottom right*).

SUMMARY

Almost a decade has passed since 3 T MR imaging of the spine was made practical with the advent of an 8-channel phased array coil. First-generation scanners were plagued by SAR and other issues that have been remedied with second-generation and third-generation systems with tailored RF sequences on systems with bores that are shorter and ultrashort (163 cm) and wide (70 cm) and that have ameliorated SAR issues and allowed neuroradiologists to obtain high-quality, detailed images on morbidly obese and large, muscular individuals such as college and professional football linemen. Increased susceptibility artifact at 3 T is greatly reduced by both traditional techniques and newer innovative sequences such as SEMAC for decreasing in-plane and out-of-plane distortion and a type of 3-point Dixon that enables adequate T1 FS despite the presence of spine hardware for both postcontrast T1-weighted imaging and T2-weighted sequences. These techniques will make susceptibility artifact associated with spine hardware less of an issue. Fourth-generation and upgrade paths for third-generation 3 T systems are recently available or will be delivered in the next months, with digital, multichannel RF transmission arranged in parallel to substantially reduce dialectic effect caused by B1 field inhomogeneities. The added SNR at 3 T permits thinner sections with higher in-plane resolution that, combined with the increased conspicuity of gadolinium agents and decreased cost, as well as increased safety margin provided by half-gadolinium agents, already makes 3 T superior to 1.5 T for routine spine imaging. In addition, all of the advanced tools (spectroscopy, diffusion, DTI, BOLD, and perfusion with dynamic susceptibility and permeability) that neuroradiologists are already accustomed to using for greater diagnostic accuracy on brain MR imaging are now available and more robust at 3 T than at 1.5 T for spine imaging. MR imaging at 7 T is in it's incipient stage of development for spine imaging. Just recently, a prototype compatible phased array spine coils were developed[40] and the first limited clinical use of 7 T for spine MR imaging was in November, 2011 with results that suggest that 3 T will remain the optimal field strength for spine MRI for the forseeable future. All of the challenges that took several years to work through for 3 T spine imaging are magnified at 7 T. In late 2011 a fourth vendor, Toshiba, announced that it is now offering a new 3 T system with ultrashort and wide bore (71 cm) with digital multichannel RF transmission from an increased number of locations. This author interprets this announcement as another positive indication that 3 T MR imaging should now be viewed as the best field strength for clinical MR imaging of the brain and spine.

ACKNOWLEDGMENTS

I would like to dedicate this article in memory of my father, Robert, a man of great integrity and intellect as well as a true scholar and my best friend in life who initiated my interest in neuroradiology and the spine. I would also like to thank Robert Quencer who is a mentor, role model, and a good friend. I also want to thank Corey Gashlin and Jason Lees; without their help I would not have been able to complete this project.

REFERENCES

1. Ross JS. The high-field strength curmudgeon. AJNR Am J Neuroradiol 2004;25:168–9.
2. Phalke V, Gujar S, Quint D. Comparison of 3T versus 1.5T MR: imaging of the spine. Neuroimaging Clin North Am 2006;16:241–8.
3. Forbes KP, Pipe JG, Bird CR, et al. PROPELLER MRI: clinical testing of a novel technique for quantification and compensation of head motion. J Magn Reson Imaging 2001;14(3):215–22.
4. Shapiro MD, Ramnath R, Hartker R. Clinical relevance of FLAIR with PROPELLER in evaluating the brain at 3T: FLAIR with PROPELLER VS ROUTINE FLAIR ASNR Proceedings. 2005.
5. Fellner C, Menzel C, Fellner FA. BLADE sagittal T2-weighted MR imaging of the cervical spine. AJNR Am J Neuroradiol 2010;31:674–81.
6. Shapiro MD. MR imaging of the spine at 3T. Magn Reson Imaging Clin North Am 2006;14(1):97–108.
7. Zhao J, Krug R, Xu D. MRI of the spine: image quality and normal–neoplastic bone marrow contrast at 3 T versus 1.5 T. AJR Am J Roentgenol 2009;192:873–80.
8. Willinek W, Kuhl C. 3.0T neuroimaging: technical considerations and clinical applications. Neuroimaging Clin North Am 2006;16:217–28.
9. Ethofer T, Mader I, Seeger U, et al. Comparison of longitudinal metabolite relaxation times in different regions of the human brain at 1.5 and 3 Tesla. Magn Reson Med 2003;50:1296–301.
10. Manka C, Traber F, Gieske J, et al. Three dimensional dynamic susceptibility-weighted perfusion MR imaging at 3.0T: feasibility and contrast agent dose. Radiology 2005;234(3):869–77.
11. Vargas MI, Nguyen D, Viallon M. Dynamic MR angiography (MRA) of spinal vascular diseases at 3T. Eur Radiol 2010;20(10):1815–6.
12. Agosta F, Valsasina P, Absinta M. Primary progressive multiple sclerosis: tactile-associated functional MR activity in the cervical spinal cord. Radiology 2009;253(1):209–15.
13. Tanenbaum L. Diffusion imaging in the spine. Appl Radiol 2011;4:1–15.
14. Porter D, Heidemann R. Multi-shot, diffusion-weighted imaging at 3T using readout-segmented EPI and GRAPPA: ISMRM Proceedings. 2006. p. 1042.
15. Alexander AL, Lee JE, Wu YC, et al. Comparison of diffusion tensor imaging measurements at 3.0 T versus 1.5 T with and without parallel imaging. Neuroimaging Clin North Am 2006;16(2):299–309.
16. Thurner M, Law M. Diffusion weighted imaging, diffusion tensor imaging and tractography of the spinal cord. Magn Reson Imaging Clin North Am 2009;17:225–44.
17. Dydak U, Schar M. MR spectroscopy and spectroscopic imaging comparing 3T versus 1.5T. Neuroimaging Clin North Am 2006;16:269–83.
18. Low RN, Austin MJ, Ma J. Fast spin-echo triple echo Dixon: initial clinical experience with a novel pulse sequence for simultaneous fat-suppressed and nonfat-suppressed T2-weighted spine magnetic resonance imaging. J Magn Reson Imaging 2011;33(2):390–400.
19. Tanenbaum L. Clinical 3T MR imaging: mastering the challenges. Magn Reson Imaging Clin North Am 2006;14:1–15.
20. Hargreaves BA, Cunningham CH, Nishimura DG, et al. Variable-rate selective excitation for rapid MRI sequences. Magn Reson Med 2004;52(3):590–7.

21. Fries P, Runge VM, Kirchin MA. Magnetic resonance imaging of the spine at 3 Tesla. Semin Musculoskelet Radiol 2008;12(3):238–51.

22. Glockner JF, Hu HH, Stanley DW, et al. Parallel MR imaging: a user's guide. Radiographics 2005;25(5): 1279–97.

23. Blaimer M, Breuer F, Mueller M, et al. SMASH, SENSE, PILS, GRAPPA: how to choose the optimal method. Top Magn Reson Imaging 2004;15(4): 223–36.

24. Melhem E, Israel D, Eustace S. MR of the spine with a fast T1-weighted fluid attenuated inversion recovery sequence. AJNR Am J Neuroradiol 1997; 18:447–54.

25. Shapiro M, Ramnath R, Williams D. T1 FLAIR vs T1FSE: the optimal T1 pulse sequence for clinical spine imaging at 3T, ASNR proceedings. 2005. p. 132.

26. Lavdas E, Vlychou M, Arikidis N. Comparison of T1-weighted fast spin-echo and T1-weighted fluid-attenuated inversion recovery images of the lumbar spine at 3.0 Tesla. Acta Radiol 2010;51(3):290–5.

27. Shapiro M, Hartker R, Williams D. Post contrast imaging of the spine at 3T: T1 FLAIR vs. T1FSE, ASNR proceedings. 2006. p. 6–7.

28. Shah L, Raghavan P, Sanderson J. Postcontrast imaging of the spine at 3 T: T1 FLAIR vs. T1 FSE RSNA Proceedings. 2006.

29. Vargas MI, Delavelle J, Kohler R. Brain and spine MRI artifacts at 3Tesla. J Neuroradiol 2009;36(2):74–81.

30. Wang M, Dai Y, Han Y. Susceptibility weighted imaging in detecting hemorrhage in acute cervical spinal cord injury. Magn Reson Imaging 2011; 29(3):365–73.

31. Shapiro M, Magee T, Williams D. The time for 3T clinical imaging is now. AJNR Am J Neuroradiol 2004; 25:1628–9.

32. Hargreaves B, Chen W, Lu W. Accelerated slice encoding for metal artifact correction. J Magn Reson Imaging 2010;31(4):987–96.

33. Cha JG, Jin W, Lee MH. Reducing metallic artifacts in postoperative spinal imaging: usefulness of IDEAL contrast-enhanced T1- and T2-weighted MR imaging–phantom and clinical studies. Radiology 2011;259(3):885–93.

34. Vernickel P, Röschmann P, Findeklee C, et al. Eight-channel transmit/receive body MRI coil at 3T. Magn Reson Med 2007;58(2):381–9.

35. Fillipi M, Rocca M. MR imaging of multiple sclerosis. Radiology 2011;259(3):259–81.

36. Poonawalla A, Hou P, Nelson F. Cervical spinal cord lesions in multiple sclerosis: T1-weighted inversion-recovery with phase-sensitive reconstruction. Radiology 2008;246(1):258–64.

37. Shapiro M, Hatton B. Sagittal 3T evaluation of cervical cord MS plaques STIR vs T2TSE FS in the detection of MS plaques in the cervical cord: 50 patient prospective study. ASNR Proceedings. 2010. p. 132.

38. Shapiro M, Lees J. Sagittal 3T evaluation of multiple sclerosis plaques of the cervical cord: STIR vs PD and T2 TSE. ASNR proceedings 2011. p. 137.

39. Shankar J, Jayakumar P, Vasudev M. CT perfusion in differentiating between neoplastic and tuberculous disease of the spine. J Neuroimaging 2009;2: 132–8.

40. Vossen M, Teeuwisse W, Reijnierse M. A radio-frequency coil configuration for imaging the human vertebral column at 7 T. J Magn Reson 2011;208: 291–7.

41. Grams AE, Kraff O, Umutlu L, et al. MRI of the lumbar spine at 7 Tesla in healthy volunteers and a patient with congenital malformations. Skeletal Radiol 2012;41(5):509–14.

Ultrahigh-Field Magnetic Resonance Imaging: The Clinical Potential for Anatomy, Pathogenesis, Diagnosis, and Treatment Planning in Brain Disease

Anja G. van der Kolk, MD*, Jeroen Hendrikse, MD, PhD, Peter R. Luijten, PhD

KEYWORDS

- MR imaging • Ultrahigh-field • Neuroradiology
- Brain anatomy

Key Points

- Main advantages of ultrahigh-field magnetic resonance (MR) imaging of the brain:
  - Higher signal-to-noise ratio (SNR)
  - Higher contrast-to-noise ratio (CNR)

These features provide higher lesion conspicuousness, spatial resolution, or faster imaging.

- Insight into normal anatomy, pathogenesis, diagnosis, and treatment can be gained for various disease categories.
- Considerations for choosing sequences for clinical application:
  - Pursue highest spatial resolution possible
  - Make use of new contrast
    - T_2*-weighted imaging
    - Phase imaging
- In a patient with suspected brain disease not seen on conventional MR imaging, and no contraindications, an ultrahigh-field MR imaging can be considered.
- Metallic implants are the most important limitation, hampering full application of ultrahigh-field MR imaging in the (acute) clinical setting.
- (Neuro)radiologists should be trained for assessment of ultrahigh-field MR images.

Disclosure statement: The authors have nothing to disclose.
Department of Radiology, University Medical Center Utrecht, Heidelberglaan 100, Postbox 85500, 3508 GA Utrecht, The Netherlands
* Corresponding author.
E-mail address: A.G.vanderKolk@umcutrecht.nl

Neuroimag Clin N Am 22 (2012) 343–362
doi:10.1016/j.nic.2012.02.004

Diagnostic Checklist

- Clinical volumetric magnetic resonance (MR) imaging sequences at 7 T show more details of cerebral disease compared with lower field strengths.
- Visualizing more details of cerebral disease can, in selected patients, help in diagnosis and treatment.
- 7 T high-resolution MR imaging protocols consisting of a dedicated series of MR imaging sequences have been developed in healthy volunteers, and first clinical patient series show their value.
- The broader range of contraindications is still a limiting factor at a field strength of 7 T, and further testing (eg, stents, clips, implants) has to be performed.

CLINICAL RECOMMENDATIONS

For clinical use, ultrahigh-field 7 T magnetic resonance (MR) imaging has (as a result of increased availability and a vast and increasing amount of clinical studies) the potential to be applied in various disease categories. Data have been obtained at 8 and even 9.4 T as well, but these systems have primarily been focused on technological developments and ex vivo measurements (eg, advanced functional MR imaging studies, ^{23}Na brain imaging).

Apart from unraveling pathogeneses of several disease entities that are not fully understood, like multiple sclerosis (MS), advantages of ultrahigh-field MR imaging regarding diagnosis and treatment are gained in many cerebral diseases, like degenerative brain diseases, tumors, and epilepsy. Choosing ultrahigh-field MR imaging for clinical diagnostics is dependent on several factors, like approximation of the added value of high-field MR imaging, the availability of ultrahigh-field sequences, and patient cooperation. Most sequences used at ultrahigh-field for clinical diagnosis are sequences with a high spatial resolution, and contrast that is substantially more pronounced at ultrahigh-field strength, namely T_2*-weighted and phase imaging. Apart from specific contraindications, ultrahigh-field MR imaging can be considered in any patient in whom a brain disease is suspected but not found on conventional MR imaging. To facilitate the dissemination of ultrahigh-field MR imaging in the high-end neuroradiology workflow, (neuro)radiologists should be trained to assess the sometimes distinctly different contrasts obtained with otherwise conventional sequences.

INTRODUCTION

Since the emergence of nuclear magnetic resonance in medicine in the 1980s, the technique has seen an evolution not surpassed by many other medical developments. From a field strength of less than 0.5 T in the beginning, MR imaging has evolved technically to a widespread use of 3 T MR imaging scanners in current clinical practice. There is abundant scientific literature on new applications and sequences of MR imaging for better diagnosis and treatment of patients. Although the larger randomized trials are mostly based on MR imaging data from more conventional field strengths like 1.5 and 3 T, there is a clear trend toward human MR imaging applications at higher and higher field strengths and the first studies at 11.7 T can be expected shortly, something few in the past would have believed possible.[1]

With all these fascinating new developments within MR imaging, it is sometimes difficult to decipher what is still clinical MR imaging and what has gone beyond clinical medicine: what is, or will be clinically relevant,[2,3] and what is not? This question is important in modern (cost-contained) health care, if a decision has to be made whether to buy a new 1.5 T or 3 T MR imaging scanner or even to contemplate acquiring a human 7 T platform. For optimal triaging of patients the question whether a 1.5 T, 3 T, or, if available, ultrahigh-field MR imaging scan would provide the best diagnostic information may become challenging. In an effort to give some suggestions and directions as to how to address ultrahigh-field MR imaging in the clinical setting, we review the current status and its clinical applicability of ultrahigh-field MR imaging of the brain, after a brief technical description of ultrahigh-field MR imaging itself. In addition, we discuss what diagnostic areas are still relatively unexplored, although several clinical caveats exist. Because the brain is the primary target for ultrahigh-field MR imaging research, as well as the anatomic area most imaged with MR imaging in the clinical setting, we focus on imaging of the brain alone, and do not go into detail about ultrahigh-field imaging of other areas of the body. To keep this review compact and synoptic, our focus is on anatomic imaging of the brain rather than including the increased functional and physiologic imaging capabilities that come with increased field strength.

Recommended Sequence Chart	

- In general: high-resolution three-dimensional (3D) imaging
- Resolution: <1 mm isotropic, with reconstructions in multiple directions
- Specific valuable MR imaging sequences: 3D fluid-attenuated inversion-recovery, 3D T_2^*, 3D time-of-flight MR angiography

ULTRAHIGH-FIELD MR IMAGING: WHAT IS IT ALL ABOUT?

There are 3 main factors to be considered that determine the design and applications of MR imaging: signal-to-noise ratio (SNR), imaging speed, and spatial resolution. Changing one of these factors has an effect on the other 2 factors, and vice versa. Within limits, one can modify these factors to make MR imaging sequences with specific advantages. For instance, when a high spatial resolution is desired, either a high SNR or a (very) long scanning time is needed. A short scanning time also requires a high SNR, because in a very short time as much signal as possible is wanted, preferably without additional noise. To get the most out of MR imaging, a high SNR is mandatory. This is one of the main reasons why ultrahigh-field MR imaging is so important, because SNR increases approximately linearly with field strength. For a certain contrast, for instance T_1, this increased SNR can be used to increase the spatial resolution, for identification of smaller pathologic lesions, to decrease scanning time, facilitating imaging of less stable patients and moving organs like the heart, or to attain better lesion conspicuousness.

Apart from a high SNR, a higher magnetic field strength also influences the relaxation times of tissues, T_1 and T_2^* in particular.[4,5] When increasing from 1.5 to 7 T, for instance, the T_1-values for gray and white matter change from 1188 milliseconds and 656 milliseconds to 2132 milliseconds and 1220 milliseconds, respectively. These prolonged relaxation times however still allow for sufficient contrast between the gray and white matter of the brain.[6] They also make exquisite time-of-flight MR angiography (TOF-MRA) possible, with a high contrast-to-noise ratio (CNR). In TOF-MRA, tissues with static spins become saturated when excited several times by radiofrequency (RF) pulses within their T_1 relaxation time. Moving spins, like in flowing blood, that enter the excited volume, have not been saturated yet and are excited for only a limited number of times (depending on the slab volume that was chosen). These spins result in a high signal on TOF-MRA. When the T_1 of tissues becomes longer, like at ultrahigh-field, the static spins relax less between pulses, resulting in a lower signal from the static spins (background) and better contrast between flowing blood and suppressed background.[7]

The shortening effects of the ultrahigh magnetic field on T_2^* relaxation (changes in T_2 are not so pronounced) are derived from the increased magnetic susceptibility effects at higher field. The magnetic susceptibility of a tissue is inherent to that particular tissue, and is the way in which the tissue becomes magnetized when put into a magnetic field. The result is that these tissue-specific magnetic fields have effects on each other, so-called magnetic susceptibility effects, which cause faster tissue relaxation. These magnetic susceptibility effects scale linearly with magnetic field strength, and have both an advantage and a disadvantage. The disadvantage is that they cause more distortion of the local magnetic field in its surroundings, causing, for a given bandwidth, image distortions or local dropouts as a result of dephasing. This distortion can be seen for instance near air-filled cavities like the sinuses, where the brain just next to the bone of these cavities becomes distorted and unrecognizable. The advantage is that these magnetic susceptibility effects can be used for generating better tissue contrast. In particular, paramagnetic and diamagnetic substances, having a high magnetic susceptibility, stand out compared with the rest of the tissue. Examples of these substances are deoxyhemoglobin (veins), calcium (calcified tumors, atherosclerotic plaque), blood degradation products like hemosiderin (microbleeds) and iron depositions.

The increased susceptibility effects at ultrahigh-field MR imaging not only influence the relaxation times of tissues but at microscopic level they also cause increased phase shifts of the individual spins. These shifts can be visualized on so-called phase images of gradient-echo sequences. Although not routinely used on lower field strengths, because of the smaller phase shifts and subsequent small signal changes on phase images, at ultrahigh-field these images show enhanced CNR between gray and white matter, for instance between white matter and deep gray nuclei.[8,9] In this way, phase images could pose a new kind of contrast for anatomic differentiation and diagnosis in many disease fields.

Because of the changed relaxation times of tissues, lower-field MR imaging sequences cannot be directly copied into ultrahigh-field MR imaging scanners without sometimes serious changes in the many different sequence parameters. For instance, until 2010 a normal fluid-attenuated inversion-recovery (FLAIR) sequence, which cannot be missed in daily clinical routine, was not even possible at ultrahigh magnetic field.[10] Only in the last couple of years have robust clinical sequences, like the already mentioned FLAIR but also standard T_1-weighted and T_2^*-weighted sequences,[11,12] been developed for ultrahigh-field MR imaging, anticipating the question for ultrahigh-field clinical MR imaging.

The advantages of higher SNR, higher spatial resolution, and changes in the relaxation times at ultrahigh-field are discussed in the next sections, including reference to several studies that show the application of these advantages in both clinical and (to a lesser extent) preclinical practice.

ANATOMY AND PATHOGENESIS

Although for clinicians the goal of imaging with MR imaging is diagnosing the patient's disease, and monitoring treatment and recurrence of this disease, a large area of research with ultrahigh-field MR imaging has focused on imaging normal anatomy and unraveling the pathogenesis of diseases. This research is not only important for our understanding of disease processes and their locations but can also give us insight into possible new screening protocols and treatment strategies. Specifically, in diseases in which the pathogenesis is not fully understood, or for which there is no effective treatment, ultrahigh-field MR imaging could make a difference, by acquiring highly detailed images with new contrasts.

Anatomy

Visualizing the in vivo normal anatomy of the brain on MR imaging is almost as important as visualizing its disease: without an idea of normal structure, one cannot discern normal brain from pathologic brain. Ultrahigh-field MR imaging has been used in this field already since its emergence, mainly using the increased spatial resolution for imaging of the small anatomic details not seen on lower field strengths. Most research has been performed on the hippocampal architecture. As discussed later, the hippocampus plays a significant role in the pathogenesis of many disease processes, including dementia and epilepsy. Visualizing the hippocampal substructures could lead to faster diagnosis of these diseases, by early recognition of small pathologic changes.

In 1999, it was already known that several lines of differing signal intensity could be seen on MR images of the hippocampus. Although at that time it was already speculated that these lines represented hippocampal substructures, Wieshmann and colleagues[13] were the first to compare ultrahigh-field MR imaging of postmortem human hippocampus at 7 T with histology. These investigators confirmed that the lines seen on MR imaging represented different layers of the hippocampal structures.[13] After this discovery, many other investigators visualized the substructures of the hippocampus on different ultrahigh-field strengths, first by using postmortem human hippocampi and temporal lobe blocks with histology comparison,[14,15] and later by imaging the hippocampus in healthy volunteers at 7 T,[16,17] resulting in a high-resolution computational atlas of the human hippocampus, derived from postmortem 9.4 T images.[18] Although not directly useful in clinical practice, these studies form the backbone of current in vivo human hippocampal imaging in patients, by showing the possibility and imaging characteristics of ultrahigh-field MR imaging of the hippocampal area (Fig. 1), and also by confirming these characteristics with histology, which is often not possible in clinical studies.

The hippocampal cortex and architecture are not the only cortex that has gained interest since the emergence of ultrahigh-field MR imaging. In 2002, Fatterpekar and colleagues[19] performed a 9.4 T MR imaging study to depict the laminar cytoarchitecture of postmortem cortex specimens and correlated the acquired images with histologic sections. These investigators showed that ultrahigh-field MR imaging could detect the laminar pattern of the isocortex, allocortex, and periallocortex, and suggested a future role for ultrahigh-field in the identification of Brodmann areas of the cortex in vivo.[19]

Next to cortical differentiation of small substructures of the hippocampus and cerebral cortex as a whole, another area where small anatomic details are sometimes effective is the arterial vessels. Specifically, the anatomy of the cerebral perforating (lenticulostriate) arteries has received some attention, because they have become associated with small vessel disease (SVD) and microbleeds.[20] The lenticulostriate arteries are the arteries penetrating and feeding the deep brain structures like the basal ganglia. The presence of lacunar infarcts in these areas is believed to be related to the pathologic state of these arteries (SVD).[20] As with cortical disease, diseases of the lenticulostriate arteries can be detected only when imaging characteristics of the nondiseased arteries are known. Zwanenburg and colleagues[21]

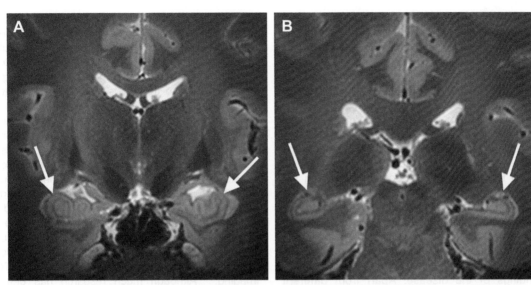

Fig. 1. Coronal 7 T MR images of a 30-year-old volunteer showing the body (*A*) and tail (*B*) of the hippocampus. Several cortical and subcortical foldings of the hippocampal area can be seen (*arrows* in *A* and *B*), as well as cortical layers. Imaging parameters were repetition time, 3158 milliseconds; echo time, 271 milliseconds; turbo spin echo factor, 181; number of signal averages, 2; resolution, $0.6 \times 0.7 \times 0.7$ mm³.

developed a magnetization-prepared anatomic reference MRA sequence to visualize both perforating arteries and related anatomy, and found its advantage over TOF-MRA in terms of visualizing possible correlation between vascular disease and tissue damage.[21] Cho and colleagues[22] and Kang and colleagues[23] also visualized and analyzed the lenticulostriate arteries with MRA at 7 T MR imaging in healthy volunteers. The results from these studies can be used for further studies investigating the role of diseased lenticulostriate arteries.

Pathogenesis

Although they are sometimes difficult to distinguish, for clinical purposes it is important to recognize studies in which the main results are related to a better understanding of the pathogenesis (or pathophysiology) of disease and studies in which the main results are (almost) directly applicable in clinical practice. We have tried to make this distinction in this section (about the first kind of studies) and the next section on diagnosis (about the second kind of studies); this does not mean that there is a clear line between the 2 kinds of studies, and others may classify studies differently. Because the main goal of this review is to create an understanding of the potential of ultrahigh-field MR imaging in the clinical setting, we believe this distinction is necessary.

MS

MS is one of the best examples of an important, frequently seen disease of which the pathogenesis is still not fully understood. Affecting relatively young patients (20–30 years), this demyelinating disease has a major impact on patients' lives during a long period of time. The pathogenesis of MS is largely unknown, and there is no cure for the demyelinating process; treatment options are limited to medicinal drugs like β-interferon. Several MS lesion types have been found, with possibly different natural courses and therapeutic options.[24] Many studies have therefore used ultrahigh-field MR imaging to further elucidate the pathophysiologic processes underlying these MS lesions. Most studies have focused on the characterization of only 1 type of MS lesion, cortical lesions, as a relatively new imaging entity in the pathogenesis of MS,[25] and have specifically tried, using these lesions, to visualize the pathophysiology of MS in vivo. Kangarlu and colleagues[26] in 2007 described several cortical types of MS lesions, by using postmortem 1.5 T and 8 T MR imaging and histology comparison, and found that 8 T ultrahigh-field MR imaging could detect more lesions than 1.5 T MR imaging because of better SNR and CNR.[26] Hammond and colleagues[27] showed the heterogeneity in characteristics of MS lesions in vivo in 19 patients with MS and found suggestions of pathologic iron content in the basal ganglia; the appearance of peripheral phase rings, which could represent iron-rich macrophages seen at histology; and vessels penetrating MS lesions.[27] The vascular involvement within MS lesions was also found by Ge and colleagues[28] using in vivo 7 T in 2 patients with MS, and by Tallantyre and colleagues[29] in 2008, who found that a central vessel (penetrating an MS lesion) was seen more often in perivascular lesions than other MS lesions. Pitt and colleagues[30] showed high accuracy for cortical lesion detection using postmortem T_2^*-weighted and white-matter-attenuated inversion-recovery T_1-weighted imaging at 7 T. Laule and colleagues[31] measured myelin water fraction using a 32-echo T_2 relaxation 7 T experiment on a postmortem specimen, visualizing fine structures such as the myelination of deep cortical layers and the hippocampus.

These studies on the pathogenesis of MS in both postmortem MS specimens and in vivo in patients with MS show the heterogeneous imaging findings of the disease. Apart from different lesion types and variable vascular involvement, we have only just begun to image the true underlying process of demyelination. Although there is increasing evidence of vascular pathogenesis in MS, mostly as a result of ultrahigh-field MR imaging, it is considered that we might be looking at differing pathogeneses within a heterogeneous disease group, called MS, instead of only 1 disease and 1 pathogenesis. The pathogenesis of MS will therefore remain a challenging topic for research into ultrahigh-field MR imaging.

Cerebrovascular diseases

Most studies on the pathogenesis of cerebrovascular diseases have focused on the effects of hypertension on the brain, for instance altered arterial anatomy and function, thereby gaining insight into hypertension-based disease. Novak and colleagues[32] showed microangiopathy and iron deposits in an asymptomatic hypertensive patient at 8.0 T, suggesting underlying pathogenic effects of hypertension even when patients do not have symptoms.[32] Kang and colleagues[33] also investigated the effect of hypertension on the lenticulostriate arteries (which have already been discussed in the section on anatomy) and showed that in hypertensive patients, the number of visible lenticulostriate arteries was smaller compared with healthy controls.[33] A case report by Biessels and colleagues[34] showed multiple microbleeds at 7 T MR imaging in a patient with a hypertensive cerebral hemorrhage and visualized a direct relationship between some of the microbleeds and a small leaking penetrating artery.[34] The results of these studies show a variable pathophysiology of hypertension-based brain disease, in which microvascularity and microbleeds show a more or less prominent role. In an era when hypertension is a common risk factor for (cerebro)vascular disease, it is important to recognize the underlying pathogenic effects of hypertension in brain disease, not only for diagnostic imaging but also for treatment decisions (eg, whether or not to treat hypertension aggressively even in asymptomatic patients).

Regarding microbleeds, next to a pathologic substrate of hypertension, they have also been associated with SVD. Imaging of microbleeds seems to depend on the spatial resolution and sensitivity to susceptibility effects of the applied magnetic field; for this reason, studies regarding microbleeds could benefit from ultrahigh-field. Conijn and colleagues[35] in 2010 visualized microbleeds at 7 T using a T_2^*-weighted double-echo sequence, and in 2011 found that microbleeds were more conspicuous at 7 T than at 1.5 T MR imaging.[36] Although much research has been carried out regarding microbleeds, real pathogenic studies are relatively lacking, which not only questions what role these microbleeds play in cerebrovascular diseases but also if what we see as numerous hypointense spots are real microbleeds or other sources of a susceptibility effect.

Two studies have focused on ischemic infarcts as a pathologic substrate of cerebrovascular diseases. One study by Chakeres and colleagues[37] studied the role of the microvascularity in lacunar infarcts in 1 patient with T_2-weighted 8 T MR imaging, compared with 1.5 T MR imaging, for better characterization of small-vessel cerebrovascular disease associated with lacunar infarctions.[37] Jouvent and colleagues[38] recently studied postmortem specimens of a patient with CADASIL (cerebral autosomal-dominant arteriopathy with subcortical infarcts and leukoencephalopathy) at 7 T and compared the results with histology. These investigators showed intracortical infarcts in this disease, and it is not known whether they are caused by different underlying mechanisms.[38] Ultrahigh-field MR imaging could provide additional pathogenic information currently not accessible by conventional imaging techniques.

Vascular malformations

Of the different vascular malformations, venous cavernomas or cerebral cavernous malformations have gained most attention. Although often incidental findings and clinically silent, these vascular malformations can also present with acute neurologic deficits, hemorrhagic stroke, or seizures. Ultrahigh-field MR imaging has been used to characterize these malformations, by taking advantage of both the high spatial resolution that can be achieved and the increased susceptibility effects of blood products. Novak and colleagues[39] visualized a venous cavernoma in vivo at 8 T MR imaging, compared with 1.5 T MR imaging, and found that at ultrahigh-field strength, the cavernoma appeared larger. This finding is of importance, because larger cavernomas tend to cause hemorrhage more often.[39] On the other hand, the greater susceptibility effect at ultrahigh-field could have caused an enlargement effect not consistent with reality. Shenkar and colleagues[40] investigated the architecture of cerebral cavernous malformations by using 9.4 T or 14.1 T proton density–weighted, T_1-weighted, T_2-weighted, and T_2^*-weighted MR imaging on excised lesions, and compared their results with histology. These investigators acquired more information regarding the biologic state of these lesions, like inflammation, angiogenesis, and production of new caverns in specific regions of the lesions.[40] Both studies give a glimpse of the pathogenesis of these sometimes clinically relevant but often overlooked malformations.

CLINICAL APPLICATIONS

After an introduction of the varying research subfields in which imaging of the normal anatomy and pathogenesis of diseases have been the primary focus, we now turn to the more directly clinically driven fields of research. There are several disease groups in which ultrahigh-field MR imaging has already provided additional diagnostic information not previously seen well on lower, conventional MR imaging field strengths. These disease groups have in common a diagnostic gap of varying size when imaging is concerned. For instance, MS may sometimes be a difficult diagnosis, especially when presented at an older age, because its characteristic lesions on conventional MR imaging (hyperintense white matter lesions) can be found in many other diseases and aging. Alzheimer disease (AD) is histologically (post mortem) relatively well defined, characterized by senile plaques and amyloid-β deposition, but using clinical MR imaging the in vivo diagnosis of dementia in general is still based on hippocampal atrophy, which is not always present in AD, especially in early-onset cases. Although classification of brain tumors has improved with the use of contrast-enhanced MR imaging, it is still difficult to distinguish between necrosis or tumor recurrence in treated glioblastoma multiforme, and often a biopsy is needed to differentiate between low-grade astrocytoma and gliomatosis cerebri, and between a lymphoma and a glioblastoma. Cryptogenic epilepsy, in which no pathologic cause can be found, still exists. These and other diseases are discussed in the following sections, in which a summary is given

of research that has been carried out at ultrahigh-field strength in an attempt to improve the diagnostic yield of imaging.

MS

The typical MR image of a patient with MS is that of a characteristic distribution of hyperintense white matter lesions on the FLAIR sequence, predominantly periventricular around the upper convex of the lateral ventricles, some of them enhancing after contrast administration. Follow-up imaging shows changing lesions, some that enhanced at first no longer enhance, although new lesions have appeared. There are few evidence-based biomarkers that can be used to predict disease course and treatment effect. As seen in the pathogenesis section, there has been new evidence that not only white matter lesions but also cortical lesions are a hallmark for MS. Furthermore, a central vessel can be found in a high percentage of MS and may at an older age distinguish between vascular-based white matter lesions and MS lesions. Mainero and colleagues[41] characterized cortical lesion types at 7 T MR imaging in 16 patients with MS, using T_2-weighted and T_2^*-weighted sequences, and compared these types of lesions in relation to clinical subtypes of MS. These investigators found that cortical MS pathology might prove a valuable tool in the assessment of the clinical course of MS.[41] Kollia and colleagues[42] also showed cortical lesions in patients with MS, which could be better visualized at 7 T than at 1.5 T, and found varying aspects of the lesions, confirming the observations of Hammond and colleagues.[27] Tallantyre and colleagues[43] focused on both imaging cortical lesions and imaging the distribution of central vessels within MS lesions.[44] These investigators found that cortical lesions were best detected when more than 1 imaging sequence was used, for instance 3 T FLAIR and 7 T magnetization-prepared rapid gradient-echo.[43] Furthermore, by using T_2^*-weighted imaging at 7 T, they showed the potential of this sequence in discriminating lesions consistent with MS and caused by vascular disease.[44] Recently, Tallantyre and colleagues[45] developed this idea by showing that a perivenous location of lesions at 7 T T_2^*-weighted imaging was predictive of the presence of demyelination, and therefore of MS, enabling discrimination between MS lesions and aging-related white matter lesions. As well as T_2^*-weighted imaging at ultrahigh-field, several other imaging sequences were used by de Graaf and colleagues[46] to show the enhanced conspicuousness of cortical and subcortical MS lesions at ultrahigh-field compared with 3 T MR imaging, even without use of contrast agents. Recently, Schmierer and colleagues[47] opened up new diagnostic possibilities by showing, with T_2-weighted 9.4 T MR imaging of a post-mortem MS specimen, that T_1 may be a predictor of neuronal density and T_2 a predictor of myelin content, when cortical gray matter was assessed quantitatively.

More detailed (also with regard to location) lesion visualization with ultrahigh-field MR imaging, specifically its association with intralesional vascular structures, could be of importance in the clinical diagnosis of MS. **Fig. 2** shows 2 cortical MS lesions in a patient with MS.

Cerebrovascular Diseases

Two diseases have received most attention for diagnosis with ultrahigh-field MR imaging, more or less consistent with research performed mainly for pathogenic purposes: ischemic stroke and SVD. Novak and colleagues[48] imaged first 1 patient with hemorrhagic stroke and subsequently 17 patients[49] with ischemic stroke using both 1.5 T and 8 T MR imaging. These investigators showed great anatomic detail of the stroke areas at ultrahigh-field and, more specifically, better visualization of microvessels than at lower field

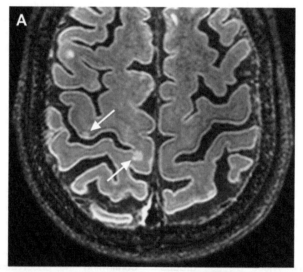

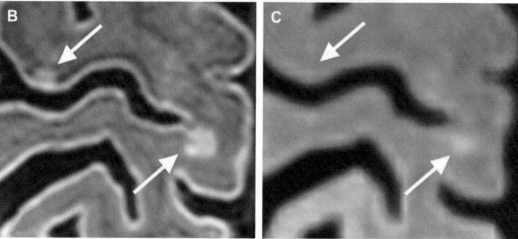

Fig. 2. 63-year-old woman with primary progressive MS with an Expanded Disability Status Score of approximately 6.0. A 7 T MR imaging scan was performed for detection of possible cortical lesions. (*A*) Axial overview and (*B*) zoomed-in image of a high parietal cortical MS lesion (*right arrow*) on axial 7 T 3D FLAIR sequence. In retrospect, this lesion could also be seen on the 3 T 3D FLAIR images, although with lower contrast-to-noise (*C*). On the other hand, the other cortical lesion (*left arrow*) could not be seen at 3 T MR imaging. Imaging parameters: 7 T 3D FLAIR as previously described[10]; 0.8-mm isotropic resolution; 3 T FLAIR 1.1-mm isotropic resolution. (*Courtesy of* W.L. de Graaf, VUmc Amsterdam, The Netherlands.)

strength.[48,49] Furthermore, additional ischemic infarcts and vascular diseases were found at ultra-high-field that were not apparent at 1.5 T.[49] **Figs. 3** and **4** show examples of small cortical and subcortical ischemic lesions in 2 clinical patients. Kang and colleagues[50] compared the number and configuration of lenticulostriate arteries between chronic stroke patients and healthy controls and found fewer arteries in the stroke group than the controls. Recent work by van der Kolk and colleagues[51] focused on visualizing the intracranial vessel wall itself (**Fig. 5**) at 7 T instead of lumen visualization, in patients with ischemic stroke or transient ischemic attack (TIA). These investigators found vessel wall lesions in several of these patients, even without causing luminal stenosis, suggesting a possible role of intracranial arterial disease in the diagnostic process and risk assessment of patients with cerebrovascular disease.[51] Based on these studies, ultrahigh-field MR imaging could play a role in better visualization of even small infarcts, making statements regarding overall vascular ischemic brain disease possible. Furthermore, visualization of lenticulostriate arteries and the intracranial arterial wall could play

a role in diagnosing patients with (chronic) ischemic brain disease, like patients with low-grade carotid artery stenosis, silent (lacunar) infarcts, and multiple infarcts for which no cause has been found.

SVD can be diagnosed only indirectly, by identification of white matter lesions and lacunar infarcts, which are believed to be imaging markers for the presence and severity of disease of the small arterial vasculature.[20] As mentioned in the section on anatomy and pathogenesis, microbleeds and disease of the lenticulostriate arteries have recently been associated with this heterogeneous disease. Only a few studies have investigated the diagnostic importance of these possible disease markers. Liem and colleagues[52] studied the luminal diameters of the lenticulostriate arteries at 7 T TOF-MRA in patients with CADASIL and compared them with luminal diameters of healthy controls. These investigators found no difference in luminal diameter between patients with CADASIL and healthy volunteers.[52] Theysohn and colleagues[53] showed a higher sensitivity for detection of microbleeds at 7 T compared with 1.5 T, although detection of white matter lesions was comparable between the 2 field

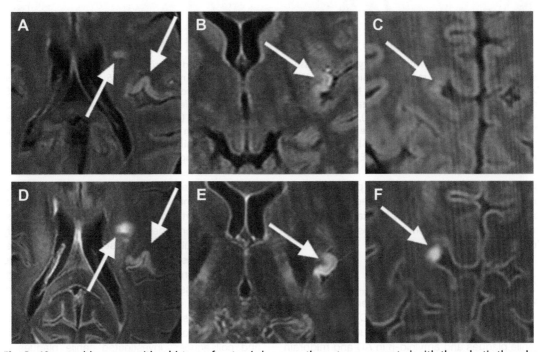

Fig. 3. 40-year-old woman with a history of systemic lupus erythematosus presented with thrombotic thrombocytopenic purpura complicated by transient motor dysphasia. (*A–C*) Axial standard clinical 1.5 T and (*D–F*) corresponding 7 T MR imaging FLAIR images, showing several small cortical and subcortical hyperintense ischemic lesions (*arrows*). Because of the higher CNR at 7 T, lesions were more conspicuous than at lower field strength, and some were seen only in retrospect at 1.5 T (*arrow* in C, compared with F). Imaging parameters as previously published [10]; 0.8-mm isotropic resolution. (*From* van der Kolk AG, Hendrikse J, Zwanenburg JJ, et al. Clinical applications of 7 Tesla MRI in the brain. Eur J Radiol 2011; doi:10.1016/j.ejrad.2011.07.007; with permission.)

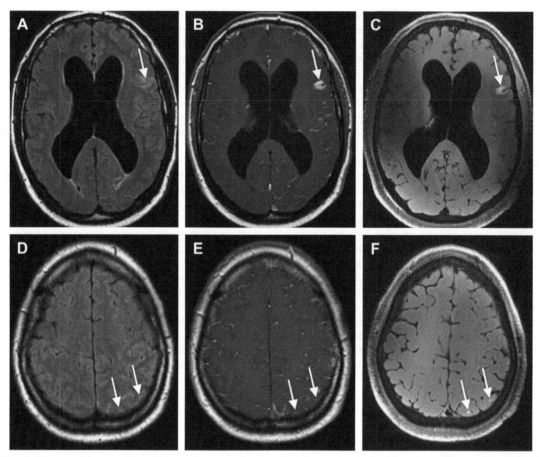

Fig. 4. 50-year-old man with a history of progressive dysphasia, suspected of primary or secondary (sarcoidosis) vasculitis. (*A, D*) Axial standard clinical 1.5 T FLAIR, (*B, E*) corresponding standard 1.5 T contrast-enhanced MRA, and (*C, F*) corresponding 7 T MR imaging contrast-enhanced inversion-recovery turbo spin echo (TSE) images, showing a relatively large area of cortical enhancement frontoparietally (*A–C*), and several small occipital foci of subcortical enhancement (*D–E*), suggestive of small ischemic lesions (*arrows*). Because of the higher CNR at 7 T also small ischemic lesions can be seen (*F*), which were not visible on the 1.5 T MR images (*D, E*). Imaging parameters: 7 T inversion-recovery TSE sequence; repetition time, 3952 milliseconds; echo time, 38 milliseconds; inversion time, 1375 milliseconds; TSE factor, 158; number of signal averages, 2; 0.8-mm isotropic resolution.

strengths. This finding suggests a possible role of ultrahigh-field MR imaging in the diagnostic workup of patients suspected of SVD. An example of micro-bleeds in a clinical patient at our institution can be found in **Fig. 6**.

Degenerative Diseases

As mentioned earlier, most degenerative diseases like AD and Parkinson disease (PD) are histologically well defined, with clear tissue markers like senile plaques and amyloid-β in AD and midbrain dopaminergic cell loss with Lewy bodies in PD. However, making a clinical diagnosis of these diseases based on imaging characteristics at MR imaging is still difficult, and one must rely on subjective and relatively nonspecific measurements of the hippocampal body, or changes in

the signal intensity of the substantia nigra. An imaging technique that could visualize the real disease underlying these degenerative diseases, or at least more specific characteristics currently unknown, would be of utmost clinical importance. Several studies have therefore used ultrahigh-field MR imaging in an attempt to develop the diagnostic process with regard to these prevalent diseases.

Most studies have used postmortem samples in their pursuit of new imaging markers. Dhenain and colleagues[54] investigated senile plaques in a postmortem human AD specimen with 11.7 T T_2*-weighted MR imaging. These investigators hypothesized that the magnetic susceptibility of senile plaques would be different from that of the surrounding tissue, making them increasingly visible at higher field strengths. They found that senile

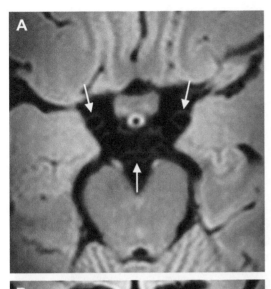

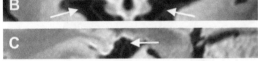

Fig. 5. 51-year-old man presented with transient paresis of the right arm and dysphasia, resolving after 1.5 hours based on a TIA of the left hemisphere. Standard 1.5 T MR imaging revealed 2 small ischemic lesions on the diffusion-weighted images (not shown). (*A*) Axial, (*B*) coronal, and (*C*) sagittal magnetization-prepared inversion-recovery turbo spin echo images, showing healthy intracranial arterial vessel wall of both distal internal carotid arteries (*A* and *B*, *upper arrows*), their bifurcation into middle and anterior cerebral artery (*B* and *C*, *arrows*), and both P1 segments of the posterior cerebral artery (*A*, *lower arrow*). Imaging parameters as previously published[51]; 0.8-mm isotropic resolution.

plaques could not be visualized in this way, suggesting a smaller (or absent) role of susceptibility effects in these plaques.[54] Van Rooden and colleagues[55] also used 7 T T_2*-weighted imaging, alongside T_2-weighted imaging, for depiction of possible differences in cortical aspects of patients with cerebral amyloid deposition. Using human brain specimens with known amyloid-β deposition, these investigators found that all specimens, when compared with healthy control specimens, showed hypointense foci or inhomogeneity of the cortex.[55] Kerchner and colleagues[56] showed, again with T_2*-weighted imaging at 7 T, that CA1 apical neuropil atrophy, a very early site of AD, could be visualized in vivo in 14 patients with AD. These studies suggest that T_2*-weighted imaging at ultrahigh-field could prove beneficial in the diagnosis of several degenerative diseases; however, much still has to be implemented in vivo before the technique can be applied clinically.

To our knowledge only 2 studies have focused on improving PD diagnosis, both within the last 2 years, so this is a relatively new field of research. Bajaj and colleagues[57] in 2010 used in vivo T_2*-weighted 7 T MR imaging to measure the relative magnetic susceptibility of the substantia nigra, specifically the pars compacta. These investigators found a difference in magnetic susceptibility of the pars compacta between patients with PD and healthy controls, suggesting an increase in iron content.[57] Oh and colleagues[58] showed, by using a comparable imaging sequence at 7 T, a difference in gross anatomic shape and quantitative so-called undulation values between patients with PD and healthy controls. These studies show 2 new imaging characteristics that seem to be specific for PD, possibly improving PD detection using MR imaging in clinical practice.

Brain Tumors

The current diagnosis of brain tumors is primarily based on MR imaging results before and after contrast administration, in which distinction of not only different types of tumors (meningioma vs astrocytoma) but also different grades (World Health Organization [WHO] grade II vs IV astrocytoma) can be made. However, a biopsy is often needed for the diagnosis and subsequent treatment. Furthermore, 2 of the most difficult diseases to discern regarding tumor treatment are tumor recurrence and necrotic tissue caused by radiation.

Several studies have tried to find new imaging markers to distinguish these different diseases with better precision, with the aim of making biopsy, with its concomitant risks, obsolete. Lupo and colleagues[59] used T_2*-weighted imaging at 7 T in 11 patients with heterogeneous brain tumors, revealing regions of calcification, microvessels, and hemorrhage. They suggested that these regions could provide better characterization of active or necrotic tumors.[59] Neovascularization is one of the hallmarks of high-grade astrocytomas, and imaging the microvasculature could help in distinguishing between low-grade and high-grade tumors, as well as in follow-up of treatment effect. Christoforidis and colleagues[60,61] and Mönninghoff and colleagues[62] focused on visualizing this microvasculature in patients with astrocytomas of different WHO grades. Christoforidis and colleagues[60] found that T_2-weighted 8 T MR imaging could identify regions of abnormal microvascularity in a glioblastoma multiforme, like tortuosity and enlargement, that were not visible with conventional techniques like 1.5 T MR imaging or digital subtraction angiography. These

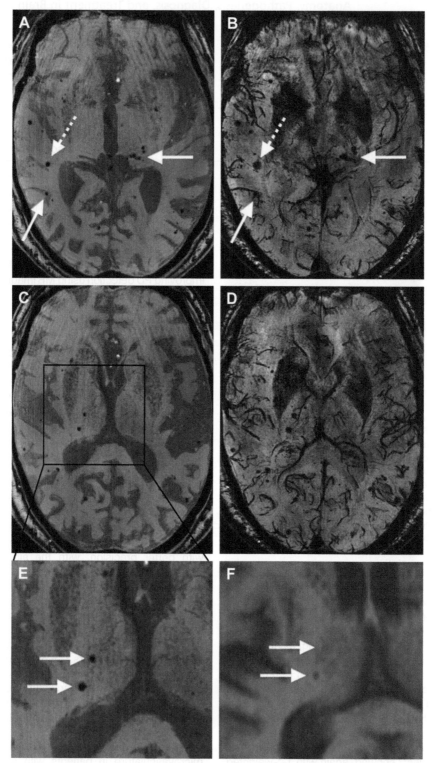

Fig. 6. 77-year-old man with a history of hypertension presented with transient dysphasia based on a TIA of the left hemisphere. (*A, C*) Axial minimal-intensity projections (minMIPs) over 10-mm-thick volumes of the first and (*B, D*) minMIPs of the second echo of 7 T T_2*-weighted images, where multiple microbleeds can be found throughout the brain (*arrows*). Some are less easily distinguished on the second echo minMIPs because of overlapping venous structures (*striped arrows*) and artifacts close to the nasal cavity. (*E*) Zoomed-in image of 7 T and (*F*) of standard clinical 1.5 T first echo minMIPs, showing better visualization of the microbleeds because of the increased susceptibility effects at 7 T compared with 1.5 T MR imaging. Imaging parameters as previously published.[35] (*Courtesy of* Dr M.M. Conijn, VUmc Amsterdam, The Netherlands.)

investigators confirmed these foci of microvascularity seen on 8 T MR imaging with histology.[61] Mönninghoff and colleagues[62] also found these results in 15 patients with astrocytoma when imaged with T_2*-weighted 7 T MR imaging, in whom necrosis was also visualized in more detail than at lower field strength. On the other hand, although more assumed microhemorrhages were seen at 7 T MR imaging within brain metastases of bronchial carcinomas, Mönninghoff and colleagues[63] found the detection of metastases themselves at 7 T equal to 1.5 T MR imaging. Delineation of a more rare tumor, a dysplastic cerebellar gangliocytoma, with respect to morphology and microstructure has also been shown to be more conspicuous at ultrahigh-field MR imaging, especially using T_2*-weighted imaging.[64] Regarding differentiation between low-grade and high-grade tumors, imaging of the microvascularity of tumors using T_2-weighted or T_2*-weighted ultrahigh-field MR imaging seems most promising. For differentiating between tumor recurrence and radiation necrosis, these sequences can also be used, as seen in 1 study, but studies on this topic are lacking. **Fig. 7** for gives 2 examples of tumor imaging at ultrahigh-field 7 T MR imaging.

Epilepsy

Cryptogenic epilepsies form a substantial amount of epilepsies in daily clinical practice. These epilepsies are believed to arise from brain lesions that are otherwise not found with the available imaging techniques. Because cryptogenic epilepsies can often be resistant to therapy, finding an imaging technique with which lesions not previously seen do appear (whether this may be because of a different energy metabolism or because of a small anatomic malformation), is important, especially when facing surgical treatment. Most studies on this topic have focused on known epilepsy-causing disease, like cavernous malformations and hippocampal sclerosis (HS), cryptogenic epilepsy (unknown cause), and for a more precise localization of already known lesions (symptomatic epilepsies **Fig. 8**). Schlamann and colleagues[65] and

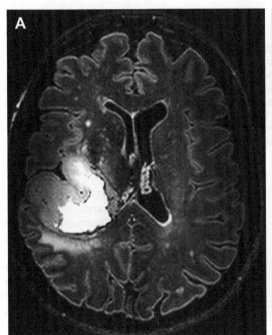
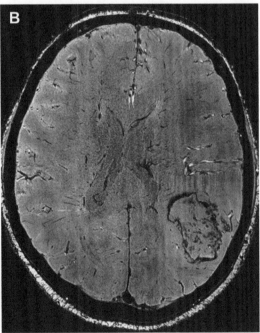

Fig. 7. Two patients with glioblastoma multiforme. A 59-year-old woman presented with an epileptic seizure based on a right-sided, inhomogeneous enhancing temporoparietal glioblastoma multiforme. (*A*) 7 T MR FLAIR image shows described tumor with a central hyperintense area suggestive of necrosis, peritumoral edema, and a slight midline shift. Because of the high CNR at 7 T, tumor as well as edema can clearly be distinguished from surrounding normal brain tissue. (*B*) Axial 7 T T_2*-weighted first echo image of a 62-year-old woman who presented with emotional and cognitive disturbances based on a left-sided parietal glioblastoma multiforme. The T_2*-weighted image (*B*) shows an irregular lesion, the rim of the lesion showing a high susceptibility effect (hypointensity). Imaging parameters for 7 T FLAIR sequence and T_2*-weighted sequence as previously published.[10,11] (*Courtesy of* D.L. Polders and A.L.H.M.W. van Lier, UMC Utrecht, The Netherlands.)

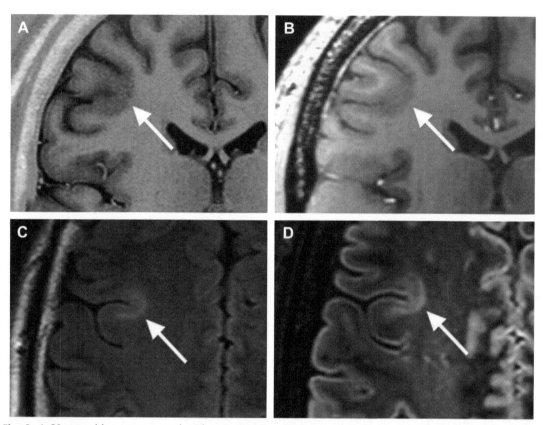

Fig. 8. A 32-year-old man presented with symptomatic therapy-resistant epilepsy characterized by recurrent partial secondary generalized seizures and recurrent status epilepticus. (A) Standard clinical 1.5 T T_1-weighted and (C) FLAIR image, with corresponding images at 7 T MR imaging (B, D). Both imaging sequences at both field strengths could visualize focal cortical dysplasia medially in the right frontal hemisphere (arrows in A–D). However, because of the higher contrast at 7 T, the focal lesion was more pronounced at the 7 T FLAIR image (D). Imaging parameters of the 7 T FLAIR sequence as previously published[10]; 7 T T_1-weighted sequence: shot interval, 3500 milliseconds, inversion time, 1200 milliseconds; TR, 7.0 milliseconds; TE, 2.9 milliseconds; 0.8-mm isotropic resolution. (Courtesy of Dr C.H. Ferrier, UMC Utrecht, The Netherlands.)

Damman and colleagues[66] assessed cerebral cavernous malformations (cavernomas) with 7 T T_2^*-weighted imaging and compared these results with images obtained at 1.5 T. Schlamann and colleagues[65] assessed 10 patients with known cavernomas, found 1 additional lesion not seen on lower field strength, and concluded that ultrahigh-field MR imaging improved the detection of cavernomas, when using T_2^*-weighted imaging. Damman and colleagues reviewed literature regarding the use of T_2^*-weighted imaging for cavernomas, and found, in their patient group, the same positive results as did Schlamann and colleagues. Damman and colleagues suggested that because of ultrahigh-field MR imaging, technical limitations of T_2^*-weighted imaging could be overcome, paving the way for clinical use of ultrahigh-field T_2^*-weighted MR imaging in diagnosing cavernomas.

Two other studies focused on HS associated with temporal lobe epilepsy. Breyer and colleagues[67] assessed the feasibility of multisequence 7 T MR imaging for identification of HS in 6 patients in whom 1.5 T had already confirmed HS. These investigators found that the increased susceptibility effects at ultrahigh-field strength increased the CNR within the hippocampus compared with lower field strength, making identification of more detailed structures possible, as well as excellent identification (on all sequences used) of HS.[67] Garbelli and colleagues[68] used surgical specimens of HS to investigate the correlation between ultrahigh-field T_2-weighted MR imaging findings at 7 T and histology. These investigators found a good correlation between abnormal cortical layering as seen on histology and MR imaging findings and suggested that ultrahigh-field could detect minute intracortical abnormalities not seen at lower fields.[68] These results and those from the cavernoma studies indicate a role of primarily ultrahigh-field T$_2$(*)-weighted MR imaging in the diagnosis of epileptic lesions.

TREATMENT PLANNING

This section discusses treatment applications of ultrahigh-field MR imaging. Treatment applications of MR imaging in general can be grossly subdivided into (novel) treatment monitoring, in which MR imaging is used as a diagnostic tool during the treatment course, identifying progression or regression of disease, and treatment planning, mostly localization-based, of which the most illustrative example is the use of MR datasets during neuronavigation-based surgery. High-intensity focused ultrasound, a relatively new noninvasive treatment modality, has to our knowledge not been used in combination with ultrahigh-field MR imaging, mostly because of its recent occurrence in the therapeutic field and the challenge of using this technique for intracranial disease. Because treatment monitoring is based on diagnosing in time, during the course of treatment, it can be deduced that all diagnostic applications of ultrahigh field reviewed in the section on diagnosis can also apply to monitoring treatment effects. Therefore we focus on the use of ultrahigh-field MR imaging in planning treatment (although the

diagnostic applications reviewed earlier are also relevant).

To our knowledge, only a few studies at ultrahigh-field MR imaging have investigated its possible use specifically for treatment planning. Mönninghoff and colleagues[69] studied a vertebrobasilar aneurysm with 7 T TOF-MRA. They found that ultrahigh-field TOF-MRA could not only identify the aneurysm with more precision but that vessel wall calcifications could also be identified using this sequence, as well as one of the posterior inferior cerebellar arteries arising from the aneurysm, not seen on lower field strength (see **Fig. 9** for an example of a small branching artery of an aneurysm patient). These investigators concluded that these findings could help in aiding endovascular and surgical therapies.[69] Two other studies focused on localizing with high precision anatomic structures used in deep brain stimulation in PD. Although most patients with PD are treated with dopamine (or analogous medication), surgical intervention in this disease has been introduced recently, and is already widely used to treat patients with advanced PD. The neurosurgical technique consists of placing a stimulating electrode within one of the target nuclei, like the subthalamic nucleus and globus pallidus, to relieve the patient's symptoms, not only of PD but also of tremor, chronic pain, and depression. The technique depends on placing

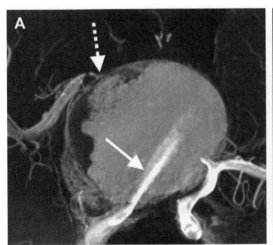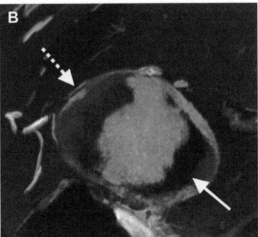

Fig. 9. 16-year-old boy presented with progressive headache and transient monocular visual field defect based on a giant fusiform aneurysm of the distal internal carotid artery. (*A*) Coronal minimal-intensity projection over 10-mm-thick volume and (*B*) sagittal image of 7 T contrast-enhanced TOF-MRA, showing the giant aneurysm extending from the internal carotid artery. A contrast agent jet can be seen inside the aneurysm (*arrow* in *A*), as well as thrombosis of part of the aneurysm (*arrow* in *B*). The branching of the middle cerebral artery (*striped arrow* in *A*) as well as of the anterior cerebral artery (*striped arrow* in *B*) can be appreciated. Imaging parameters as previously published [78]; resolution 0.25 × 0.30 × 0.40 mm, 60-mm slab, feet-head coverage 60 mm. (*Courtesy of* E H J. Voormolen, UMC Utrecht, The Netherlands.)

the electrode at the exact location, which in turn depends on detailed visualization of the target nuclei. Two studies, by Rijkers and colleagues[70] and Cho and colleagues,[71] have used ultrahigh-field MR imaging for this purpose. Rijkers and colleagues[70] used 9.4 T MR imaging on a postmortem human brain sample to obtain three-dimensional (3D) reconstructions of the subthalamic nucleus and found a new reference point based on these detailed images, which might be used for targeting the nucleus. Cho and colleagues[71] used in vivo 7 T MR imaging to visualize several targets for deep brain stimulation, like the subthalamic nucleus and internal globus pallidus, and compared their results with images obtained at 3 T and 1.5 T MR imaging, in both healthy volunteers and 1 patient with PD. These investigators found ultrahigh-field MR imaging to be superior in visualizing the stimulation targets compared with lower field strengths, mainly caused by significantly improved tissue contrast.

Based on these preliminary studies on applicability in treatment planning, ultrahigh-field MR imaging could have a significant value in the visualization of anatomic structures during surgery, like target nuclei and small arteries originating from aneurysms. However, this application could well be just the tip of the iceberg for clinical treatment applicability of ultrahigh-field.

LIMITATIONS IN CLINICAL USE
Technical Issues

As discussed earlier, a high magnetic field strength causes larger magnetic susceptibility effects for a given receiver bandwidth, resulting in signal dropouts and distortion of images. Furthermore, a severe inhomogeneity in the applied transmit field (RF field) is seen at ultrahigh-field. Because of this inhomogeneity, the pulse angle achieved varies between different locations in the brain, resulting in a spatially varying SNR.[72] More importantly for clinical imaging is that, depending on the sequence used, it might lead to deviation of the contrast obtained from different locations in the image.[7] For instance, when obtaining a T_1-weighted image, several areas of the brain will show on the image with a different contrast, sometimes even T_2 contrast instead of T_1 contrast. These effects are most pronounced in the cerebellum and the temporal lobes of the brain, which makes assessment of anatomy and disease in these areas more difficult. By developing improved pulse sequences and new hardware approaches, a more homogeneous transmit field might be attained, reducing the purely technical limitations to a minimum.

Safety

Apart from causing spatially varying SNR,[72] the inhomogeneous transmit field mentioned earlier also causes specific absorption rate (SAR) restrictions. This finding is in addition to the global SAR (mean SAR over a certain volume) increase, which increases with the square of the applied magnetic field strength. Like SNR, the SAR is also less homogeneously distributed over the brain[73] because of the inhomogeneous transmit field, causing larger differences between areas and high SAR peaks at certain places. These increases in SAR impose stringent limitations on the duty cycle of applied sequences.

Metallic objects are currently a contraindication in the area of ultrahigh-field MR imaging. Apart from causing image distortions and artifacts for a given bandwidth, more than at lower field strengths, because of the larger susceptibility effects, potential temperature effects in conducting implant material are another limitation for the use of ultrahigh-field MR imaging in clinical practice. Although these effects cause strict safety measures also at lower field strengths, at high-field strength they may be more pronounced and, from a practical point of view, specific tests to determine safety at ultrahigh-field are still in their infancy. Increased concern for safety at ultrahigh-field is related to the shorter RF wavelength at higher field strength that matches more easily with metallic objects, possibly causing resonance and heating.[7] Although it is not clear what effect metallic implants have when they are placed in an ultrahigh magnetic field strength, because most studies on this topic have been performed on lower field strengths, safety precautions regarding imaging at 7 T, for instance, state that nothing metallic should enter the bore.[7]

It is easy to see the implications of these metallic safety precautions on the implementation of ultrahigh-field MR imaging in the clinical setting. Patients generally are older people who have had surgery, after which metallic implants are sometimes left behind. Examples are patients with atherosclerotic-related diseases, who often have clips or stents in the heart, lower extremity vessels, or carotid arteries. Although sometimes surgical reports can be checked stating the implantation (or not) of metallic objects (and which metallic objects, and whether they have been tested for safety), in most patients this is not the case, and often patients themselves are not fully informed of the presence and location of metallic implants after surgery. Even if older people have been healthy their whole lives, they often have dental implants that prohibit scanning at ultrahigh-field.

To illustrate this problem, in a recent study of patients with ischemic stroke and TIA, 173 of 611 eligible patients had to be excluded because of contraindications for 7 T MR imaging caused by metallic implants.[51] Furthermore, although young and healthy people could in theory readily be scanned at ultrahigh-field, even in this group the increased use of (permanent) dental braces poses a challenge for implementing ultrahigh-field MR imaging in the clinical workup. Decreasing the list of contraindications is therefore mandatory if ultrahigh-field MR imaging is to be used in clinical practice.

Learning Curve for the Radiologist

It is not only a question of having the right techniques and sequences at hand, and overcoming limitations that are still hampering ultrahigh-field MR imaging from being implemented in clinical routine. With the new MR imaging contrasts and details found at ultrahigh-field MR imaging, radiologists should learn to interpret them. We cannot just assume that assessment of anatomy and disease at higher-field MR images will be the same at lower-field MR imaging. Ultrahigh-field images should be validated with known pathology as seen on lower field strengths like 1.5 T or 3 T MR imaging. With higher anatomic detail comes the chance of finding unexpected lesions, like very small aneurysms or developmental venous anomalies. Furthermore, new artifacts, related to the increased sensitivity for susceptibility and RF inhomogeneities present at ultrahigh-field MR imaging, can easily lead to false-positive findings. To get the best out of this new MR imaging application, radiologists need to be trained in assessing these new images.

DISCUSSION

Using ultrahigh-field has many advantages over lower field strengths, because of its higher achievable spatial resolution and increased susceptibility effects. These advantages enable us to see many things in different diseases that have not previously been seen on lower fields, as well as more detailed anatomic structures. However, how do we know that what we see as disease is accurate? A few studies have tried to answer this question using postmortem specimens. Yao and colleagues[74] investigated the validity of T_2*-weighted contrast in the detection of iron and found that it was a valid indicator of iron content in iron-rich brain regions. On the other hand, de Reuck and colleagues[75] found that at 7 T T_2*-weighted imaging, in a postmortem brain specimen of patients with dementia, only quantification of cerebral microbleeds in the

corticosubcortical regions is reliable. This finding means that we have to be careful with diagnosing pathologic lesions, without having histologic comparison. This last issue can be a challenge, because opinions are varied regarding the use of fixed or nonfixed specimens for MR imaging and histology correlation. Dashner and colleagues[76] found unfixed specimens to show microvascularity better than fixed specimens, in which no vessels could be found at all. On the other hand, Garbelli and colleagues[68] showed superior MR contrast between cortical layers in completely fixed specimens compared with recently excised samples.

Furthermore, although there is a trend toward higher field strengths, with associated higher spatial resolution, even these ultrahigh-field techniques have a maximum resolution that can be realistically attained. For instance, using 8 T MR imaging, visualization of deoxygenated small vessels was excellent down to a resolution of about 100 μm, but these studies were performed using a human cadaver brain, and the question remains whether this high resolution can be achieved in vivo.[77] Also, the additional value of ultrahigh-field MR imaging in diagnosis and treatment compared with lower field strengths has not been studied extensively.

However, regardless of these critical remarks, it is clear that ultrahigh-field MR imaging can improve diagnosis by finding disease that has not been found at lower field strengths. For example, in some patients with cryptogenic epilepsy (from our own clinical experience with 7 T MR imaging), we do find lesions when we move to ultrahigh field. This application of ultrahigh-field MR imaging has such implications for these patients that it is too important to neglect. Another clinical example is that of patients with an aneurysm. One of the questions when planning surgery for an aneurysm is if there are any small branching arteries that arise from the aneurysm itself. If the aneurysm is clipped or coiled and a small important branching artery arises from the aneurysm, it is blocked from flow and can cause an ischemic infarct.

In current practice, ultrahigh-field MR imaging can officially be used only for clinical research purposes. When it becomes available for human clinical use, choosing sequences will in the beginning be at least partially dependent on which sequences are already available at ultrahigh-field MR imaging sites. Sequences should be successfully tested in healthy volunteers, so that any technical errors have already been dealt with. Furthermore, the sequence should not be long, because motion artifacts may reduce image quality. Most additional diagnostic value will probably be gained from using either high-resolution 3D sequences or T_2*-weighted imaging.

When different diseases are considered, it is clear that T_2^*-weighted imaging is most promising in degenerative diseases and epilepsy. FLAIR imaging has proved to be important in visualizing MS lesions, but can be used for all brain diseases, as is current clinical practice on lower magnetic fields.

REFERENCES

1. Vaughan T, DelaBarre L, Snyder C, et al. 9.4T human MRI: preliminary results. Magn Reson Med 2006;56: 1274–82.
2. Cha S, Gore JC. Clinical applications of ultra-high field 7T MRI—moving to FDA/EU approval. In: Proceedings of the ISMRM 19th Annual Meeting & Exhibition. Montreal, May 11, 2011.
3. Ladd ME, van Buchem MA, Rinck PA. Hot Topics Debate "Can 7T go clinical?". In: Proceedings of the ISMRM 18th Annual Meeting & Exhibition. Stockholm, May 5, 2010.
4. Bottomley PA, Foster TH, Argersinger RE, et al. A review of normal tissue hydrogen NMR relaxation times and relaxation mechanisms from 1-100 MHz: dependence on tissue type, NMR frequency, temperature, species, excision, and age. Med Phys 1984;11:425–48.
5. Li TQ, Yao B, van GP, et al. Characterization of T(2)* heterogeneity in human brain white matter. Magn Reson Med 2009;62:1652–7.
6. Rooney WD, Johnson G, Li X, et al. Magnetic field and tissue dependencies of human brain longitudinal 1H2O relaxation in vivo. Magn Reson Med 2007;57:308–18.
7. van der Kolk AG, Hendrikse J, Zwanenburg JJ, et al. Clinical applications of 7 Tesla MRI in the brain. Eur J Radiol 2011. DOI:10.1016/j.ejrad.2011.07.007.
8. Abduljalil AM, Schmalbrock P, Novak V, et al. Enhanced gray and white matter contrast of phase susceptibility-weighted images in ultra-high-field magnetic resonance imaging. J Magn Reson Imaging 2003;18:284–90.
9. Budde J, Shajan G, Hoffmann J, et al. Human imaging at 9.4 T using T(2) *-, phase-, and susceptibility-weighted contrast. Magn Reson Med 2011;65:544–50.
10. Visser F, Zwanenburg JJ, Hoogduin JM, et al. High-resolution magnetization-prepared 3D-FLAIR imaging at 7.0 Tesla. Magn Reson Med 2010;64: 194–202.
11. Zwanenburg JJ, Versluis MJ, Luijten PR, et al. Fast high resolution whole brain T2* weighted imaging using echo planar imaging at 7T. Neuroimage 2011;56(4):1902–7.
12. Van de Moortele PF, Auerbach EJ, Olman C, et al. T1 weighted brain images at 7 Tesla unbiased for Proton Density, T2* contrast and RF coil receive B1

sensitivity with simultaneous vessel visualization. Neuroimage 2009;46:432–46.
13. Wieshmann UC, Symms MR, Mottershead JP, et al. Hippocampal layers on high resolution magnetic resonance images: real or imaginary? J Anat 1999; 195(Pt 1):131–5.
14. Chakeres DW, Whitaker CD, Dashner RA, et al. High-resolution 8 Tesla imaging of the formalin-fixed normal human hippocampus. Clin Anat 2005; 18:88–91.
15. Augustinack JC, van der Kouwe AJ, Blackwell ML, et al. Detection of entorhinal layer II using 7Tesla [corrected] magnetic resonance imaging. Ann Neurol 2005;57:489–94.
16. Thomas BP, Welch EB, Niederhauser BD, et al. High-resolution 7T MRI of the human hippocampus in vivo. J Magn Reson Imaging 2008;28:1266–72.
17. Theysohn JM, Kraff O, Maderwald S, et al. The human hippocampus at 7 T–in vivo MRI. Hippocampus 2009;19:1–7.
18. Yushkevich PA, Avants BB, Pluta J, et al. A high-resolution computational atlas of the human hippocampus from postmortem magnetic resonance imaging at 9.4 T. Neuroimage 2009;44:385–98.
19. Fatterpekar GM, Naidich TP, Delman BN, et al. Cytoarchitecture of the human cerebral cortex: MR microscopy of excised specimens at 9.4 Tesla. AJNR Am J Neuroradiol 2002;23:1313–21.
20. Wardlaw JM. Blood-brain barrier and cerebral small vessel disease. J Neurol Sci 2010;299:66–71.
21. Zwanenburg JJ, Hendrikse J, Takahara T, et al. MR angiography of the cerebral perforating arteries with magnetization prepared anatomical reference at 7 T: comparison with time-of-flight. J Magn Reson Imaging 2008;28:1519–26.
22. Cho ZH, Kang CK, Han JY, et al. Observation of the lenticulostriate arteries in the human brain in vivo using 7.0T MR angiography. Stroke 2008;39: 1604–6.
23. Kang CK, Park CW, Han JY, et al. Imaging and analysis of lenticulostriate arteries using 7.0-Tesla magnetic resonance angiography. Magn Reson Med 2009;61:136–44.
24. Lucchinetti C, Bruck W, Parisi J, et al. Heterogeneity of multiple sclerosis lesions: implications for the pathogenesis of demyelination. Ann Neurol 2000;47: 707–17.
25. Rudick RA, Trapp BD. Gray-matter injury in multiple sclerosis. N Engl J Med 2009;361:1505–6.
26. Kangarlu A, Bourekas EC, Ray-Chaudhury A, et al. Cerebral cortical lesions in multiple sclerosis detected by MR imaging at 8 Tesla. AJNR Am J Neuroradiol 2007;28:262–6.
27. Hammond KE, Metcalf M, Carvajal L, et al. Quantitative in vivo magnetic resonance imaging of multiple sclerosis at 7 Tesla with sensitivity to iron. Ann Neurol 2008;64:707–13.

28. Ge Y, Zohrabian VM, Grossman RI. Seven-Tesla magnetic resonance imaging: new vision of microvascular abnormalities in multiple sclerosis. Arch Neurol 2008;65:812–6.

29. Tallantyre EC, Brookes MJ, Dixon JE, et al. Demonstrating the perivascular distribution of MS lesions in vivo with 7-Tesla MRI. Neurology 2008; 70:2076–8.

30. Pitt D, Boster A, Pei W, et al. Imaging cortical lesions in multiple sclerosis with ultra-high-field magnetic resonance imaging. Arch Neurol 2010; 67:812–8.

31. Laule C, Kozlowski P, Leung E, et al. Myelin water imaging of multiple sclerosis at 7 T: correlations with histopathology. Neuroimage 2008;40: 1575–80.

32. Novak V, Abduljalil A, Kangarlu A, et al. Intracranial ossifications and microangiopathy at 8 Tesla MRI. Magn Reson Imaging 2001;19:1133–7.

33. Kang CK, Park CA, Lee H, et al. Hypertension correlates with lenticulostriate arteries visualized by 7T magnetic resonance angiography. Hypertension 2009;54:1050–6.

34. Biessels GJ, Zwanenburg JJ, Visser F, et al. Hypertensive cerebral hemorrhage: imaging the leak with 7-T MRI. Neurology 2010;75:572–3.

35. Conijn MM, Geerlings MI, Luijten PR, et al. Visualization of cerebral microbleeds with dual-echo T2*-weighted magnetic resonance imaging at 7.0 T. J Magn Reson Imaging 2010;32:52–9.

36. Conijn MM, Geerlings MI, Biessels GJ, et al. Cerebral microbleeds on MR imaging: comparison between 1.5 and 7T. AJNR Am J Neuroradiol 2011; 32:1043–9.

37. Chakeres DW, Abduljalil AM, Novak P, et al. Comparison of 1.5 and 8 tesla high-resolution magnetic resonance imaging of lacunar infarcts. J Comput Assist Tomogr 2002;26:628–32.

38. Jouvent E, Poupon C, Gray F, et al. Intracortical infarcts in small vessel disease: a combined 7-T postmortem MRI and neuropathological case study in cerebral autosomal-dominant arteriopathy with subcortical infarcts and leukoencephalopathy. Stroke 2011;42:e27–30.

39. Novak V, Chowdhary A, Abduljalil A, et al. Venous cavernoma at 8 Tesla MRI. Magn Reson Imaging 2003;21:1087–9.

40. Shenkar R, Venkatasubramanian PN, Zhao JC, et al. Advanced magnetic resonance imaging of cerebral cavernous malformations: part I. High-field imaging of excised human lesions. Neurosurgery 2008;63: 782–9.

41. Mainero C, Benner T, Radding A, et al. In vivo imaging of cortical pathology in multiple sclerosis using ultra-high field MRI. Neurology 2009;73:941–8.

42. Kollia K, Maderwald S, Putzki N, et al. First clinical study on ultra-high-field MR imaging in patients with multiple sclerosis: comparison of 1.5T and 7T. AJNR Am J Neuroradiol 2009;30:699–702.

43. Tallantyre EC, Morgan PS, Dixon JE, et al. 3 Tesla and 7 Tesla MRI of multiple sclerosis cortical lesions. J Magn Reson Imaging 2010;32:971–7.

44. Tallantyre EC, Morgan PS, Dixon JE, et al. A comparison of 3T and 7T in the detection of small parenchymal veins within MS lesions. Invest Radiol 2009;44:491–4.

45. Tallantyre EC, Dixon JE, Donaldson I, et al. Ultra-high-field imaging distinguishes MS lesions from asymptomatic white matter lesions. Neurology 2011;76:534–9.

46. de Graaf WL, Visser F, Wattjes MP, et al. 7 Tesla 3D-FLAIR and 3D-DIR: high sensitivity in cortical regions in multiple sclerosis. In: Proceedings of the ISMRM 18th Annual Meeting & Exhibition [abstract 409]. Montreal, May 1–7, 2010.

47. Schmierer K, Parkes HG, So PW, et al. High field (9.4 Tesla) magnetic resonance imaging of cortical grey matter lesions in multiple sclerosis. Brain 2010;133: 858–67.

48. Novak V, Kangarlu A, Abduljalil A, et al. Ultra high field MRI at 8 Tesla of subacute hemorrhagic stroke. J Comput Assist Tomogr 2001;25:431–5.

49. Novak V, Abduljalil AM, Novak P, et al. High-resolution ultrahigh-field MRI of stroke. Magn Reson Imaging 2005;23:539–48.

50. Kang CK, Park CA, Park CW, et al. Lenticulostriate arteries in chronic stroke patients visualised by 7 T magnetic resonance angiography. Int J Stroke 2010;5:374–80.

51. van der Kolk AG, Zwanenburg JJ, Brundel M, et al. Intracranial vessel wall imaging at 7.0 Tesla MRI. Stroke 2011;42:2478–84.

52. Liem MK, van der GJ, Versluis MJ, et al. Lenticulostriate arterial lumina are normal in cerebral autosomal-dominant arteriopathy with subcortical infarcts and leukoencephalopathy: a high-field in vivo MRI study. Stroke 2010;41(12): 2812–6.

53. Theysohn JM, Kraff O, Maderwald S, et al. 7 tesla MRI of microbleeds and white matter lesions as seen in vascular dementia. J Magn Reson Imaging 2011;33:782–91.

54. Dhenain M, Privat N, Duyckaerts C, et al. Senile plaques do not induce susceptibility effects in T2*-weighted MR microscopic images. NMR Biomed 2002;15:197–203.

55. van Rooden S, Maat-Schieman ML, Nabuurs RJ, et al. Cerebral amyloidosis: postmortem detection with human 7.0-T MR imaging system. Radiology 2009;253:788–96.

56. Kerchner GA, Hess CP, Hammond-Rosenbluth KE, et al. Hippocampal CA1 apical neuropil atrophy in mild Alzheimer disease visualized with 7-T MRI. Neurology 2010;75:1381–7.

57. Bajaj N, Schafer A, Wharton S, et al. PATH53 magnetic susceptibility of substantia nigra in Parkinson's disease: a 7-T in vivo MRI study. J Neurol Neurosurg Psychiatry 2010;81:e22.

58. Oh SH, Kim JM, Park SY, et al. Direct visualization of Parkinson's disease by in vivo human brain imaging using 7.0T MRI. In: Proceedings of the ISMRM 19th Annual Meeting & Exhibition [abstract 421]. Montreal, May 7–13, 2011.

59. Lupo JM, Banerjee S, Hammond KE, et al. GRAPPA-based susceptibility-weighted imaging of normal volunteers and patients with brain tumor at 7 T. Magn Reson Imaging 2009;27:480–8.

60. Christoforidis GA, Grecula JC, Newton HB, et al. Visualization of microvascularity in glioblastoma multiforme with 8-T high-spatial-resolution MR imaging. AJNR Am J Neuroradiol 2002;23:1553–6.

61. Christoforidis GA, Kangarlu A, Abduljalil AM, et al. Susceptibility-based imaging of glioblastoma microvascularity at 8 T: correlation of MR imaging and postmortem pathology. AJNR Am J Neuroradiol 2004;25:756–60.

62. Mönninghoff C, Maderwald S, Theysohn JM, et al. Imaging of adult astrocytic brain tumours with 7 T MRI: preliminary results. Eur Radiol 2010;20:704–13.

63. Mönninghoff C, Maderwald S, Theysohn JM, et al. Imaging of brain metastases of bronchial carcinomas with 7T MRI–initial results. Rofo 2010;182:764–72.

64. Mönninghoff C, Kraff O, Schlamann M, et al. Assessing a dysplastic cerebellar gangliocytoma (Lhermitte-Duclos disease) with 7T MR imaging. Korean J Radiol 2010;11:244–8.

65. Schlamann M, Maderwald S, Becker W, et al. Cerebral cavernous hemangiomas at 7 Tesla: initial experience. Acad Radiol 2010;17:3–6.

66. Dammann P, Barth M, Zhu Y, et al. Susceptibility weighted magnetic resonance imaging of cerebral cavernous malformations: prospects, drawbacks, and first experience at ultra-high field strength (7-Tesla) magnetic resonance imaging. Neurosurg Focus 2010;29:E5.

67. Breyer T, Wanke I, Maderwald S, et al. Imaging of patients with hippocampal sclerosis at 7 Tesla: initial results. Acad Radiol 2010;17:421–6.

68. Garbelli R, Zucca I, Milesi G, et al. Combined 7-T MRI and histopathologic study of normal and dysplastic samples from patients with TLE. Neurology 2011;76:1177–85.

69. Mönninghoff C, Maderwald S, Wanke I. Pre-interventional assessment of a vertebrobasilar aneurysm with 7 tesla time-of-flight MR angiography. Rofo 2009;181:266–8.

70. Rijkers K, Temel Y, Visser-Vandewalle V, et al. The microanatomical environment of the subthalamic nucleus. Technical note. J Neurosurg 2007;107:198–201.

71. Cho ZH, Min HK, Oh SH, et al. Direct visualization of deep brain stimulation targets in Parkinson disease with the use of 7-tesla magnetic resonance imaging. J Neurosurg 2010;113:639–47.

72. Vaughan JT, Garwood M, Collins CM, et al. 7T vs. 4T: RF power, homogeneity, and signal-to-noise comparison in head images. Magn Reson Med 2001;46:24–30.

73. Collins CM, Liu W, Wang J, et al. Temperature and SAR calculations for a human head within volume and surface coils at 64 and 300 MHz. J Magn Reson Imaging 2004;19:650–6.

74. Yao B, Li TQ, Gelderen P, et al. Susceptibility contrast in high field MRI of human brain as a function of tissue iron content. Neuroimage 2009;44:1259–66.

75. De Reuck J, Auger F, Cordonnier C, et al. Comparison of 7.0-T T*-magnetic resonance imaging of cerebral bleeds in post-mortem brain sections of Alzheimer patients with their neuropathological correlates. Cerebrovasc Dis 2011;31:511–7.

76. Dashner RA, Chakeres DW, Kangarlu A, et al. MR imaging visualization of the cerebral microvasculature: a comparison of live and postmortem studies at 8 T. AJNR Am J Neuroradiol 2003;24:1881–4.

77. Dashner RA, Kangarlu A, Clark DL, et al. Limits of 8-Tesla magnetic resonance imaging spatial resolution of the deoxygenated cerebral microvasculature. J Magn Reson Imaging 2004;19:303–7.

78. Hendrikse J, Zwanenburg JJ, Visser F, et al. Noninvasive depiction of the lenticulostriate arteries with time-of-flight MR angiography at 7.0 T. Cerebrovasc Dis 2008;26:624–9.

Ultrahigh-Field Magnetic Resonance Imaging: The Clinical Potential for Anatomy, Pathogenesis, Diagnosis and Treatment Planning in Neck and Spine Disease

Lale Umutlu, MD[a],*, Michael Forsting, MD[a],
Mark E. Ladd, PhD[a,b]

KEYWORDS

- 7 tesla MR imaging • Neck and spine imaging
- Ultrahigh-field MR imaging • 7 T spine MR imaging
- 7 T neck MR imaging

Key Points

- Ultrahigh-field magnetic resonance (MR) imaging of the neck and spine is an emerging promising imaging technique; the increased signal/noise ratio (SNR) at 7 T can be used to achieve higher spatio-temporal resolution imaging than at lower field strengths
- Initial ultrahigh-field radiofrequency (RF) coil concepts have enabled the successful demonstration of high-resolution nonenhanced MR angiography of the carotid arteries and structural imaging of the spine and parotid gland
- Further developments in RF coil design, pulse sequences, and shimming strategies are needed before the full diagnostic potential of ultrahigh-field MR imaging of the neck and spine can be assessed

---

ULTRAHIGH-FIELD MR IMAGING OF THE NECK AND SPINE

MR imaging has evolved to become the diagnostic modality of choice for spine imaging and, because of its excellent soft tissue contrast, also the preferred diagnostic modality for neck imaging. Indications to perform MR imaging of the neck and spine range from suspected vertebral disk herniation to spinal cord tumors, as well as

---

Financial disclosure/conflict of interest: Mark E. Ladd receives research support from Siemens Healthcare, Erlangen, Germany. Lale Umutlu is a consultant and speaker for Bayer Healthcare, Berlin, Germany.
[a] Department of Diagnostic and Interventional Radiology and Neuroradiology, University Hospital Essen, Hufelandstr. 55, D-45122 Essen, Germany
[b] Erwin L. Hahn Institute for Magnetic Resonance Imaging, University of Duisburg-Essen, UNESCO World Cultural Heritage Zollverein, Arendahls Wiese 199, D-45141 Essen, Germany
* Corresponding author.
E-mail address: Lale.Umutlu@uk-essen.de

Neuroimag Clin N Am 22 (2012) 363–371
doi:10.1016/j.nic.2012.02.014

Diagnostic Checklist

- Owing to recent advancements in RF coil design and construction, 7 T MR imaging has established its initial feasibility for neck and spine applications
- The increase in the magnetic field strength to ultrahigh-field yields potentially advantageous as well as disadvantageous changes in physical effects
- The increase in SNR associated with 7 T can be transitioned into imaging at high spatial resolution, allowing for detailed anatomic depictions
- 7 T MR imaging allows nonenhanced, high-resolution MR angiography of the carotid arteries and high-quality cross-sectional plaque assessment
- The exacerbation of artifacts affiliated with the increase in the magnetic field strength may impede the diagnostic quality of 7 T MR imaging and necessitates imaging sequence and parameter modification
- Imaging of large fields of view (FOVs) at 7 T, as is often required in spine imaging, remains challenging because of RF field inhomogeneities
- Specific absorption rate (SAR) limitations, especially with respect to local SAR, need particular consideration
- Medical implants, metallic devices in general (eg, piercings), and tattoos have to be handled with caution when scanning at ultrahigh-field strength to prevent potential harm
- Further optimization of imaging sequences, shim techniques, and RF coil concepts is needed to make imaging at 7 T competitive with the diagnostic ability of neck and spine imaging at low to high-field strength

assessment of possible neoplastic or inflammatory disease of the cervical soft tissue.

Although 1.5 T MR systems are still considered the clinical standard, 3 T imaging has established its place in clinical diagnostics within the last few years.[1–11] A further increase in field strength to 7 T has shown initial benefits for clinically oriented neuroimaging[12–16]; however, potential diagnostic benefits for extracranial imaging are yet to be shown.

This article reviews the current status of ultrahigh-field MR imaging in the neck and spine. Ultrahigh-field is defined here as imaging at more than 3 T but, because 7 T is emerging as the next standard field strength beyond 3 T, the article focuses on work at 7 T.

INCREASE OF THE MAGNETIC FIELD STRENGTH: BENEFITS

The urge to increase the magnetic field strength is based on potentially beneficial physical properties. The increase of the SNR is considered one of the most desirable physical effects associated with the increase of the field strength, because the higher SNR can be transformed into imaging at higher spatial or temporal resolution, or both.[17–20] Various ultrahigh-field studies, mainly neuroskeletal and musculoskeletal MR imaging, have shown the successful transformation of the associated higher SNR into a higher spatiotemporal resolution, enabling an improvement in the assessment of anatomic details as well as increased accuracy for the depiction of pathologic findings.[12–15,21–24]

INCREASE OF THE MAGNETIC FIELD STRENGTH: CHALLENGES

Despite the anticipated gain in SNR, an increase in the magnetic field strength is also accompanied by various physical effects that can lead to an impairment of image quality and confound the expected advantages. Apart from an increase of magnetic susceptibility and chemical shift artifacts, RF field alterations and increased deposition of RF energy are considered major disadvantages of high-field MR imaging.[4,8,17–20,25–28]

The energy deposition in tissue, measured by the SAR, scales with the square of the magnetic field, with the square of the flip angle, and is proportional to the duty cycle of the RF pulse, which is particularly problematic for the adequate acquisition of RF-intense turbo-spin-echo (TSE) and fat-saturated sequences. To mitigate the associated SAR increase and preclude potentially harmful heating of the human body, parallel imaging can be applied to reduce the number of RF excitations, or various flip angle modulation techniques can be used. However, the application of parallel imaging as well as the reduction of flip angles may result in an SNR penalty.[17–19,27]

With increasing field strength, maintenance of the homogeneity of the RF magnetic field also becomes more challenging. The wave frequency scales linearly with increasing magnetic strength, leading to a shortening of the RF wavelengths applied for tissue excitation (53 cm at 1.5 T, 27 cm at 3 T, 14–15 cm at 7 T),[17,26] which may result in alterations of the RF energy distribution in tissue and so-called B_1 inhomogeneity, which is particularly pronounced in high-field body applications when a large FOV (eg, abdomen) is imaged. Hence, ultrahigh-field body imaging requires multi-channel RF transmit systems that enable RF shimming. One example of an add-on system for RF shimming[29] consists of an RF amplifier with 8 individual modules, modified to split the excitation signal of the conventional single-channel system into 8 independent channels. Optimized sets of amplitudes and phase shifts thus enable more uniform excitation of specific body regions, as shown in recent ultrahigh-field abdominal studies.[30,31]

Notwithstanding these challenges, the exacerbation of certain artifacts caused by an increase in field strength may also be useful for diagnostics. Magnetic susceptibility effects are known to increase with increasing field strength, resulting in image distortion and signal loss at interfaces of soft tissue and bowel gas in abdominal MR imaging.[8,20,32] However, increased sensitivity to susceptibility differences may also improve the conspicuity of possible microbleeds in the brain, because paramagnetic substances such as hemosiderin may be superiorly detected at higher magnetic field strength.[16]

ULTRAHIGH-FIELD SPINE IMAGING

MR imaging of the spine benefits from an increase of the magnetic field strength from 1.5 T to 3 T, resulting in an improved delineation of soft tissue, cerebrospinal fluid, vertebral discs, and bone interfaces.[33,34] In a comparison study in the spine in patients with isolated syndrome suggesting multiple sclerosis, the imaging results revealed an improved diagnostic accuracy for 3 T MR imaging.[34] With the benefits of increased field strength being shown for 3 T spinal cord imaging, even higher field strengths such as 7 T and greater may be able to improve the diagnostic accuracy, or may even may be able to provide earlier diagnosis of spinal disease.[35]

Initially hampered by the lack of dedicated RF coils, recent advancements in RF coil design have created opportunities for scientific research in 7 T spine imaging.[36–38] In an initial technical approach Wu and colleagues[38] designed and built transceiver arrays with coil geometries of different coil size and number. Their preliminary results showed the feasibility of in vivo human spine imaging using a microstrip loop design with adjustable inductive decoupling, offering large image coverage and satisfactory B_1 penetration and parallel imaging performance.

Using an alternative design approach, Kraff and colleagues[36] recently introduced a prototype of a custom-built 8-channel transmit coil for spine imaging at 7 T (Fig. 1). The combined transmit/receive RF array is constructed of 8 square surface loop coils, with neighboring elements being

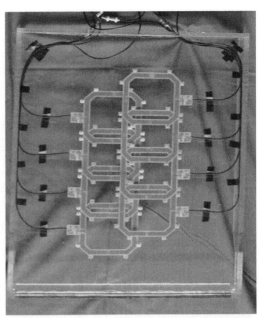

Fig. 1. A spine array designed for 7 T showing the arrangement of the 8 transmit/receive coil elements.

overlapped to decrease the mutual inductance. The assembled spine array is connected to a set of 8 preamplifiers and T/R switches to provide controlled independent tissue excitation for maximum excitation uniformity and coverage. Imaging results revealed a reasonably homogeneous excitation along the spine for a coverage of a 40-cm FOV, providing good delineation of anatomic details including the vertebral bodies, longitudinal ligaments, and the venous drainage through the vertebrae (Fig. 2). Residual signal alterations caused by B_1 inhomogeneity and inconsistent contrast between cerebrospinal fluid and myelin (caused by flip angle variations) were noted as impairing limitations.[36]

This combined transmit/receive RF spine array was used by Grams and colleagues[39] to perform a clinical study to evaluate the feasibility of common clinical sequences for imaging of the lumbar spine at ultrahigh-field strength. After sequence adjustments and modifications for 7 T, T2-weighted (T2w) TSE, three-dimensional (3D) double-echo steady-state (DESS), 3D constructive interference in steady-state (CISS), and 3D volumetric interpolated breath hold examination (VIBE) sequences were acquired. T2w TSE imaging in 5 healthy volunteers was strongly limited in its penetration depth, yielding sufficient signal homogeneity in only 2 slim volunteers. Hence, qualitative image analysis of T2w TSE imaging was rated as poor. In contrast, 3D VIBE MR imaging provided the best imaging results,

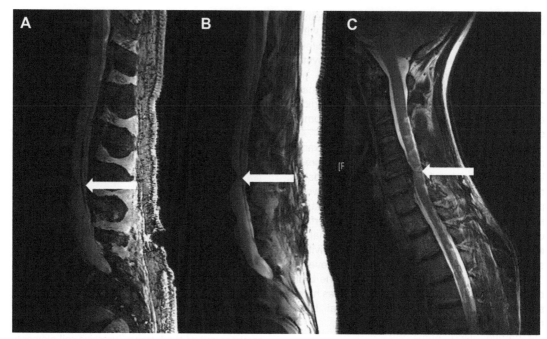

Fig. 2. Nonenhanced two-dimensional fluorescence in situ hybridization (FLASH) sagittal image (*A*) revealing slight protrusion of the intervertebral disk L3/L4 (*arrows*) with concomitant T2-weighted (T2w) TSE image (*B*). Arrow in (*C*) points at intervertebral disk protrusion (C5/6) in the cervical spine in T2w imaging. Note strong medulla spinalis signal alterations, impeding the detection of possible myelopathy.

enabling the highest spatial resolution with 0.57 isotropic imaging. Gradient-echo sequences are generally less susceptible to flip angle variations than spin-echo sequences.[40] Nevertheless, VIBE imaging also showed limitations in terms of signal loss in portions of the spine more distant from the coil, as well as an impaired delineation of the caudal fibers and the intraforaminal structures. 3D CISS and 3D DESS MR imaging yielded comparable imaging results in terms of anatomic display, with slightly better conspicuity of intraforaminal structures in CISS imaging and slightly better conspicuity of the facet joints in DESS MR imaging. In terms of quantitative image analysis, T2w TSE imaging achieved the highest mean values of all the assessed sequences for the contrast ratio between the cerebrospinal fluid and the vertebral body, as well as between the cerebrospinal fluid and the spinal cord. The best contrast ratio between vertebral disc and body was rated for 3D CISS MR imaging. Despite these promising initial imaging results of ultrahigh-field spine imaging, none of the assessed sequences, all of which are established in 1.5 T and 3 T clinical imaging, could provide sufficient conspicuity of all assessed anatomic structures or compete with the diagnostic ability of clinical spine imaging at low to high-field strength. Hence, the routine clinical

application of ultrahigh-field spine MR imaging is not yet possible.[39]

Vossen and colleagues[37] examined ultrahigh-field spine imaging for assessing the complete human spinal column within an acceptable scanning time. For image acquisition, they used a dedicated quadrature transmit, 8-channel receive array RF coil. Large FOV scanning allowed sagittal spine imaging in 2 or 3 stations within a total scan time of 10 to 15 minutes. In addition to initial clinical findings such as signs of osteochondrosis as well as small dislocations in the disks, their study results also revealed the efficiency of using an anterior coil for transmission of RF energy combined with a posterior receive array.

In conclusion, these first approaches toward dedicated 7 T spine MR imaging reveal the potential benefits as well as challenges of ultrahigh-field spine imaging. Further optimization of RF sequences, shim techniques, and dedicated RF coil concepts are expected to better cope with the physical effects affiliated with high magnetic field strength, enabling clinically oriented studies at 7 T. The first commercial RF coils for the spine are becoming available and include a dedicated cervical spine coil that is constructed in a 2 × 2 channel arrangement and is compatible with MR systems with both a single transmitter or 4 individual transmitters for parallel excitation applications such as Transmit SENSE.[41,42]

ULTRAHIGH-FIELD NECK IMAGING

Within the last decade, MR imaging of the neck has established itself as an excellent alternative to computed tomography based on the omission of ionizing radiation and its excellent inherent soft tissue contrast. It has emerged as the imaging modality of choice for head and neck imaging, yielding improved delineation and assessment of possible neoplastic diseases.[43] Despite the expected benefits of an increased magnetic field strength, the published research regarding ultrahigh-field neck imaging is limited to a few contributions, mainly because of the lack of dedicated RF coil concepts.[44–48]

One publication by Kraff and colleagues[47] shows promising imaging results of high-resolution 7 T MR imaging of the parotid gland. In a comparison trial of 1.5 T MR imaging versus 7 T MR imaging of the parotid gland, numerous gradient-echo and TSE sequences, including T2*-weighted multiecho data combination (MEDIC), 3D DESS, double-echo proton density and T2w TSE sequence (PD/T2), and T2w short TI inversion recovery (STIR), were optimized for ultrahigh-field strength and evaluated in a total of 8 subjects (including 4 healthy volunteers and 4 patients). Imaging results were correlated qualitatively and quantitatively (SNRs, contrast/noise ratios). Despite the basic coil design using a single 10-cm-diameter loop coil (RAPID Biomedical, Rimpar, Germany) for image acquisition (Fig. 3), 7 T MR imaging yielded excellent image contrast and high-quality resolution of the parotid gland and duct. MEDIC and DESS MR imaging in particular provided excellent assessment of the duct and branches, confirmed by qualitative and quantitative analysis. In contrast, PD/T2 TSE yielded the best evaluation of the gland tissue in patients with tumors. Quantitative analysis revealed a strong SNR increase for the MEDIC sequence at 7 T, whereas TSE imaging showed only comparable or less SNR at ultrahigh-field strength. This finding was attributed to a combination of physical effects at 7 T including B_1 inhomogeneities, the limited penetration depth of the loop coil, as well as the 8-fold higher spatial resolution. Nevertheless, these initial parotid imaging results at 7 T show the diagnostic potential of ultrahigh-field MR imaging as a noninvasive imaging method.[47]

As previously described, the lack of dedicated RF coils is still a major limiting factor for

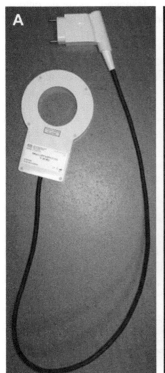
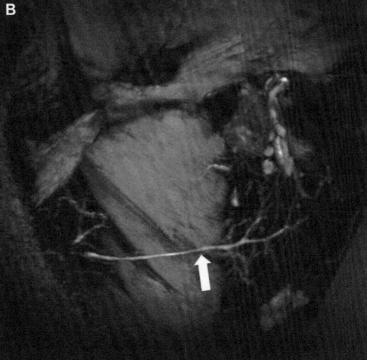

Fig. 3. (*A*) Ten-centimeter-diameter transmit/receive single-loop coil used for imaging of the parotid. (*B*) MEDIC maximum-intensity projection in a healthy volunteer yielding excellent conspicuity of the duct for its full extent (*arrow*).

ultrahigh-field MR imaging. Hence, apart from modification of imaging sequences and protocols, the development of dedicated RF coils is a mandatory cornerstone for high-quality ultrahigh-field imaging. Kraff and colleagues[48] were one of the first groups to endeavor to construct a dedicated RF coil for carotid imaging at 7 T (Fig. 4). The custom-built RF phased-array coil was constructed of 2 coil clusters, each consisting of 4 overlapping surface loop elements. For validation of the coil construction, maps of the transmit B_1 field were correlated between simulation and measurement. To evaluate the feasibility of in vivo imaging, sets of high-spatial-resolution nonenhanced 3D fluorescence in situ hybridization (FLASH) MR imaging (isotropic voxel size of 0.54 mm) and a pulse-triggered PD/T2w TSE sequence were obtained in a healthy volunteer and a patient (ulcerating plaque and a 50% stenosis of the right internal carotid artery; Fig. 5). The acquisition of high-resolution nonenhanced MR angiography of the carotid arteries as well as assessment of the atherosclerotic plaque at 7 T were feasible because of an inherently hyperintense signal intensity of the arterial vasculature.[48] This phenomenon has been shown in various settings of intracranial and extracranial ultrahigh-field MR imaging studies[24,30,31,49]; nevertheless, the cause is still incompletely. A combination of steady-state and inflow effects as well as the use of local transmit coil

systems at 7 T seems to be accountable. The use of local transmit/receive RF coils at ultrahigh-field strength precludes a presaturation by RF pulses outside the imaging region. Thus, inflowing fresh spins may contribute to the inherently increased vessel signal.[31] Grinstead and colleagues[49] conducted a study of magnetization prepared rapid gradient-echo (MPRAGE) imaging at 3 T and 7 T, using local transmit coils for ultrahigh-field imaging, and compared the signal intensity of arterial vessels. Their imaging results confirmed the consequence of local transmit coils at 7 T, and this implies that a nonselective inversion recovery pulse is effectively a slab-selective pulse.[49]

In a further refinement of RF coil design, Koning and colleagues[46] recently introduced a 6-channel radiative transmit array, constructed with elements designed for low RF power deposition and uniform B_1 using RF phase shimming. The transmit array was combined with a dedicated 16-channel small-element receive coil. In initial in vivo imaging studies, high-resolution TSE images could be obtained to evaluate carotid vessel wall integrity.[46]

Research in ultrahigh-field imaging is being designed to maximize the potential gain in SNR. Piccirelli and colleagues[44] and Wiggins and colleagues[45] introduced modified coil concepts to fully exploit the improved SNR at 7 T. Wiggins and colleagues[45] assessed several different transmit array configurations in simulations. A

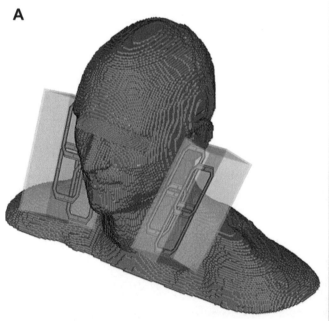

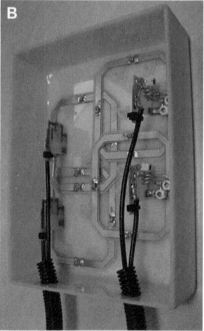

Fig. 4. (A) An inhomogeneous tissue model for numerical simulations to determine SAR exposure during carotid imaging. (B) The corresponding RF coil with 4 geometrically overlapping RF transmit/receive loop coil elements.

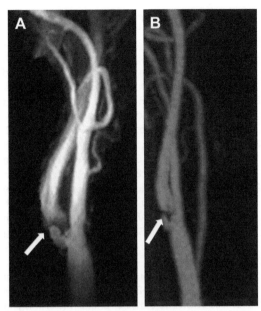

Fig. 5. Concomitant maximum-intensity projection images of the (A) nonenhanced 7 T 3D FLASH sequence and the 1.5 T contrast-enhanced image (B). Note the homogeneously hyperintense signal of the nonenhanced vasculature in 7 T T1-weighted imaging (A). Both images provide good delineation of an ulcerated atherotic plaque and 50% stenosis in the right internal carotid artery (arrows).

dedicated 8-channel array model achieved up to 77% of the ultimate SNR. In the study by Piccirelli and colleagues,[44] an anatomically shaped receive-only surface coil was introduced to address the SNR potential. The geometry of the coil was designed to optimally adapt to an average adult's anatomy in the bifurcation region, providing improved SNR and high-quality imaging of the carotid bifurcation and vertebral artery. Furthermore, phase-contrast imaging was assessed, enabling flow imaging at 7 T field strength.

Despite the demonstration of successful high-resolution MR angiography of the carotid arteries and high-quality, cross-sectional, high-resolution plaque assessment at 7 T, imaging results thus far have also underlined the importance of further improvements in RF coil concepts to take full advantage of the expected benefits and enable contrast-enhanced MR angiography applications.

SUMMARY AND OUTLOOK

With the successful implementation of commercial 7 T whole-body scanners within the last few years, ultrahigh-field MR imaging has made considerable progress in overcoming initial hurdles and is rapidly evolving in its diagnostic capacities. The increase of the magnetic field strength has been shown to be beneficial for multiple facets of intracranial und musculoskeletal imaging, providing high-resolution anatomic display and higher diagnostic accuracy for disease detection.[12–15,21,22,24,50,51] Owing to recent advancements in RF coil design and construction, 7 T MR imaging has also established its feasibility for whole-body applications.[30,52–57] Initial studies of neck and spine imaging have revealed promising imaging results, showing the successful transformation of the increased SNR into higher spatiotemporal resolution and indicating the potential benefits and challenges of ultrahigh-field MR imaging.[36–38,44,46] Nevertheless, imaging outside the brain at 7 T is still in its infancy, demanding further improvements and optimization of RF sequences, shim techniques, and dedicated RF coil concepts. In accordance with these technical advances, future research should focus on patient studies and comparison studies to lower field strengths to evaluate the clinical diagnostic value of ultrahigh-field MR imaging.

REFERENCES

1. Edelman RR. MR imaging of the pancreas: 1.5T versus 3T. Magn Reson Imaging Clin North Am 2007;15(3):349.
2. Fenchel M, Nael K, Deshpande VS, et al. Renal magnetic resonance angiography at 3.0 Tesla using a 32-element phased-array coil system and parallel imaging in 2 directions. Invest Radiol 2006;41(9): 697–703.
3. Kuhl CK, Träber F, Gieseke Jr, et al. Whole-body high-field-strength (3.0-T) MR imaging in clinical practice part II. Technical considerations and clinical applications. Radiology 2008;247(1):16–35.
4. Kuhl CK, Träber F, Schild HH. Whole-body high-field-strength (3.0-T) MR imaging in clinical practice part I. Technical considerations and clinical applications. Radiology 2008;246(3):675–96.
5. Kukuk GM, Gieseke Jr, Weber S, et al. Focal liver lesions at 3.0 T: lesion detectability and image quality with T2-weighted imaging by using conventional and dual-source parallel radiofrequency transmission. Radiology 2011;259(2):421–8.
6. Lauenstein TC, Salman K, Saar B, et al. MR colonography: 1.5T versus 3T. Magn Reson Imaging Clin North Am 2007;15(3):395–402.
7. Morakkabati-Spitz N, Gieseke J, Kuhl C, et al. MRI of the pelvis at 3 T: very high spatial resolution with sensitivity encoding and flip-angle sweep technique in clinically acceptable scan time. Eur Radiol 2006; 16(3):634–41.
8. Ramalho M, Altun E, Heredia V, et al. Liver MR imaging: 1.5T versus 3T. Magn Reson Imaging Clin North Am 2007;15(3):321–47.

9. Ramalho M, Herédia V, Tsurusaki M, et al. Quantitative and qualitative comparison of 1.5 and 3.0 tesla MRI in patients with chronic liver diseases. J Magn Reson Imaging 2009;29(4):869–79.

10. Schindera ST, Merkle E. MR cholangiopancreatography: 1.5T versus 3T. Magn Reson Imaging Clin North Am 2007;15(3):355–64.

11. Tsurusaki M, Semelka RC, Zapparoli M, et al. Quantitative and qualitative comparison of 3.0 T and 1.5 T MR imaging of the liver in patients with diffuse parenchymal liver disease. Eur J Radiol 2009; 72(2):314–20.

12. Kollia K, Maderwald S, Putzki N, et al. First clinical study on ultra-high-field MR imaging in patients with multiple sclerosis: comparison of 1.5T and 7T. AJNR Am J Neuroradiol 2009;30(4):699–702.

13. Moenninghoff C, Maderwald S, Theysohn J, et al. Imaging of adult astrocytic brain tumours with 7 T MRI: preliminary results. Eur Radiol 2010;20(3): 704–13.

14. Mönninghoff C, Maderwald S, Theysohn JM, et al. Imaging of brain metastases of bronchial carcinomas with 7 T MRI - initial results. Rofo 2010; 182(19):764–72.

15. Mönninghoff C, Maderwald S, Theysohn JM, et al. Evaluation of intracranial aneurysms with 7 T versus 1.5 T time-of-flight MR angiography- initial experience. Rofo 2009;181(1):16–23.

16. Theysohn JM, Kraff O, Maderwald S, et al. 7 Tesla MRI of microbleeds and white matter lesions as seen in vascular dementia. J Magn Reson Imaging 2011;33(4):782–91.

17. Akisik FM, Sandrasegaran K, Aisen AM, et al. Abdominal MR imaging at 3.0 T. Radiographics 2007;27(5):1433–44.

18. Bernstein MA, Huston J III, Ward H. Imaging artifacts at 3.0T. J Magn Reson Imaging 2006;24(4): 735–46.

19. Chang KJ, Kamel IR, Macura KJ, et al. 3.0-T MR imaging of the abdomen: comparison with 1.5 T1. Radiographics 2008;28(7):1983–98.

20. Merkle EM, Dale BM. Abdominal MRI at 3.0 T: the basics revisited. Am J Roentgenol 2006;186(6): 1524–32.

21. Banerjee S, Krug R, Carballido-Gamio J, et al. Rapid in vivo musculoskeletal MR with parallel imaging at 7T. Magn Reson Med 2008;59(3):655–60.

22. Behr B, Stadler J, Michaely H, et al. MR imaging of the human hand and wrist at 7 T. Skeletal Radiol 2009;38(9):911–7.

23. Kraff O, Theysohn JM, Maderwald S, et al. MRI of the knee at 7.0 Tesla. Rofo 2007;179(12):1231–5.

24. Maderwald S, Ladd S, Gizewski E, et al. To TOF or not to TOF: strategies for non-contrast-enhanced intracranial MRA at 7 T. Magnetic resonance materials in physics. Biol Med 2008;21(1): 159–67.

25. Ladd M. High-field-strength magnetic resonance: potential and limits. Top Magn Reson Imaging 2007;18(2):139–52.

26. Moser E, Stahlberg F, Ladd M, et al. 7-T MR—from research to clinical applications? NMR Biomed 2011. DOI:10.1002/nbm.1794. [Epub ahead of print].

27. Barth MM, Smith MP, Pedrosa I, et al. Body MR imaging at 3.0 T: understanding the opportunities and challenges. Radiographics 2007;27(5):1445–62.

28. Soher BJ, Dale BM, Merkle E. A review of MR physics: 3T versus 1.5T. Magn Reson Imaging Clin North Am 2007;15(3):277–90.

29. Bitz A, Brote I, Orzada S, et al. An 8-channel add-on RF shimming system for whole-body 7 Tesla MRI including real-time SAR monitoring [abstract: 4767]. Proceedings of the ISMRM 17th Scientific Meeting & Exhibition. Honolulu (HI), April 18–24, 2009.

30. Umutlu L, Kraff O, Orzada S, et al. Dynamic contrast-enhanced renal MRI at 7 Tesla: preliminary results. Invest Radiol 2011;46(7):425–33.

31. Umutlu L, Orzada S, Kinner S, et al. Renal imaging at 7 Tesla: preliminary results. Eur Radiol 2010; 21(4):841–9.

32. Merkle EM, Dale BM, Paulson EK. Abdominal MR Imaging at 3T. Magn Reson Imaging Clin North Am 2006;14(1):17–26.

33. Nelles M, Königig RS, Gieseke Jr, et al. Dual-source parallel RF transmission for clinical MR imaging of the spine at 3.0 T: intraindividual comparison with conventional single-source transmission. Radiology 2010;257(3):743–53.

34. Wattjes MP, Harzheim M, Kuhl CK, et al. Does high-field MR imaging have an influence on the classification of patients with clinically isolated syndromes according to current diagnostic MR imaging criteria for multiple sclerosis? AJNR Am J Neuroradiol 2006; 27(8):1794–8.

35. Bakshi R, Thompson AJ, Rocca MA, et al. MRI in multiple sclerosis: current status and future prospects. Lancet Neurol 2008;7(7):615–25.

36. Kraff O, Bitz A, Kruszona S, et al. An eight-channel phased array RF coil for spine MR imaging at 7 T. Invest Radiol 2009;44(11):734–40.

37. Vossen M, Teeuwisse W, Reijnierse M, et al. A radiofrequency coil configuration for imaging the human vertebral column at 7 T. J Magn Reson 2011;208(2):291–7.

38. Wu B, Wang C, Krug R, et al. 7T human spine imaging arrays with adjustable inductive decoupling. IEEE Trans Biomed Eng 2010;57(2):397–403.

39. Grams A, Kraff O, Umutlu L, et al. MRI of the lumbar spine at 7 Tesla in healthy volunteers and a patient with congenital malformations. Skeletal Radiol 2011. [Epub ahead of print].

40. Wang D, Heberlein K, Laconte S, et al. Inherent insensitivity to RF inhomogeneity in FLASH imaging. Magn Reson Med 2004;52(4):927–31.

41. Available at: http://www.rapidbiomed.com/pages/english/human-coils/head-and-neck/cervical-spine-array.php. Accessed February 24, 2012.

42. Katscher U, Bornert P. Parallel magnetic resonance imaging. Neurotherapeutics 2007;4(3):499–510.

43. Phillips C, Gay S, Newton R, et al. Gadolinium-enhanced MRI of tumors of the head and neck. Head Neck 1990;12(4):308–15.

44. Piccirelli M, DeZanche N, Nordmeyer-Massner J, et al. Carotid artery imaging at 7T: SNR improvements using anatomically tailored surface coils [abstract: 735]. Proceedings of the ISMRM 16th Scientific Meeting & Exhibition. Ontario (Canada), May 3–9, 2008.

45. Wiggins G, Zhang B, Duan Q, et al. 7 Tesla transmit-receive array for carotid imaging: simulation and experiment [abstract: 394]. Proceedings of the ISMRM 17th Scientific Meeting & Exhibition. Honolulu (HI), April 18–24, 2009.

46. Koning W, Langenhuizen E, Raaijmakers A, et al. 6 Channel radiative transmit array with a 16 channel surface receiver array for improved carotid vessel wall imaging at 7T [abstract: 327]. Proceedings of the ISMRM 19th Annual Meeting & Exhibition. Québec (Canada), May 7–13, 2011.

47. Kraff O, Theysohn JM, Maderwald S, et al. High-resolution MRI of the human parotid gland and duct at 7 Tesla. Invest Radiol 2009;44(9):518–24.

48. Kraff O, Bitz AK, Breyer T, et al. A transmit/receive radiofrequency array for imaging the carotid arteries at 7 Tesla: coil design and first in vivo results. Invest Radiol 2011;46(4):246–54.

49. Grinstead JW, Rooney W, Laub G. The origins of bright blood MPRAGE at 7 Tesla and a simultaneous method for T1 imaging and non-contrast MRA. Proc Intl Soc Magn Reson Med 2010;18:1429.

50. Nordmeyer-Massner JA, Wyss M, Andreisek G, et al. In vitro and in vivo comparison of wrist MR imaging at 3.0 and 7.0 tesla using a gradient echo sequence and identical eight-channel coil array designs. J Magn Reson Imaging 2011;33(3):661–7.

51. Polders DL, Leemans A, Hendrikse J, et al. Signal to noise ratio and uncertainty in diffusion tensor imaging at 1.5, 3.0, and 7.0 Tesla. J Magn Reson Imaging 2011;33(6):1456–63.

52. Orzada S, Maderwald S, Poser BA, et al. RF excitation using time interleaved acquisition of modes (TIAMO) to address B1 inhomogeneity in high-field MRI. Magn Reson Med 2010;64(2):327–33.

53. Maderwald S, Orzada S, Schäfer LC, et al. 7T Human in vivo cardiac imaging with an 8-channel transmit/receive array [abstract: 2723]. Proceedings of the ISMRM 17th Scientific Meeting & Exhibition. Honolulu (HI), April 18–24, 2009.

54. Snyder CJ, DelaBarre L, Metzger GJ, et al. Initial results of cardiac imaging at 7 tesla. Magn Reson Med 2009;61(3):517–24.

55. Umutlu L, Maderwald S, Kraff O, et al. Dynamic contrast-enhanced breast MRI at 7 Tesla utilizing a single-loop coil: a feasibility trial. Acad Radiol 2010;17(8):1050–6.

56. Vaughan JT, Snyder CJ, DelaBarre LJ, et al. Whole-body imaging at 7T: preliminary results. Magn Reson Med 2009;61(1):244–8.

57. von Knobelsdorff-Brenkenhoff F, Frauenrath T, Prothmann M, et al. Cardiac chamber quantification using magnetic resonance imaging at 7 Tesla—a pilot study. Eur Radiol 2010;20(12):2844–52.

Current Status and Future Perspectives of Magnetic Resonance High-Field Imaging: A Summary

Vivek Prabhakaran, MD, PhD[a],*, Veena A. Nair, PhD[b],
Benjamin P. Austin, PhD[c,d], Christian La, BA[e],
Thomas A. Gallagher, MD[f], Yijing Wu, PhD[g],
Donald G. McLaren, PhD[h,i], Guofan Xu, MD, PhD[j],
Patrick Turski, MD[k], Howard Rowley, MD[a]

KEYWORDS

- Magnetic resonance imaging • High-field MR imaging
- Current status • Future perspectives

There are several magnetic resonance (MR) imaging techniques that benefit from high-field MR imaging. This article features a range of novel techniques that are currently being used clinically or will be used in the future for clinical purposes as they gain popularity. These techniques include functional MR (fMR) imaging, diffusion tensor imaging (DTI), cortical thickness assessment, arterial spin labeling (ASL) perfusion, white matter hyperintensity (WMH) lesion assessment, and advanced MR angiography (MRA).

fMR imaging and DTI are currently being used for presurgical planning in brain tumors, vascular lesions, and patients with epilepsy, and several

This work was supported by Grant No. 1RC1MH090912-01, KL2 RR025012, R21 EB009441, 5 T32 HL007936-10, from the National Institutes of Health.
[a] Division of Neuroradiology, Department of Radiology, University of Wisconsin, 600 Highland Avenue, Madison, WI 53792-3252, USA
[b] Department of Radiology, University of Wisconsin, 600 Highland Avenue, Madison, WI 53792-3252, USA
[c] The UW Cardiovascular Research Center, Department of Medicine, University of Wisconsin, 2500 Overlook Terrace, Madison, WI 53705, USA
[d] Department of Veterans Affairs, Geriatric Research, Education and Clinical Center, D-4211, 2500 Overlook Terrace, Madison, WI 53705, USA
[e] Neuroscience Training Program, Wisconsin Institutes for Medical Research, University of Wisconsin, 1111 Highland Avenue, Madison, WI 53705, USA
[f] Division of Neuroradiology, Department of Radiology, Northwestern Memorial Hospital, Northwestern University, 676 North Saint Clair, Chicago, IL 60611, USA
[g] Department of Medical Physics, Wisconsin Institutes for Medical Research, University of Wisconsin, 1111 Highland Avenue Room 1125, Madison, WI 53705, USA
[h] Geriatric Research, Education and Clinical Center, ENRM VA Medical Center, 200 Springs Road, Bedford, MA 01730, USA
[i] Department of Neurology, Massachusetts General Hospital and Harvard Medical School, 149 Thirteenth Street, Room 2671, Charlestown, MA 02129, USA
[j] Nuclear Medicine Program, Nuclear Medicine, UW Hospital and Clinics, University of Wisconsin, 600 North Highland Avenue, Madison, WI 53792, USA
[k] Department of Radiology, Division of Neuroradiology, Wisconsin Institutes for Medical Research, University of Wisconsin, 1111 Highland Avenue, Room 1316, Madison, WI 53705, USA
* Corresponding author.
E-mail address: vprabhakaran@uwhealth.org

Neuroimag Clin N Am 22 (2012) 373–397
doi:10.1016/j.nic.2012.02.012
1052-5149/12/$ – see front matter

Key Points

- High-field intraoperative magnetic resonance (MR) imaging (functional MR imaging and diffusion tensor imaging) systems offer the possibility of integration of presurgical data with neuronavigation systems, which could change the face of functional neuroradiology.

- Differences in cortical thickness in different brain regions may have the potential to serve as biomarkers in different patient populations such as those with schizophrenia, dementia, and depression.

- White matter hyperintensities (WMHs) are associated with age and cardiovascular risk factors and are characterized by regional hypoperfusion. Extensive WMH load increases risk for stroke and detrimentally affects cognition, especially in older adults.

- WMH burden can be assessed using qualitative visual rating scales or quantitative computer-based techniques. Quantitative methods range from manual region-of-interest to fully automated techniques that are capable of providing reliable volumetric assessments of WMH load.

- In the future, WMH burden as assessed by MR fluid-attenuated inversion-recovery imaging may be helpful in predicting cognitive decline, perfusion deficits, and disease development.

- Arterial spin labeling (ASL) is a noninvasive method for quantitative assessment of cerebral perfusion or cerebral blow flow. This imaging method offers the possibility to detect perfusion deficit in clinical populations.

- Signal from ASL perfusion MR is highly reliable and reproducible within session and across sessions at a later time, making it suitable for longitudinal and replication studies.

- ASL is now used in various clinical setting including cerebrovascular diseases, central nervous system neoplasms, and neurodegenerative diseases such as Alzheimer disease, and has been proved to show similar perfusion deficits as observed in dynamic susceptibility contrast (DSC) perfusion imaging, positron emission tomography and single-photon emission computed tomography.

- Although DSC perfusion imaging still offers the most thorough evaluation of perfusion, ASL perfusion MR imaging provides a noninvasive MR perfusion method able to depict similar perfusion abnormalities and deficits without the need of injection of exogenous tracers.

- Advanced MR angiographic techniques have the potential to provide standard information about flow, stenosis with increased spatiotemporal resolution and signal-to-noise ratio as well as additional novel measures such as pressure gradient and wall shear stress.

studies have suggested clinical benefits from use of these techniques.[1–4] Current procedural terminology (CPT) codes are already in place for clinical reimbursement of fMR imaging. Cortical thickness assessment tools are gaining popularity in the research sector. This technique is used clinically for dementia assessment in some institutions. WMH lesion assessment is used in the research sector for assessing lesion load in normal aging, vasculopathies, and patients with dementia as well as other white matter (WM) diseases such as demyelinating conditions (eg, multiple sclerosis). These quantitative assessment tools may gain ground clinically because clinicians are demanding more than a qualitative assessment of these lesions. ASL perfusion has been added to complement the clinical protocol in several institutions when investigating brain tumors, vascular disease, and patients with epilepsy. This noncontrast perfusion method may replace the gadolinium-based perfusion method given the increasing concerns with contrast-based perfusion methodology. MRA in its current state

provides adequate evaluation of flow, obstruction, and stenosis of the intracranial and extracranial vasculature, but forthcoming advanced MRA techniques are capable of providing high-resolution images along with information such as shear stress, and plaque characterization with the aid of high-field strength imaging. Overall, several of these techniques will benefit from the increase in signal-to-noise ratio (SNR) as well as spatial resolution that high-field MR imaging readily allows. Temporal resolution can be increased sacrificing SNR and spatial resolution given this benefit, which may be advantageous for some of the more dynamic methods.

HIGH-FIELD CLINICAL fMR IMAGING

fMR imaging is a noninvasive technique widely used to study brain function in humans. Blood oxygenation level-dependent (BOLD) fMR imaging takes advantage of the different magnetic properties of oxygenated (oxy-Hb) and deoxygenated (deoxy-Hb) hemoglobin to generate image

---

Diagnostic Checklist

fMR Imaging

- Preoperative fMR imaging at high-field scanner strength can provide reliable estimates of the spatial relationship of eloquent cortex with respect to brain tumor or lesion and is recommended to facilitate the risk-benefit assessment and decision regarding surgery with the aim of minimizing postoperative deficits.

- The use of noninvasive BOLD fMR imaging is recommended especially for language mapping because of the high concordance rates between fMR imaging and the traditionally accepted albeit invasive Wada test.

DTI

- Preoperative DTI at high-field scanner strength can provide reliable estimates of the spatial relationship of eloquent networks with respect to brain tumor or lesion and is recommended to facilitate the risk-benefit assessment and decision regarding surgery with the aim of minimizing postoperative deficits.

Cortical Thickness

- Cortical thickness measures can provide an assessment of whether an individual is at risk for dementia compared with normal aging-related thickness changes.

ASL Perfusion

- ASL perfusion offers a complementary clinical diagnosis tool to DSC perfusion and other MR imaging techniques.

- An alternative when patient has a contraindication to gadolinium (eg, allergy to gadolinium or renal insufficiencies).

WMH

- WMH burden can be accurately assessed using T2-weighted FLAIR sequences, especially at higher scanner strength (3 T and greater) and when acquired in 3D.

- The use of T2 FLAIR sequences to quantify WM disease is recommended to potentially assess increased risk of stroke and decreased cognitive performance, especially in older adults.

Advanced MRA

- Advanced MRA techniques can provide additional diagnostic information such as pressure gradient and shear stress as well as increased spatiotemporal resolution and SNR compared with current standard clinical MRA sequences.

---

contrast. Neuronal activity increases local cerebral oxygen consumption, leading to an initial decrease in local oxy-Hb concentration and an increase in the deoxy-Hb in the functional area. Within a few seconds, there is an increase in blood flow in the capillaries and draining veins, with the result that deoxy-Hb is gradually washed out, leading to a reduction of local field inhomogeneity and an increase in the BOLD signal in T2*-weighted MR images.[1] The technique thus takes advantage of the differences in magnetic properties of oxy-Hb and deoxy-Hb to generate image contrast. A typical fMR imaging scan involves 20 to 30 seconds of task phase alternating with rest phase while a subject is presented with visual or auditory stimuli in the scanner. After preprocessing steps including removal of motion-related artifacts, and coregistration with the structural scan, images are generated that show areas of activation (ie, brain areas engaged during the specific task). These images are routinely reported with statistical thresholds that are applied to optimize the specificity and sensitivity of the functional activation. High sensitivity in identifying different functional areas and its noninvasiveness, obviating injection of any contrast, has led to increasing use of this technique in presurgical planning. Because of its high spatial and temporal resolution compared with other neuroimaging methods that use radioactive tracers, fMR imaging is used to identify areas of functional relevance or eloquent cortex as part of presurgical planning in patients with brain tumors, epilepsy, and vascular lesions[2–4] to reduce the risk of morbidity associated with different treatment options. Patients with lesions are scanned while performing tasks that activate appropriate regions of the cortex, and the relative distance between the lesion and the activation areas provides a measure of risk involved in surgery.

The last decade has seen a proliferation of high-field MR scanners (3–4 T) and very high-field scanners (>4 T) throughout major research centers in the world. This situation is primarily a result of the linear relationship between the magnetic field strength (B_0) and the SNR, with more protons aligned with the main magnetic field. The use of improved pulse sequences and high SNR coils also yields increased spatial resolution, which allows for the scanning of deeper subcortical structures. Several factors have contributed to the growing use of 3 T scanners: the more than doubled increase in T2* sensitivity at 3 T compared with 1.5 T leads to greater dephasing of the proton signal, in turn leading to better visualization of blood oxygen changes at the vascular level.[5] 3 T also facilitates acquisition of images with higher resolution at an accelerated rate because of the application of parallel imaging. Parallel imaging reduces the number of steps necessary in image acquisition as a result of the use of multiple radiofrequency (RF) receiving coils, each of which can acquire images faster and at shorter echo times (TEs), reducing artifacts and noise.[6] Important scan sequences can therefore be performed more routinely in a 3 T than in a 1.5 T scanner. Although several other factors including magnetic field inhomogeneities and RF flip angle govern the observed SNR, the signal to noise gain is approximately doubled (about 1.7–1.8 times)[7] from a 1.5 T to a 3 T scanner. Although the increase in field strength is accompanied by increase in SNR, high-field imaging has some limitations, the most important being the increased sensitivity of the images to magnetic field inhomogeneities, leading to geometric distortion in the images and nonuniform intensity.[8] The differing susceptibility of neighboring tissues and poor shimming effects leads to these field inhomogeneities. The susceptibility effect can be large in areas of air-bone and air–soft tissue interface and may lead to signal loss in those regions.

However, the advances in scan sequences and software, the use of echo-planar imaging (EPI), and the acquisition of field maps representing the field inhomogeneity across the images to correct for distortions in the EPI scans have led to improvement in the quality of the images.

Several clinical functional imaging studies in recent years have provided evidence that fMR imaging at 3 T provides high-quality activation maps with a high degree of confidence in the localization of functional areas.[9] There is evidence that the increase in field strength from 1.5 T to 3 T increases the percent signal change as a result of the BOLD effect, for example, from 1% to 2% to 3% to 4% for motor paradigms.[10] Clinical fMR imaging can contribute effectively to preoperative decision making; fMR imaging maps can inform surgeons about the risk-benefits involved in surgery, contribute to making recommendations regarding patients suitable for invasive intraoperative mapping, and select an optimal surgical route to resect the tumor (Fig. 1).[11] More recent advances in clinical functional imaging include the availability of fully integrated fMR imaging systems that can handle the complete pipeline from data acquisition and paradigm delivery to technologist-driven streamlined processing.[12] These systems offer a set of task paradigms for language and motor mapping that elicit reliable activations in the corresponding functional areas. With growing advances in pulse sequences and parallel imaging techniques, 3 T imaging has seen increased application in pediatric patients.[13] The increased spatial resolution provides pediatric scans with superior anatomic details, leading to better visualization of small structures such as nerves and vessels.[7] This advantage is especially useful in imaging children with epilepsy because it allows for better visualization of hippocampi and cortical dysplasia.[7] The shorter scan time is especially useful in children, who may not be able to hold still for a long time.

Because of the large number of studies that have shown the usefulness of fMR imaging in the

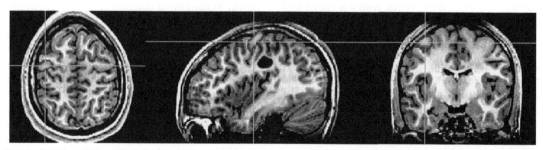

Fig. 1. fMR imaging activation images, overlaid on T1 anatomical, for a patient with tumor in the right hemisphere. Images show regions engaged during the left finger-tapping task. Images are shown in radiologic convention with left of the patient to the right (see Table 1 for representative scan parameters).

mapping of eloquent cortex as well as language lateralization, the last couple of years have seen increased efforts in the development and advancement of high-field intraoperative MR imaging.[14] The usefulness of integrating functional data with neuronavigational systems, availability of neuronavigational tools that help to update the brain position intraoperatively, the ability to operate with routine surgical instruments, and also the ability to confirm complete resection have made intraoperative MR imaging increasingly attractive to neurosurgeons and neuroradiologists alike. Although few studies have used intraoperative fMR imaging for presurgical planning, there is some evidence that in patients with brain tumors, this holds promise in terms of achieving total resection in most patients and is associated with improved postoperative outcomes.[15]

A relatively recent development in functional neuroimaging is the discovery that spontaneous low-frequency fluctuations occur in the BOLD fMR imaging signal during the resting condition in the absence of any explicit task performance or stimulation.[16,17] Individuals are typically asked to rest with their eyes closed or open or fixating on a crosshair. The BOLD fMR imaging signal is recorded and analyzed to identify correlations between different brain area and is referred to as resting-state functional-connectivity MR (rs-fcMR) imaging. These rs-fcMR imaging maps have shown that brain regions with similar function, such as the right and left motor cortices, show coherent BOLD fluctuations even in the absence of any motor movements (Fig. 2).[17] Although few studies have specifically examined the effect of high-field strength on rs-fcMR imaging correlations, similar to task fMR imaging, high-field-strength systems could provide increased SNR,[18,19] which also allows for detailed investigation of temporal fluctuations in rs-fcMR imaging, which may be important in specific neurologic disorders (eg, epilepsy[20]).

Given that rs-fcMR imaging studies require minimal patient compliance and can be used in different patient populations (eg, brain neoplasms, epilepsy, autism, schizophrenia, Alzheimer disease (AD), patients under anesthesia), several recent studies have used an rs-fcMR imaging approach to study different neurologic and psychiatric conditions.[21,22] The motivation for applying rs-fcMR imaging to patients also stems from the differences in SNR in task versus resting states. Although the resting human brain consumes 20% of the energy of the body, task-related increase in neuronal metabolism is smaller (<5%).[23] In addition, differences in task-related changes between healthy volunteers and diseased populations is still smaller (<1%). Furthermore, investigations into SNRs derived from task versus resting fMR imaging has shown that rs-fcMR imaging may have approximately 3 times the SNR as task-based fMR imaging.[24] Therefore spontaneous fluctuations in the resting brain may be a rich source of disease-related signal changes (Table 1).

HIGH-FIELD DTI

DTI is a clinically useful, model-based technique that attempts to characterize the three-dimensional (3D) diffusion profile in a voxel. Exponential signal decay related to dephasing from Brownian motion is sampled in many different directions and corresponding diffusion coefficients are calculated.[25–28] These directionally specific diffusion coefficients are entered into a 3 × 3 diffusion tensor matrix and resolved into the eigenvalues and eigenvectors that define the 3 principle directions of diffusion in a voxel. Scalar metrics such as fractional anisotropy (FA) are derived from the eigenvalues of the diffusion tensor matrix.[29] Ranging from 0 to 1, FA provides a quantitative measure of difference between the 3 eigenvalues in a given voxel. Higher FA (approaching 1) corresponds to a larger difference and alludes to the dominant orientation of diffusion in a voxel. Because intact axons are believed to be the main determinant of anisotropic diffusion in the

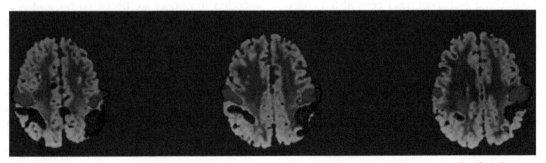

Fig. 2. Resting-state functional networks in a patient with epilepsy, representing primary motor (*red*) and sensory (*blue*) cortices, overlaid on T2-weighted postcontrast FLAIR Cube volume. Left is on right.

Table 1
Recommended MR sequences and protocols for clinical fMR imaging

Procedure	Recommended MR Imaging Research Scan Parameters	Duration (Min)
3 plane localizer, 2D gradient echo, fast	FOV, 24.0 cm; slice thickness, 10.0 mm; slice spacing, 2.5 mm Freq, 256; phase 128, NEX, 1.00; phase FOV, 1.00 cm	2
Calibration scan 2D gradient echo, fast	FOV, 30.0 cm; slice thickness, 6.0 mm; slice spacing, 0.0 mm; number of echoes, 1	~10 seconds
3D Ax gradient echo StealthBravo (with and without contrast)	TR, 9.228 ms; TE, 3.716 ms; slice thickness, 1.2 mm; slice spacing, 1.2 mm; acquisition matrix, 256 × 256; flip angle, 13;	~3
EPI BOLD scan: gradient echo (4 task blocks alternating with 4 control blocks, each block = 20 s)	TE, 30 ms; TR, 2000 ms; flip angle, 75; FOV, 24.0 cm; freq, 256; phase, 256; freq DIR, R/L; slice thickness, 4.0 mm; slice spacing, 0.0 mm;	3
DTI	56 directions; FOV, 25.6 cm; slice thickness, 2 mm; spacing, 0 mm; matrix, 128 × 128; NEX, 1; b-value, 2000; TE, 76.6 ms; TR, 9000 ms	

Abbreviations: Ax, axial; DIR, direction; FOV, field of view; Freq, frequency; L, left; NEX, number of excitations; R, right; TE, echo time; TR, repetition time; 2D, two-dimensional.

brain, further influenced by the presence or absence of myelin,[30] directionally encoded color FA maps of the brain can resolve the orientation of the major WM highways in the brain[31] and are commonly interpreted alongside BOLD fMR imaging for preoperative planning. Diffusion tensor tractography can also be performed to render a certain WM tract in 3 dimensions. With certain caveats, metrics such as FA, mean diffusivity (MD), and other scalar metrics such as axial and radial diffusivity have been studied as tools to smoke out disease otherwise covert or wholly nonspecific on conventional MR imaging.

In the brain, DTI has significant improvements when performed at higher field strengths, and these benefits come mostly as gains in signal to noise. Using 8-channel head coils at 3 T, Alexander and colleagues,[32] showed near 100% increase in SNR for DTI performed at 3 T over 1.5 T. These investigators emphasized that the increased sensitivity provided by multiple coils was necessary to harness full 3 T potential. Improved signal leads to more accurate calculation of directionally specific diffusion coefficients, which in turn leads to more reliable determination of eigenvalues and FA. Because single-shot EPI (SS-EPI) techniques remain the workhorse for functional imaging, the challenges of higher B_o acquisitions in this setting begin to surface. The

gains in signal to noise with DTI at 3 T or even 7 T must be pitted against greater geometric distortions and off-resonance effects in areas prone to susceptibility artifact.[26,33,34] Further, long echo train lengths in the absence of refocusing pulses in SS-EPI predispose the image to off-resonance effects and blurring. Novel methods of filling k-space such as periodically rotated overlapping parallel lines with enhanced reconstruction (PROPELLER), when combined with SS-EPI, have been shown to reduce these effects in DTI at 3 T by shortening acquisition time while oversampling the center of k-space relative to the periphery,[35] improving image contrast. In addition, parallel imaging techniques such as SENSE (sensitivity encoding) and ASSET (array spatial sensitivity encoding technique) are becoming necessities to an armory of techniques keeping susceptibility effects, geometric distortion, and off-resonance effects at bay. The goal of parallel imaging is to shorten acquisition time by reducing the number of required phase encode steps. This goal is accomplished with multichannel coils, each positioned in parallel so to listen to its own small field of view (FOV). However, the small FOV per receiver element also has the result of intentional aliasing, from which valuable secondary information, in the setting of different coil sensitivities, can be obtained. Taking into account all of the primary and secondary (aliased) information from the different receiver elements, a system of linear equations is used to assemble a full FOV image with fewer phase encode steps. The result is a faster acquisition, a shorter echo train, and a sharper image with less geometric distortion at higher field strengths. Although parallel techniques have a small fundamental loss of SNR because they operate with fewer phase encode steps (SNR decrease in the order of 19% per Alexander and colleagues[32]), the gains in image quality and overall SNR at higher field strengths make them worth this small price (Figs. 3–5).

These improvements of DTI at 3 T translate into increased reliability of the tool in the clinical setting, particularly with regard to quantitative measures such as FA or MD as well as fiber tractography. For example, Song and colleagues[36] showed differences between axial (the largest eigenvalue) and radial diffusivity (the mean of the 2 less eigenvalues of the diffusion tensor) in disorders of myelination. Improved SNR will improve reliability and consistency of such metrics. Several groups have also found significant benefits of parallel imaging and 3 T DTI in the spinal cord, a notoriously difficult structure to image given its narrow (1-cm) width, surrounding cerebrospinal fluid (CSF) pulsations, and susceptibility imposed by the bony spinal column. In particular, Hesseltine and colleagues[37]

found significant differences in FA in the dorsal, lateral, and central spinal cords of patients with MS compared with those the more anterior changes common to degenerative disease. Newer, reduced FOV diffusion-weighted image techniques[38] have shown even better image quality, and along with cardiac gating, these techniques may further improve 3 T DTI acquisitions of the spinal cord.[39] Although changes in FA have been applied to many different disease states (it remains a nonspecific measure), perhaps one of its greatest benefits will be as an indicator of occult disease, otherwise invisible on conventional MR imaging.[40] This benefit could be particularly relevant to patients with multiple sclerosis who have clinical symptoms despite negative conventional imaging. Information of this nature could affect clinical decision making, especially if baseline quantitative studies differed from those of the acute phase. Reliable interpretation of FA, particularly changes in FA, should be as standardized as possible. Different MR scanners may produce different FA results, even within the same vendor.[41]

Upadhyay and colleagues[42] applied an innovation to DTI called diffusion tensor spectroscopy (DTS) to investigate differences in architecture of the right versus left arcuate fasciculus. Although DTI most commonly focuses on molecular

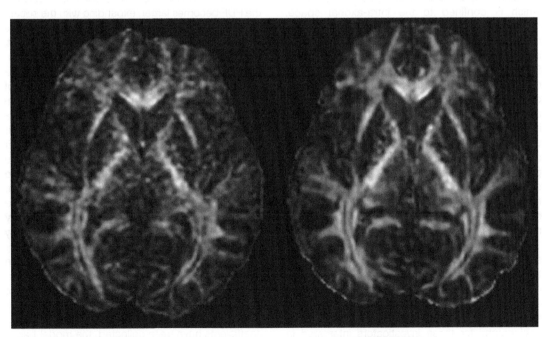

FA at 1.5 T   FA at 3 T

Fig. 3. Clear benefits from increased signal to noise at 3 T (*right*) are evident in these FA maps. Notice the sharper outline of the hyperintense WM tracts at 3 T. (*From* Alexander AL, Lee JE, Wu YC, et al. Comparison of diffusion tensor imaging measurements at 3.0 T versus 1.5 T with and without parallel imaging. Neuroimag Clin North Am 2006;16(2):299–309; with permission.)

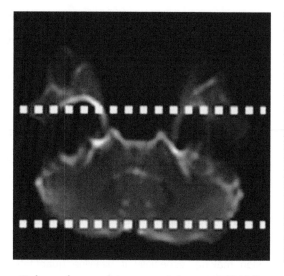
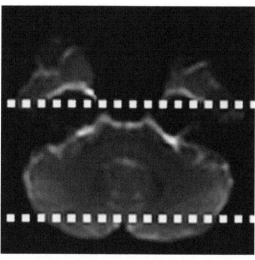

Echo planar image without SENSE   Echo planar image with SENSE

Fig. 4. Notice reduced geometric distortions of the brainstem and cerebellum (*right*) with application of parallel imaging techniques. (*From* Alexander AL, Lee JE, Wu YC, et al. Comparison of diffusion tensor imaging measurements at 3.0 T versus 1.5 T with and without parallel imaging. Neuroimag Clin North Am 2006;16(2):299–309; with permission.)

diffusion of water, which is found in both intra-axonal and extra-axonal compartments, these investigators used DTS to specifically seek out diffusion properties of *N*-acetylaspartate (NAA), which is confined to the intra-axonal space. Images were acquired at 3 T using SENSE parallel imaging. Conventional DTI was first performed to isolate the arcuate fasciculus as a target for DTS. DTS was then performed with point-resolved spectroscopy (TE 135 milliseconds) combined with diffusion-sensitizing gradients to obtain directionally specific water and NAA spectra and diffusion information. Both NAA and water diffusion tensors were filled and respective eigenvalues were obtained, from which scalars including trace apparent diffusion coefficient, FA, radial, and axial diffusivities were calculated. The investigators found asymmetrically increased radial diffusivity of NAA in the left arcuate fasciculus, suggesting increased axonal diameters.

Although there are significant improvements in signal to noise and image quality at 3 T, it is necessary to revisit a fundamental concept in DTI to understand its limitation, regardless of the perfect acquisition at even the highest field strengths. These limitations are particularly relevant assessing FA as well as for tractography for those investigators interested in functional connectivity of the brain. Again, DTI is a model-based technique that is rooted in probability theory. The model assumes, in the absence of barriers that might constrain diffusion, that a spherical probability density function (PDF) would emerge.

Specifically, the PDF is a 3D Gaussian distribution reflecting the proportion of water molecules displaced from the origin outward to a certain radius after a certain time. As time passes, the radius of the PDF becomes larger, expanding with the square root of time following stochastic theory and the Einstein equation $r = \sqrt{6Dt}$ (D = diffusion coefficient, t = time). Each concentric layer of the sphere essentially represents a probability isosurface at a certain displacement or radius (ie, the proportion of water molecules diffusing outward from the origin to a certain distance). At more distant radii, a given isosurface is more sparsely populated by water molecules. The highest proportion of water molecules have traveled the smallest radius and congregate near the origin. Along with time and temperature, the diffusion coefficient D of water (or whatever the molecule happens to be) is also a contributor to its displacement. For clinical neuroimaging, temperature is essentially body temperature.

A diffusion tensor demands at least 6 diffusion coefficients to compute the eigenvalues and eigenvectors necessary to characterize the 3 principle directions of diffusion in a voxel. Even although 6 (or potentially 20–30) directionally specific diffusion coefficients have been collected, the model-based constraints of DTI distill this information down to 3 principal orientations. These directions can be visually rendered as color-coded probability isosurfaces, or ellipsoids, which are essentially spheres molded by the eigenvalues and eigenvectors

A

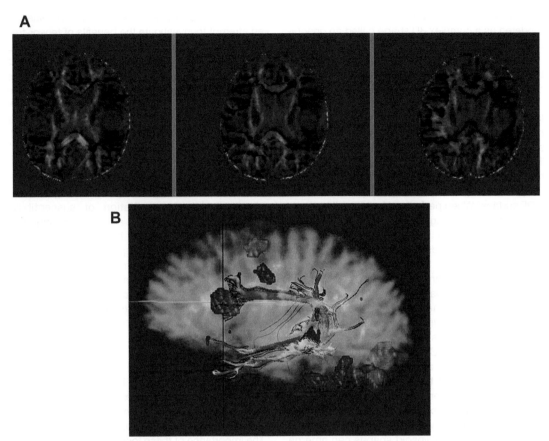

B

Fig. 5. (A) Axial color DTI images in a patient with a tumor in the left frontal lobe. Left corticospinal tracts and superior longitudinal fasciculus seem to be affected by mass effect from the tumor. X, Y, and Z directions are red, green, and blue, respectively. Any other direction is assigned a combination of red, green, and blue. (B) fMR imaging/DTI of normal subject. Diffusion tractography demonstrating superior longitudinal fasciculus of a patient connecting functional areas (Broca and Wernicke area, noted by fMR imaging activation). (Courtesy of A. Field.)

specific to a voxel. Of these isosurfaces, 3 dominant shapes can arise: (1) prolate (cigar-shaped) (2) oblate (UFO-shaped or saucer-shaped), or (3) spherical. DTI tractography methods such as fiber assignment by continuous tractography[43,44] attempt to link dominant eigenvector orientations, voxel to voxel, beginning from multiple points within a seed voxel. Although a family of resultant fiber tracts can arise from different geometric orientations borne in the seed voxel, the ultimate fiber tract is something of a summary of a summary. The largest eigenvector summarizes the principal direction of diffusion within a single voxel, and DTI tractography methods summarize diffusion patterns across several contiguous voxels. DTI tractography is most robust in areas populated by prolate tensors and concordantly these areas feature intrinsically higher FA. When a growing tract encounters progressively lower FA regions, or if the FA constraints on the growing tract are lowered, a wider array of tracts emerge. Further, as a fundamental limitation of the tensor model, intravoxel crossing WM tracts cannot be resolved by DTI. Despite idealized conditions (no motion, no noise) and even the highest field strengths, a symmetric intersection of 3 orthogonal WM tracts is imaged as a spherical tensor with FA = 0. As a result, tractography methods may generate nonphysiologic pathways, begging a careful approach to choosing seed points and a working knowledge of the anatomy.[45]

To break free of these limitations, model-free methods of high angular resolution WM imaging were developed, notably diffusion spectrum imaging (DSI)[46,47] and q-ball imaging (QBI).[48,49] Using higher b-values and novel schemes of filling q-space (a 3D repository organizing diffusion-weighted images obtained at varying b-values in different directions), these methods attempt to more directly characterize molecular displacement (radii) in many different directions. For example, more than 500 directions are sampled in DSI and more than 60 directions are common in QBI. With these techniques, a more realistic representation of intravoxel diffusion can be rendered as a complex 3D shape called an orientation distribution function (ODF).

When studying diffusion along 1 particular direction, the distribution of water molecules can be depicted as a histogram, with higher density of water molecules near the origin and more sparsely populated at further distances. Summing the entire histogram (integrating under the curve) provides a measure of overall diffusion in that direction.[50] This area is translated into a specific diffusion radius, which can be thought of as a strut of a specific length supporting its portion of the ODF surface. When performed in many directions, many struts of varying lengths are produced, and are used to construct the final ODF. Although analogous to the ellipsoids of DTI in that they reflect diffusion patterns in 3D, the ODFs of DSI and QBI are distinctly more complex shapes that can depict intravoxel crossing fibers. To understand the difference, imagine a simple orthogonal intersection of 2 fiber bundles within a given voxel. DTI would image this arrangement as a saucer, whereas DSI and QBI would attempt to render a cruciate object like a 4-leaf clover. The orientation of the leaves of the object, now visible and defined, can be incorporated into growing fiber tracts through this voxel and beyond. In contrast to *model-based* DTI, where essentially only three dominant, predicted ellipsoid shapes can emerge from the analysis, *model-free* DSI and QBI can render distinctly unique shapes that cannot be predicted by a model. QBI at 3 T has recently confirmed a more complex organization of the arcuate fasciculus,[51] the principal language-processing WM highway in the brain. Until recently, the arcuate fasciculus was believed to essentially connect Broca and Wernicke language centers; however, DTI and high-angular resolution QBI techniques have shown that language connections also run alongside the classic arcuate fasciculus, such as in the extreme capsule, and have terminations in different areas of cortex, particularly the intraparietal region. Further, relay stations in the premotor area via Geschwind fibers have been elucidated in better detail.

Given minute difference in diffusion trends within a voxel, estimation of specific struts (radii) for the ODF demands exquisite SNR and high b-values. In an attempt to investigate the benefits of tensor-free techniques at ultrahigh-fields, Mukherjee and colleagues[33] imaged supratentorial crossing tracts with QBI at 3 T and 7 T in healthy volunteers. These investigators reported 79.5% and 38.6% boosts in SNR at b = 3000 s/mm^2 and b = 6000 s/mm^2, respectively, with the 7 T acquisition. Higher b-values (6000 s/mm^2) at 7 T, although not showing as high a gain in SNR compared with b = 3000 s/ mm^2, helped sculpt the ODF, which improved high-angular resolution. Despite these gains in SNR and refinement in the ODF, the investigators did emphasize the exacerbation of susceptibility effects near the skull base at 7 T, suggesting that the greatest advantage of the ultrahigh-field QBI technique may come in imaging supratentorial tracts with application of parallel imaging techniques.

It seems that advancements in study of brain connectivity at higher field strengths will evolve alongside refinements in techniques such as multichannel parallel imaging (**Table 2**).

CORTICAL THICKNESS

High-resolution structural imaging coupled with advances in image processing has enabled researchers to investigate properties of the cortical thickness or surface at submillimeter resolution.[52] The importance of these tools has recently been underscored in a review by Van Essen and Dierker,[53] who concluded that cortical surface analysis can be invaluable for investigating cortical changes in individuals, improves localization of results, and provides a framework to compare results (eg, integrate information from previous studies to a single patient in a clinic). These ideas are driving surface-based analyses in the Human Connectome Project (http://humanconnectome.org/).

In the past, several free software packages have been used to create cortical surface representations, including FreeSurfer (http://surfer.nmr.mgh. harvard.edu/), CARET (http://brainvis.wustl.edu/ wiki/index.php/Caret:About), and SUMA (http:// afni.nimh.nih.gov/afni/suma). Currently, FreeSurfer and CARET dominate the research world. CARET has now changed to using FreeSurfer to create its cortical surfaces as well, although the

Table 2		
Recommended MR sequences and protocols for functional clinical imaging DTI		
Procedure	**Recommended MR Imaging Research Scan Parameters**	**Duration (Min)**
DTI	56 directions; FOV, 25.6 cm; slice thickness, 2 mm; spacing, 0 mm; matrix, 128 × 128; frequency, direction right/left; NEX, 1; b-value, 2000; TE, minimum; repetition time, 9000 ms	5–10

registration methods differ (see later discussion). In addition, similar methods have been commercially developed. One such package, NeuroQuant developed by CorTech Labs (http://www.cortechs.net/), is almost identical to FreeSurfer. NeuroQuant is now approved by the US Food and Drug Administration (FDA) for use in diagnostic imaging. Thus, from a research perspective, methodology can be freely developed using FreeSurfer and then migrated to a commercial FDA-approved platform such as NeuroQuant.

Cortical surface analysis requires 3 steps: segmentation, surface creation, and normalization. The failure or inaccuracies in any 1 step propagate through the processing stream to the final metrics. For example, if the segmentation misclassifies the tissue as CSF instead of gray matter (GM), then the computed pial surface is in the middle of the cortical ribbon along the edge of GM and CSF based on the segmentation.

The FreeSurfer segmentation has developed over time, but still requires manual intervention to produce the highest-quality segmentations.[54] The T1-weighted MR image is transformed to the Talairach atlas.[55] Next, the main body of WM is identified by atlas location, intensity, and neighbors, and the variation in intensity across WM is used to correct the B1 bias in the image. The image is then skull stripped leaving only the brain. The remaining voxels are classified as WM or non-WM based on intensity and neighbor constraints.

The FreeSurfer surface creation has also been refined over time, but in principle has not changed.[56] First, the cerebellum, pons, and brainstem are removed and the hemispheres are split. Then, for each hemisphere, an initial surface is created along the edge of the WM and refined to follow the WM/GM intensity gradient. Next, this surface is pushed outward until the intensity gradient between GM and CSF is reached, or the pial surface. In CARET, the midthickness of the pial and GM/WM surface is used and is computed by averaging the 2 FreeSurfer surfaces.

The FreeSurfer normalization process can be divided into 2 parts.[57,58] First, the surface is inflated into a sphere. Next, the sulcal and gyral pattern is aligned to FreeSurfer average surface. After normalization, the surface is resampled into a common reference space, with the same number of nodes, or points, on the surface to analyze the results across individuals node by node or regionally.

The CARET normalization process similarly involves 2 steps.[59] First, the surface is inflated into a sphere. Next, 6 core landmarks that have the most consistency across individuals (calcarine sulcus, central sulcus, anterior half of the superior temporal gyrus, sylvian fissure, and the dorsal and ventral parts of the medial wall boundary) are identified. These landmarks are aligned to the PALS (population-average, landmark and surface-based) atlas landmarks. After normalization, the surface is resampled into a common reference space, with the same number of nodes, or points, on the surface to analyze the results across individuals node by node or regionally.

Both FreeSurfer and CARET report increased overlap of cortical areas compared with volume registration,[59,60] validating the need for surface-based methodology. In comparing these 2 programs, Zhong and colleagues concluded that if one wants to preserve curvature/gyral estimates, then CARET should be used, whereas if one wants to use cortical parcellation to interrogate the data, then FreeSurfer should be used.[61]

Both FreeSurfer and CARET have revealed important scientific and clinical findings related to brain morphology. For example, CARET was used to show that the olfactory sulcus was shallower in patients with Williams syndrome compared with healthy controls.[62] Results from FreeSurfer typically focus on cortical thickness and have shown effects in patients with AD,[63-65] Parkinson disease,[66,67] depression,[68] attention-deficit/hyperactivity disorder,[69] epilepsy,[70] schizophrenia,[71] and many others. Differences have also been reported based on age,[72] genotype,[73] and amyloid deposition.[74] Most studies focus on identifying group differences or correlations; however, Dickerson and colleagues[75] used the difference between patients with AD and healthy controls to show that thinner cortices in areas of group differences predict the conversion to AD. Theses investigators termed this difference the Alzheimer signature. Future work will likely investigate which areas are predictive of different diseases or disorders. Currently, only T1-weighted images are typically used in these packages; however, FreeSurfer has recently developed a surface-based tractography tool, TRACULA, which is now publicly available.[76] The integration of DTI and other modalities could be used in preoperative planning. Although cross-sectional studies are potentially more useful in the clinic, FreeSurfer also has a longitudinal processing stream that enables atrophy to be tracked over time. The use of longitudinal imaging has potential as a biomarker in clinical trials.

Surface-based analysis has been shown to have clinical implications from both a basic science perspective and from a treatment perspective. The use of surface-based image analysis clinically and in research will bring many benefits to patients (**Fig. 6, Table 3**).

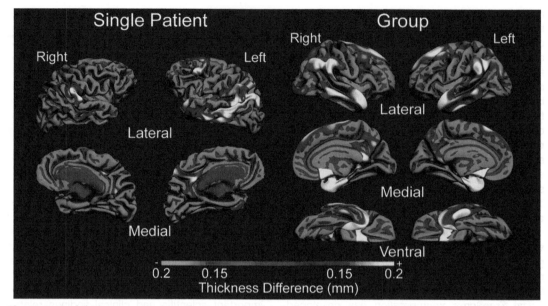

Fig. 6. Cortical thickness results from FreeSurfer. (*Left*) A single patient with probable AD compared with a group of age-matched normal adults. All surface nodes with more than 0.15 mm atrophy are shown in red or yellow. (*Right*) A group of patients with probable AD compared with a group of age-matched normal adults. Cortical thickness differences are shown for nodes with atrophy greater than 0.15 mm. The regions shown in this figure are those that can be used to aid in making a diagnostic decision and have been termed the AD cortical signature. NeuroQuant, from CorTech Labs, provides the percentile, based on the patient's age, of the cortical thickness or volume for regions that are atrophic in AD. (*Courtesy of* Dr Brad C. Dickerson.)

ASL PERFUSION

Arterial spin labeling (ASL) is a noninvasive MR imaging method for the measuring of cerebral perfusion or cerebral blow flow (CBF), a measure quantified in units of mL/g/min. CBF reflects the volume of flow per unit brain mass per unit time. Two commonly adopted methods for the measuring of brain perfusion include the dynamic susceptibility contrast (DSC) approach, in which an intravascular contrast agent such as gadolinium is injected into the blood stream, and ASL, in which arterial blood water works as the endogenous tracer.

DSC perfusion MR imaging is the current method of choice for clinical use as it provides the most thorough evaluation of perfusion. DSC perfusion not only provides information regarding blood flow, but blood volume and transit time as well. However, the use of gadolinium-based contrast agents has raised concerns as it has been recently associated with nephrogenic systemic fibrosis, a new and rare disease of unknown cause that affects patients with significant renal insufficiency.[77–79] Alternatively, ASL offers gadolinium-free method for conducting perfusion MR imaging with no injection of exogenous tracers, but with magnetically labeled arterial blood water serving as the endogenous flow tracer.

ASL typically works by magnetically tagging the arterial blood just upstream of the area of interest

Table 3		
Recommended MR sequences and protocols for cortical thickness		
Procedure	**Recommended MR Imaging Research Scan Parameters**	**Duration (Min)**
3D TR-weighted, Ax FSPGR BRAVO (high-resolution structural images)	Flip angle, 12; FOV, 25.6 cm; repetition time, 8.2; TR, 450 ms; TE, 3.2 ms (ARC on); number of echoes, 1; slice thickness, 1.0 mm; frequency, 256; phase, 256; frequency direction, right/left; NEX, 1; phase FOV, 1 cm	~4

using RF, followed by an image acquisition of the tagged arterial blood in the plane or volume of interest.[80] The effects of ASL are generated by a pair-wise subtraction of the image acquired from magnetically labeled arterial blood water and the image acquired from a nonmagnetized blood water control condition. **Fig. 7** presents the ASL perfusion images from a patient with bilateral occipital lobe ischemic stroke (top) compared with the aged-matched control (bottom). Not only is a perfusion deficit observed in the area of the stroke but also an overall reduction of brain perfusion is recorded in the patient's perfusion image. The intensity scale of the 2 sets of images is identical (8–80 mL/g/min) (see **Fig. 7**).

Labeling of the arterial blood can be achieved with numerous strategies. With the continuous arterial spin labeling (CASL) technique, continuous RF of weak intensity is applied in conjunction with a gradient in the direction of flow, allowing the signal to reach steady state.[80,81] Pulsed arterial spin labeling (PASL) technique is another approach. In this method, a single, well-defined RF pulse is employed instead.[82,83] Theoretically and experimentally, studies[84–86] have demonstrated that the use of CASL allows for a stronger perfusion contrast than pulsed ASL. However, the impracticality of its hardware implementation considerably reduce it's potential benefits.[87] A new approach has been characterized as pseudocontinuous ASL (PCASL), employs rapidly repeated RF pulses to mimic CASL and achieve high labeling efficiency. With PCASL, a 50% SNR gain compared with PASL and a 30% efficiency gain compared with CASL were readily achievable.[88–90] In addition, the use of pseudocontinuous inversion is compatible with most current clinical and research scanners without the need of any additional hardware.[90]

The extensive work on the optimization of ASL MR perfusion imaging techniques has permitted the introduction of such technique in an increasing number of clinical settings, including cerebrovascular disease, central nervous system (CNS) neoplasms, epilepsy, aging and development, neurodegenerative and neuropsychiatric disorders. In 2000, studying 15 patients within 24 hours of acute stroke symptom onset, Chalela and colleagues[91] reviewed the detectability of perfusion deficits and perfusion/diffusion mismatches in acute ischemic stroke using continuous ASL perfusion imaging. Of the 11 patients with perfusion deficits, 8 showed perfusion-diffusion mismatches, ranging from small diffusion with large perfusion abnormalities to large diffusion with small perfusion abnormalities.[91] In a subsequent study, Wolf and colleagues[92] performed a direct comparison between DSC and continuous ASL MR perfusion imaging in patients

with known cerebrovascular disease. Of the 10 individuals showing an abnormality, 9 showed complete or partial agreement in regions of apparent perfusion deficit between CASL perfusion images and DSC time-to-peak (TTP) maps. After removal of patients with major transit delay, CASL CBF correlated best with DSC relative CBF. Transit delay has been know to cause issues in the qualitative interpretation of perfusion deficit, but with post-labeling delay, and techniques involving multiple inversion times, a reduction of transit time sensitivity is readily achievable.[93]

The implementation of ASL perfusion MR imaging can also be found in CNS neoplasm studies. Gaa and colleagues[94] were the first group to report the use of ASL in imaging brain tumors. Using a specific ASL technique (EPISTAR), these investigators reported agreement between tumor vascularity obtained through single-photon emission computed tomography (SPECT) and through the use of the ASL perfusion technique. Meningiomas were shown to have the highest EPISTAR tumor/white matter contrast, and low-grade astrocytomas the lowest. Warmuth and colleagues[95] conducted a comparison of perfusion differences in patients with brain tumors between the methods of DSC and ASL perfusion MR imaging. Both approaches offered distinction between high-grade and low-grade gliomas. In a later study by Weber and colleagues,[96] 79 patients with first detection of brain neoplasm on enhanced computed tomography (CT) scans were examined. Both, DSC and pulsed ASL perfusion MR imaging showed higher diagnostic performance and better discrimination of glioblastomas from metastases, CNS lymphomas, and other gliomas than spectroscopic MR imaging.

In the field of aging and degenerative disease, ASL perfusion MR imaging is also readily implemented, but the impact of normal development and aging processes on brain perfusion need to be accounted for. In adults, global CBF decreases with age, and so does the SNR of the ASL signal.[97] Parkes and colleagues[98] reported a decrease of 0.45% per year in gray matter perfusion in their study. The study by Sandson and colleagues[99] was among the first studies applying ASL methodology in neurodegenerative illness. Using the EPISTAR technique, 11 patients with AD and 8 age-matched control individuals, significantly lower ASL signal changes in two regions (parietal-occipital and temporal-occipital) were found. Similarly, Alsop and colleagues[100] compared 18 patients with probable AD with 11 age-matched controls using a multislice CASL perfusion method and found significant decreases in CBF in temporal, parietal, frontal, and posterior cingulated

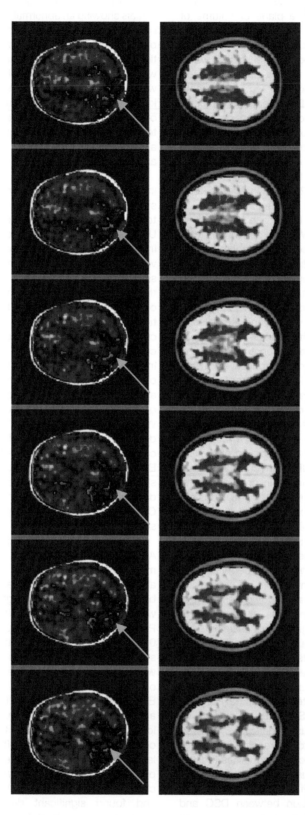

Fig. 7. ASL perfusion of imaging of a patient with bilateral occipital lobe ischemic stroke (*top*) versus aged-matched control (*bottom*). Same intensity scale is used for both set of images with low of 8 mL/g/min and high of 80 mL/g/min.

cortices for the patients compared with controls. Posterior parietal and posterior cingulate (no temporal) decreases were significantly correlated with clinical severity of disease measured by the Mini-Mental State Examination.[100] In a more recent study with 22 patients with AD, 18 with MCI, and 23 control normal individuals, Johnson and colleagues[101] investigated the regional cerebral hypo-perfusion in subjects with AD and mild cognitive impairment (MCI), and found decreased perfusion in the right inferior parietal lobe and bilateral middle frontal gyri in the AD group compared to controls. Similar areas were previously depicted in fluorodeoxyglucose positron emission tomography (PET) and hexamethylpropylene-amineoxine SPECT studies. To a lesser extent but still significant ($P = .046$), ASL perfusion was also able to show regional perfusion deficit in the MCI group compared with normal controls, more specifically in the right inferior parietal lobe, the same area that showed the greatest perfusion deficit in AD.[101]

Many research groups have been working in improving the sensitivity of ASL and its image acquisition, and it played a major part in ASL perfusion MR development for the last 10 to 20 years. As the magnetic field increases not only does image SNR increase in proportion to the field, but T1 also lengthens, allowing more spin label to accumulate.[86] Transitioning from PASL/CASL at 1.5 T field strength to higher field strength of 3 or 4 T allows for a 2-fold signal gain.[86,102] Wang and colleagues[86] found SNR of 2.3:1.4:1 in the gray matter and contrast-to-noise (CNR) of 2.7:1.1:1 between the gray matter and white matter for the difference perfusion images acquired using 4 T PASL, 1.5 T CASL, and 1.5 T PASL, respectively.

A secondary and complementary approach for improving SNR in ASL perfusion MR imaging is the use of phased with optimization for parallel imaging. With this technique, image acquisition time is significantly shorter. And although parallel imaging suffers from a reduction in SNR, much of this SNR cost can be regained through shorter TE along with reduced distortion from susceptibility artifact.[103,104] The array coil also provided 3 times the average SNR increase and higher temporal stability for the perfusion-weighted images compared to the standard volume coil, even with the 3-fold acceleration.[103] In addition, slab excitation and a prolonged image acquisition window of fast 3-dimensional sequences have been introduced to improve image quality.[104] The 3D sequence also reduces the image distortion arising from magnetic field inhomogeneity compared with routine 2D gradient-echo EPI.[104] With ASL imaging sequences incorporating parallel imaging, high-field,

pseudo-CASL technique, and 3D imaging with background suppression, sensitivity for imaging CBF have the potential of providing an approximate 10-fold increase.[105]

Though not receiving much attention comparatively, the approach of perfusion-based fMR imaging offers distinct advantages over BOLD fMR imaging such as the ability of quantifying CBF at rest and with task activation, and eliminating the obstacle of low-frequency drift effects.[106] In addition, ASL perfusion MR imaging has demonstrated to be a robust and reliable method for the quantification of CBF in normal as well as in clinical populations. Ongoing development of new ASL perfusion MR imaging technique, the standardization of high-field MR scanner and other hardware and software developments, the applications of ASL in research and clinical settings seem favorable and promising (**Box 1**).

WMHs

WMHs are regions of high signal intensity in cerebral WM as frequently observed on T2-weighted fluid-attenuated inversion-recovery (FLAIR) MR imaging scans. Often considered to be lesions of the WM, WMHs are consistently associated with age,[107] hypertension, and other cardiovascular risk factors,[108] but their functional significance remains unclear. WMH disease, often referred to as leukoariosis when WMHs are extensively distributed around the ventricles,[109] is considered to be a part of the spectrum of vascular-related injury.[110–113] WMH is reported to involve a loss of vascular integrity, which may, in turn, detrimentally affect blood-brain barrier integrity.[114] These lesions are believed to reflect small vessel vascular disease[115] and have been shown through perfusion-weighted MR imaging studies to show a decline in blood flow compared with regions of normal-appearing WM.[116–118]

Individuals with extensive WMHs have been shown to have increased risk for future stroke.[119–121] In a longitudinal MR imaging study of 3293 participants, it was reported that individuals with high WMH burden (grades of ≥5 on a 0–9 scale) showed increased risk of stroke 4 to 5 times greater than that shown by individuals with low WMH burden (grades 0–1), independent of traditional stroke risk factors.[122] Risk for stroke may also be influenced by the location of WMHs, which are commonly divided into 2 categories: periventricular WMH (PVWMH), which lie in the WM surrounding the ventricles, and deep WMH (DWMH), which lie in deeper subcortical WM regions (**Fig. 8**).[123–129] The Rotterdam Scan Study[130] found that individuals in the highest tertile of WMH distribution showed a greater risk of

Box 1
Recommended MR sequences and protocols for 3D PCASL

Procedure	Recommended MRI Research Scan Parameters

3D pcASL:
  Pseudo-continuous labeling technique[89]
	Pseudo-continuous labeling[86]:
	  Repeated selective saturation
	  Slab selective inversion
	  Pseudo-continuous labeling
	  Saturation plus non-selective inversion
	  After-labeling saturation and inversion

Fast spin echo acquisition[106]	Fast spin echo acquisition:
	  Interleaved stack of spiral readout
	  8 spiral arms with 512 sampling points
	  TR of 6 seconds
	  Echo train length of 40
	  Echo spacing 7 ms
	  Effective echo time of 21 ms
	  FOV of 24 x 24 x 16 cm
	  64 x 64 x 40 matrix after Fourier Transform

stroke for PVWMH (4.7-fold) compared with DWMH (3.6-fold). Furthermore, worsening of WMH load has been associated with declined cognitive performance on the Mini-Mental State Examination and the Digit-Symbol Substitution test.[131]

WMHs have also been reported to affect cognition in otherwise healthy older adults[132] as well as individuals with MCI and dementia, including AD.[133–144] In normal older adults, WMHs are associated with reductions in memory, processing speed, and executive function. Similarly, WMHs are associated with symptoms of MCI, including memory loss and conversion to dementia.[133–144] In addition, WMH severity is reported to be more extensive in AD, but this finding is not consistent.

Measuring WMH burden has received considerable attention as MR imaging technology has advanced over the past 2 decades. Generally, WMH load can be assessed using qualitative or quantitative scales, which vary in degree of automaticity. Qualitative assessments of WMH load

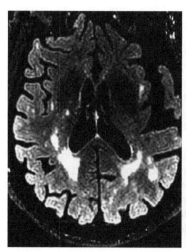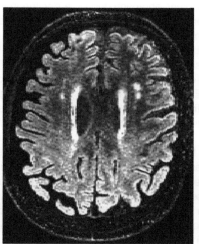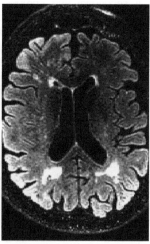

Fig. 8. Representative T2 FLAIR Cube axial images in 3 different patients with cerebral vascular disease showing WMH lesions.

use visual rating scales to describe WMH severity and are usually described by a single value.[145–151] Such qualitative scales require a well-trained rater to assign a measure of WMH burden based on an operationally defined rating scale.[151,152] Visual rating scales offer several advantages over quantitative assessments of WMH: they are easier to use and they are insensitive to the many imaging artifacts that often limit quantitative methods. However, such qualitative methods are subject to considerable disadvantages, namely, that (1) categorical ratings are restricted by a range of values that limit the power of association, (2) visual ratings are inherently subjective, which limits both intrarater and interrater reliability,[151] and (3) such scales are poor discriminators of absolute lesion volume. In a study comparing 13 different visual rating scales, Mäntylä and colleagues[151] reported that some of the inconsistencies in previous studies of WMHs are caused by differences in visual rating scales and that some of these scales were limited by ceiling effects.

Such limitations in qualitative measures of WMH burden have spurred the development of quantitative methods to assess WMH load. Quantitative assessments, which use computer-based techniques to obtain volumetric measures of WMH burden,[153–162] range from manual outlining techniques to fully automatic detection of WMHs. Manual techniques are commonly referred to as region-of-interest (ROI) methodologies. This method requires a reviewer to manually trace regions of WMH on FLAIR images using a mouse and cursor. Typically, this procedure is performed on a slice-by-slice basis, and after ROIs are defined, the computer is able to calculate ROI volume (by adding the volume of pixels residing within the traced area throughout multiple slices) and total WMH volume (by adding together the volume of ROIs). Manual techniques such as this provide reliable volumetric assessments of WMH burden but are time consuming and require computer-based digital imaging and a well-trained reviewer.[162] In turn, semiautomated and fully automated techniques have seen significant advancements in recent years because they are able to measure WMH volume more consistently and require less time. Automated techniques are based on computer algorithms and are typically designed to first segment WM from CSF and GM and then to identify WMHs using voxel intensity value thresholds. Threshold values can be defined simply or by using global and local intensity histograms. One popular semiautomated method, JIM,[163] is provided by Java Image software and applies local thresholding techniques to FLAIR images. JIM is a medical image display package for various medical imaging technologies (eg, MR

imaging, radiography, CT) that allows for easy viewing and analysis and has been used successfully to delineate WMHs from normal-appearing WM and similarly appearing lacunar infarcts [eg, Refs.[164–166]].

An example of a fully automated WMH analysis is that used by Charles DeCarli and colleagues at the University of California at Davis. A summary of this technique follows,[167–172] and further details can be found in Yoshita and colleagues.[133]

The WMH analysis requires 2 sequences: a T1-weighted 3D spoiled gradient-recalled echo acquisition and a FLAIR sequence. To segment, or extract, WMH locations from the FLAIR images, 3D volume images are first reoriented to ensure that brain regions are delineated using common internal landmarks, nonbrain elements are removed by manual tracing, and image intensity nonuniformity correction is applied. Then, WMH segmentation is performed using inhouse computer algorithms and other programs. Specifically, CSF-brain matter segmentation is performed by defining a pixel intensity threshold that represents the intersection of the CSF-modeled Gaussian distribution with the brain-matter–modeled Gaussian distribution, then a pixel intensity histogram of the brain-matter–only FLAIR image is modeled as a normal Gaussian distribution, and pixel intensities of 3.5 standard deviations more than the mean are identified as WMHs. The second part of the analysis involves deforming individual patients' templates into a common template space for cross-sectional comparison and group statistics and can be summarized by the following steps: (1) align and reslice FLAIR image to T1 image and transform WMH map onto T1, (2) use WMH map to reset corresponding T1 voxel intensities to reduce normalization matching errors, (3) apply high-dimensional cubic B-spline warp of minimal deformation template (MDT) to T1, then use parameters to deform WMH map to MDT, (4) construct WMH population composite map in MDT, and (5) create WMH composite frequency distribution map for separate groups using MDT and define specific ROIs as needed for group comparisons.

Similar to this method, fully automated techniques often define voxels as being a WMH ("Yes") or not being a WMH ("No"). This categorical method is suitable for many analyses but limits statistical inferences.[133] Thus, WMH analysis techniques, such as that being developed by Sterling Johnson, Vikas Singh and colleagues at the University of Wisconsin at Madison, are designed to assign probabilistic values to each voxel as a measure of proven WMH likeliness. The computer algorithm used in this method implements a 3D version of random walker (RW)-based segmentation of Grady's[173] two-dimensional

Table 4 Recommended MR sequence for T2 FLAIR Cube	
Name of Sequence	Sagittal Cube FLAIR
Thickness (mm)	2
Gap (mm)	0 (2-mm spacing between slices)
TE (ms)	124.31
Repetition time (ms)	6000
Inversion time (ms)	1866
Echo train length	140
FOV (mm)	256 × 256 × 144
Acquisition matrix (voxels)	256 × 256 × 72
Acquisition voxel size (mm)	1 × 1 × 2
Flip angle	90
Percent phase FOV (%)	90
Bandwidth	122.07
Plane	Sagittal
Number of slices	144
Pulse sequence	3D fast spin echo

implementation[174] and provides a graphical user interface to segment 3D images. This is a semisupervised method in which a user places foreground and background seeds interactively in the image to provide the algorithm with boundary conditions. Based on these boundary conditions, the RW algorithm simulates a random walk process from each voxel under analysis to assign it with the highest probability of being a part of either the foreground or background (ie, being a WMH or not). The outcome is a probability map of the region under analysis, which can easily be thresholded to produce a binary mask of WMHs. The RW model is used to generate initial training data for a support vector machine that is learned on the training data and can be used to automatically segment WMHs in FLAIR images.

Although much progress has been made in automating WMH detection, there still exists a need for developing analyses that are able to accurately measure the distribution of WMHs across subjects.[133] The variability in size and location of WMHs should be taken into consideration, although debate exists as to whether categorical distinctions between PVWMH and DWMH are arbitrary[175] or whether the two WMH subtypes differ in functional significance. Nonetheless, further research is needed to investigate distribution patterns of WMHs to determine if differences exist between otherwise healthy older adults, patients with vasculopathies, and individuals with MCI and dementia. If significant

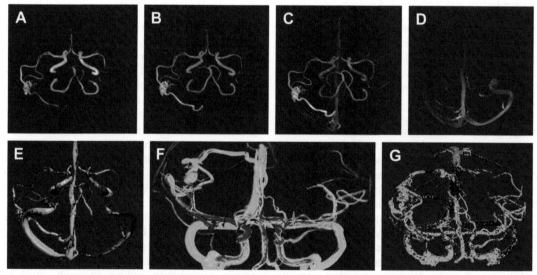

Fig. 9. An example of the HYPRFlow study from a patient with brain arteriovenous malformation. (A–D) Selected time frames from high-resolution four-dimensional MRA, showing the early arrival of the contrast at the feeding artery and the nidus, and the rapid shunting to the drainage vein. (E) Increased wall shear stress in the feeding arteries relative to the contralateral arteries. (F, G) The complex flow condition, shown using streamlines (F) and pressure gradient map (G).

methodological advancements are developed and group differences can be further distinguished, it is possible that MR imaging FLAIR scans can eventually be used to predict risk of stroke and disease development and provide further insights on the effects of WMH on perfusion and cognition (see **Fig. 8, Table 4**).

ADVANCED MRA

Cerebrovascular MRA requires high spatial and high temporal resolution because of the small size of intracranial vessels and the rapid flow of blood through the brain. However, achieving high temporal and spatial resolution simultaneously is difficult because of the tradeoffs between temporal resolution, spatial resolution, and the SNR. HYPRFlow[176,177] technique is able to achieve subsecond temporal resolution, submillimeter isotropic spatial resolution, and physiologic parameters such as pressure gradient and wall shear stress by using the VIPR[178] (vastly undersampled imaging with projections) acquisition and HYPR[179,180] (highly constrained back projection) reconstruction methods. High-field strength boosts the SNR of images and improves visualization of distal vessels and accuracy of the quantitative measurements of physiologic parameters.

HYPRFlow involves 2 sequential scans: a time-resolved fast acquisition (2 frames/s) during the first pass of the contrast to capture the contrast kinetics and a high resolution (0.68 × 0.68 × 0.68 mm³) postcontrast phase contrast scan to measure the flow dynamics and serve as a spatial constraint for the first-pass time-resolved scan.

Both scans use VIPR (undersampled 3D radio) trajectory to achieve high acceleration factor with minimum undersampling artifacts. The final high-resolution 4-dimensional MRA is reconstructed using the HYPR reconstruction method, which inherits the high temporal resolution from the first scan and high spatial resolution and high SNR from the second scan. Physiologic parameters can be calculated using the 3D velocity fields and the boundaries of the vessels derived from PC VIPR data.[181] HYPRFlow, for the first time, splits the task of acquiring high temporal and spatial resolution and high SNR images into 2 scans and uses HYPR reconstruction to obtain a series of images with all of these features. HYPRFlow is able to provide both morphologic and hemodynamic information of cerebral vasculature (**Fig. 9, Box 2**).

REFERENCES

1. Ogawa S, Lee TM, Kay AR, et al. Brain magnetic resonance imaging with contrast dependent on blood oxygenation. Proc Natl Acad Sci U S A 1990;87(24):9868–72.
2. Moritz CH, Rowley HA, Haughton VM, et al. Functional MR imaging assessment of a non-responsive brain injured patient. Magn Reson Imaging 2001;19(8):1129–32.
3. Sailor J, Meyerand ME, Moritz CH, et al. Supplementary motor area activation in patients with frontal lobe tumors and arteriovenous malformations. AJNR Am J Neuroradiol 2003;24(9):1837–42.
4. Nelson L, Lapsiwala S, Haughton VM, et al. Preoperative mapping of the supplementary motor area in patients harboring tumors in the medial frontal lobe. J Neurosurg 2002;97(5):1108–14.
5. Di Salle F, Esposito F, Elefante A, et al. High field functional MRI. Eur J Radiol 2003;48(2):138–45.
6. Bakshi R, Thompson AJ, Rocca MA, et al. MRI in multiple sclerosis: current status and future prospects. Lancet Neurol 2008;7(7):615–25.
7. Barth MM, Smith MP, Pedrosa I, et al. Body MR imaging at 3 T: understanding the opportunities and challenges. Radiographics 2007;27(5):1445–62.
8. Chavhan GB, Babyn PS, Singh M, et al. MR imaging at 3 T in children: technical differences, safety issues, and initial experience. Radiographics 2009;29(5):1451–66.
9. Hutton C, Bork A, Josephs O, et al. Image distortion correction in fMRI: a quantitative evaluation. Neuroimage 2002;16(1):217–40.
10. van Westen D, Skagerberg G, Olsrud J, et al. Functional magnetic resonance imaging at 3T as a clinical tool in patients with intracranial tumors. Acta Radiol 2005;46(6):599–609.

> **Box 2**
> **Recommended MR sequences and protocols for HYPRFlow**
>
> *HYPRFlow protocol*
>
> ME VIPR: FOV = 22 × 22 × 22 cm³, repetition time (TR)/TE = 3.0/0.4 ms, BW = 125 kHz, frame time = 0.5 s. Readout matrix, 128 points per projection.
>
> PC VIPR: FOV = 22 × 22 × 22 cm³, TR/TE = 12.5/4.8 ms, VENC = 80 cm/s, BW = 62.5 kHz; Readout matrix, 320 points per projection, spatial resolution for the composite image is 0.7 × 0.7 × 0.7 mm³, 7000 projections were acquired within 5 minutes.
>
> Contrast agent (eg, gadobenate dimeglumine [MultiHance, Bracco Diagnostics, Princeton, NJ]) injected at 3 mL/s and contrast dose was 0.1 mm/kg followed by 20 mL saline flush.
>
> *Abbreviations:* BW, band width; ME, multi-echo; PC, phase contrast; VENC, velocity encoding.

11. Yang Y, Wen H, Mattay VS, et al. Comparison of 3D BOLD functional MRI with spiral acquisition at 1.5 and 4.0 T. Neuroimage 1999;9(4):446–51.

12. Lee CC, Ward HA, Sharbrough FW, et al. Assessment of functional MR imaging in neurosurgical planning. AJNR Am J Neuroradiol 1999;20(8): 1511–9.

13. Prism Clinical, Prism Clinical Imaging. Milwaukee (WI): Medical College of Wisconsin; 2005.

14. Dagia C, Ditchfield M. 3 T MRI in paediatrics: challenges and clinical applications. Eur J Radiol 2008; 68(2):309–19.

15. Pillai JJ. The evolution of clinical functional imaging during the past 2 decades and its current impact on neurosurgical planning. AJNR Am J Neuroradiol 2010;31(2):219–25.

16. Krishnan R, Raabe A, Hattingen E, et al. Functional magnetic resonance imaging-integrated neuronavigation: correlation between lesion-to-motor cortex distance and outcome. Neurosurgery 2004;55(4): 904–14 [discussion: 914–5].

17. Fox MD, Raichle ME. Spontaneous fluctuations in brain activity observed with functional magnetic resonance imaging. Nat Rev Neurosci 2007;8(9): 700–11.

18. Biswal B, Yetkin FZ, Haughton VM, et al. Functional connectivity in the motor cortex of resting human brain using echo-planar MRI. Magn Reson Med 1995;34(4):537–41.

19. Bandettini P. Functional MRI today. Int J Psychophysiol 2007;63(2):138–45.

20. Kruger G, Kastrup A, Glover GH. Neuroimaging at 1.5 T and 3 T: comparison of oxygenation-sensitive magnetic resonance imaging. Magn Reson Med 2001;45(4):595–604.

21. Morgan VL, Price RR, Arain A, et al. Resting functional MRI with temporal clustering analysis for localization of epileptic activity without EEG. Neuroimage 2004;21(1):473–81.

22. Zhang D, Raichle ME. Disease and the brain's dark energy. Nat Rev Neurol 2010;6(1):15–28.

23. Fox MD, Greicius M. Clinical applications of resting state functional connectivity. Front Syst Neurosci 2010;4:19.

24. Raichle ME, Mintun MA. Brain work and brain imaging. Annu Rev Neurosci 2006;29:449–76.

25. Stejskal EO, Tanner JE. Spin diffusion measurements: spin echoes in the presence of time-dependent field gradient. J Chem Phys 1965; 42(1):288–92.

26. Moseley ME, Cohen Y, Kucharczyk J, et al. Diffusion-weighted MR imaging of anisotropic water diffusion in cat central nervous system. Radiology 1990;176:439–45.

27. Moseley ME, Kucharczyk J, Asgari HS, et al. Anisotropy in diffusion weighted MRI. Magn Reson Med 1991;19(2):321–6.

28. Le Bihan D, Mangin JF, Poupon C, et al. Diffusion tensor imaging: concepts and applications. J Magn Reson Imaging 2001;13:534–46.

29. Pierpaoli C, Basser PJ. Toward a quantitative assessment of diffusion anisotropy. Magn Reson Med 1996;36:893–906.

30. Beaulieu C, Allen PS. Determinants of anisotropic water diffusion in nerves. Magn Reson Med 1994b;31:394–400.

31. Pajevic S, Pierpaoli C. Color schemes to represent the orientation of anisotropic tissues from diffusion tensor data: application to white matter fiber tract mapping in the human brain. Magn Reson Med 1999;42:526–40.

32. Alexander AL, Lee JE, Wu YC, et al. Comparison of diffusion tensor imaging measurements at 3.0 T versus 1.5 T with and without parallel imaging. Neuroimag Clin North Am 2006;16(2):299–309.

33. Mukherjee P, Chung SW, Berman JI, et al. Diffusion tensor MR imaging and fiber tractography: theoretic underpinnings. AJNR Am J Neuroradiol 2008;29:632–41.

34. Mukherjee P, Chung SW, Berman JI, et al. Diffusion tensor MR imaging and fiber tractography: technical considerations. AJNR Am J Neuroradiol 2008;29:842–52.

35. Wang FN, Huang TY, Lin FH, et al. PROPELLER EPI: an MRI technique suitable for diffusion tensor imaging at high field strength with reduced geometric distortions. Magn Reson Med 2005;54: 1232–40.

36. Song SK, Sun SW, Ramsbottom MJ, et al. Dysmeylination revealed through MRI as increased radial (but unchanged axial) diffusion of water. Neuroimage 2002;17:1429–36.

37. Hesseltine SM, Law M, Babb J, et al. Diffusion tensor imaging in multiple sclerosis: assessment of regional differences in the axial plane within normal-appearing cervical spinal cord. AJNR Am J Neuroradiol 2006;27:1189–93.

38. Zaharchuk G, Saritas EU, Andre JB, et al. Reduced field-of-view diffusion imaging of the human spinal cord: comparison with conventional single-shot echo-planar imaging. AJNR Am J Neuroradiol 2011;32:813–20.

39. Saritas EU, Zaharchuk G, Shankaranarayanan A, et al. High-resolution DTI tractography of the spinal cord with reduced-FOV single-shot EPI at 3T [abstract]. Presented at: 17th Annual Meeting of the International Society for Magnetic Resonance in Medicine. Honolulu (HI), 2009.

40. Ge Y, Law M, Johnson G, et al. Preferential occult injury of corpus callosum in multiple sclerosis measured by diffusion tensor imaging. J Magn Reson Imaging 2004;20:1–7.

41. Vollmar C, O'Muircheartaigh J, Barker GJ, et al. Identical, but not the same: intra-site and inter-site

reproducibility of fractional anisotropy measures on two 3 T scanners. Neuroimage 2010;51:1384–94.

42. Upadhyay J, Hallock K, Ducros M, et al. Diffusion tensor spectroscopy and imaging of the arcuate fasciculus. Neuroimage 2008;39:1–9.

43. Mori S, Crain BJ, Chacko VP, et al. Three-dimensional tracking of axonal projections in the brain by magnetic resonance imaging. Ann Neurol 1999;45:265–9.

44. Conturo TE, Lori NF, Cull TS, et al. Tracking neuronal fiber pathways in the living human brain. Proc Natl Acad Sci U S A 1999;96:10422–7.

45. Jones DK. Studying connections in the living human brain with diffusion MRI. Cortex 2008;44:936–52.

46. Wedeen VJ, Hagmann P, Tseng WY, et al. Mapping complex tissue architecture with diffusion spectrum magnetic resonance imaging. Magn Reson Med 2005;54:1377–86.

47. Wedeen VJ, Wang RP, Schmahmann JD, et al. Diffusion spectrum magnetic resonance imaging (DSI) tractography of crossing fibers. Neuroimage 2008;41:1267–77.

48. Tuch DS, Reese TG, Wiegell MR, et al. Diffusion MRI of complex neural architecture. Neuron 2003;40:885–95.

49. Tuch DS. qBall imaging. Magn Reson Med 2004;52(6):1358–72.

50. Hagmann P, Jonasson L, Maeder P, et al. Understanding diffusion MR imaging techniques: from scalar diffusion-weighted imaging to diffusion tensor imaging and beyond. Radiographics 2006;26:205–23.

51. Frey S, Campbell JS, Pike GB, et al. Dissociating the human language pathways with high angular resolution diffusion fiber tractography. J Neurosci 2008;28(45):11435–44.

52. Fischl B, Dale AM. Measuring the thickness of the human cerebral cortex from magnetic resonance images. Proc Natl Acad Sci U S A 2000;97:11050–5.

53. Van Essen DC, Dierker DL. Surface-based and probabilistic atlases of primate cerebral cortex. Neuron 2007;56:209–25.

54. Dale AM, Fischl B, Sereno MI. Cortical surface-based analysis. I. Segmentation and surface reconstruction. Neuroimage 1999;9:179–94.

55. Talairach J, Tournoux P. Co-planar stereotaxic atlas of the human brain. New York: Thieme; 1988.

56. Van Essen DC, Drury HA, Dickson J, et al. An integrated software suite for surface-based analyses of cerebral cortex. J Am Med Inform Assoc 2001;8:443–59.

57. Fischl B, Sereno MI, Dale AM. Cortical surface-based analysis. II: Inflation, flattening, and a surface-based coordinate system. Neuroimage 1999;9:195–207.

58. Fischl B, Sereno MI, Tootell RB, et al. High-resolution intersubject averaging and a coordinate system for the cortical surface. Hum Brain Mapp 1999;8:272–84.

59. Van Essen DC. A population-average, landmark- and surface-based (PALS) atlas of human cerebral cortex. Neuroimage 2005;28:635–62.

60. Fischl B, Rajendran N, Busa E, et al. Cortical folding patterns and predicting cytoarchitecture. Cereb Cortex 2008;18:1973–80.

61. Zhong J, Phua DY, Qiu A. Quantitative evaluation of LDDMM, FreeSurfer, and CARET for cortical surface mapping. Neuroimage 2011;52:131–41.

62. Van Essen DC, Dierker D, Snyder AZ, et al. Symmetry of cortical folding abnormalities in Williams syndrome revealed by surface-based analyses. J Neurosci 2006;26:5470–83.

63. Julkunen V, Niskanen E, Koikkalainen J, et al. Differences in cortical thickness in healthy controls, subjects with mild cognitive impairment, and Alzheimer's disease patients: a longitudinal study. J Alzheimers Dis 2011;21:1141–51.

64. Im K, Lee JM, Seo SW, et al. Variations in cortical thickness with dementia severity in Alzheimer's disease. Neurosci Lett 2008;436:227–31.

65. Dickerson BC, Bakkour A, Salat DH, et al. The cortical signature of Alzheimer's disease: regionally specific cortical thinning relates to symptom severity in very mild to mild AD dementia and is detectable in asymptomatic amyloid-positive individuals. Cereb Cortex 2009;19:497–510.

66. Jubault T, Gagnon JF, Karama S, et al. Patterns of cortical thickness and surface area in early Parkinson's disease. Neuroimage 2011;55:462–7.

67. Lyoo CH, Ryu YH, Lee MS. Cerebral cortical areas in which thickness correlates with severity of motor deficits of Parkinson's disease. J Neurol 2011;258(10):1871–6.

68. Koolschijn PC, van Haren NE, Schnack HG, et al. Cortical thickness and voxel-based morphometry in depressed elderly. Eur Neuropsychopharmacol 2011;20:398–404.

69. Almeida LG, Ricardo-Garcell J, Prado H, et al. Reduced right frontal cortical thickness in children, adolescents and adults with ADHD and its correlation to clinical variables: a cross-sectional study. J Psychiatr Res 2011;44:1214–23.

70. Bernhardt BC, Bernasconi N, Concha L, et al. Cortical thickness analysis in temporal lobe epilepsy: reproducibility and relation to outcome. Neurology 2011;74:1776–84.

71. Murakami M, Takao H, Abe O, et al. Cortical thickness, gray matter volume, and white matter anisotropy and diffusivity in schizophrenia. Neuroradiology 2011;53(11):859–66.

72. Salat DH, Buckner RL, Snyder AZ, et al. Thinning of the cerebral cortex in aging. Cereb Cortex 2004;14:721–30.

394 Prabhakaran et al

73. Gutierrez-Galve L, Lehmann M, Hobbs NZ, et al. Patterns of cortical thickness according to APOE genotype in Alzheimer's disease. Dement Geriatr Cogn Disord 2009;28:476–85.

74. Becker JA, Hedden T, Carmasin J, et al. Amyloid-beta associated cortical thinning in clinically normal elderly. Ann Neurol 2011;69:1032–42.

75. Dickerson BC, Stoub TR, Shah RC, et al. Alzheimer-signature MRI biomarker predicts AD dementia in cognitively normal adults. Neurology 2011;76:1395–402.

76. Yendiki A, Panneck P, Stevens A, et al. Automated reconstruction of white-matter pathways constrained by the underlying anatomy: application to schizophrenia. Washington, DC: Society for Neuroscience Annual Meeting; 2011.

77. Marckmann P, Skov L, Rossen K, et al. Nephrogenic systemic fibrosis: suspected causative role of gadodiamide used for contrast-enhanced magnetic resonance imaging. J Am Soc Nephrol 2006;17:2359–62.

78. Perazella MA. Current status of gadolinium toxicity in patients with kidney disease. Clin J Am Soc Nephrol 2009;4:461–9.

79. Sadowski EA, Bennett LK, Chan MR, et al. Nephrogenic systemic fibrosis: risk factors and incidence estimation. Radiology 2007;243:148–57.

80. Williams DS, Detre JA, Leigh JS, et al. Magnetic resonance imaging of perfusion using spin inversion of arterial water. Proc Natl Acad Sci U S A 1992;89:212–6.

81. Detre JA, Alsop DC. Perfusion magnetic resonance imaging with continuous arterial spin labeling: methods and clinical applications in the central nervous system. Eur J Radiol 1999;30:115–24.

82. Kwong KK, Chesler D, Weisskoff RM, et al. MR perfusion studies with T1-weighted echo planar imaging. Magn Reson Med 1995;34:878–87.

83. Edelman RR, Siewert B, Darby DG, et al. Qualitative mapping of cerebral blood flow and functional localization with echo-planar MR imaging and signal targeting with alternating radio frequency. Radiology 1994;192:513–20.

84. Buxton RB, Frank LR, Wong EC, et al. A general kinetic model for quantitative perfusion imaging with arterial spin labeling. Magn Reson Med 1998;40:383–96.

85. Wang J, Zhang Y, Wolf RL, et al. Amplitude modulated continuous arterial spin-labeling 3.0-T perfusion MR imaging with a single coil: feasibility study. Radiology 2005;235:218–28.

86. Wang J, Alsop DC, Li L, et al. Comparison of quantitative perfusion imaging using arterial spin labeling at 1.5 and 4.0 Tesla. Magn Reson Med 2002;48:242–54.

87. Wong E, Buxton RB, Frank LR. A theoretical and experimental comparison of continuous and pulsed arterial spin labeling techniques for quantitative perfusion imaging. Magn Reson Med 1998;40:348–55.

88. Garcia DM, de Bazelaire C, Alsop DC. Pseudo-continuous flow driven adiabatic inversion for arterial spin labeling. In: Proceeding of the 13th Annual Meeting of ISMRM [abstract 9]. Miami Beach (FL), May 7–13, 2005.

89. Wu WC, Fernandez-Seara D, Detre JA, et al. A theoretical and experimental investigation of the tagging efficiency of pseudo-continuous arterial spin labeling. Magn Reson Med 2007;58:1020–7.

90. Dai W, Garcia D, de Bazelaire C, et al. Continuous flow-driven inversion for arterial spin labeling using pulsed radio frequency and gradient fields. Magn Reson Med 2008;60:1488–97.

91. Chalela JA, Alsop DC, Gonzalez-Atavales JB, et al. Magnetic resonance perfusion imaging in acute ischemic stroke using continuous arterial spin labeling. Stroke 2000;31:680–7.

92. Wolf RL, Alsop DC, McGarvey ML, et al. Susceptibility contrast and arterial spin labeled perfusion MRI in cerebrovascular disease. J Neuroimaging 2003;13:17–27.

93. Alsop DC, Detre JA. Reduced transit-time sensitivity in noninvasive magnetic resonance imaging of human cerebral blood flow. J Cereb Blood Flow Metab 1996;16:1236–49.

94. Gaa J, Warach S, Wen P, et al. Noninvasive perfusion imaging of human brain tumors with EPISTAR. Eur Radiol 1996;6:518–22.

95. Warmuth C, Gunther M, Zimmer C. Quantification of blood flow in brain tumors: comparison of arterial spin labeling and dynamic susceptibility-weighted contrast-enhanced MR imaging. Radiology 2003;228:523–32.

96. Weber MA, Zoubaa S, Schlieter M, et al. Diagnostic performance of spectroscopic and perfusion MRI for distinction of brain tumors. Neurology 2006;66:1899–906.

97. Wang J, Licht DJ, Jahng GH, et al. Pediatric perfusion imaging using pulsed arterial spin labeling. J Magn Reson Imaging 2003;18:404–13.

98. Parkes LM, Rashid W, Chard DT. Normal cerebral perfusion measurements using arterial spin labeling: reproducibility, stability, and age and gender effects. Magn Reson Med 2004;51:736–43.

99. Sandson TA, O'Connor M, Sperling RA, et al. Noninvasive perfusion MRI in Alzheimer's disease: a preliminary report. Neurology 1996;47:1339–42.

100. Alsop DC, Detre JA, Grossman M. Assessment of cerebral blood flow in Alzheimer's disease by spin-labeled magnetic resonance imaging. Ann Neurol 2000;47:1339–42.

101. Johnson NA, Jahng GH, Weiner MW, et al. Pattern of cerebral hypoperfusion in Alzheimer disease and mild cognitive impairment measured with

arterial spin-labeling MR imaging: initial experience. Radiology 2005;234:851–9.

102. Yongbi MN, Fera F, Yang Y, et al. Pulsed arterial spin labeling: comparison of multisection baseline and functional MR imaging perfusion signal at 1.5 and 3 T: initial results in six subjects. Radiology 2002;222:569–75.

103. Wang Z, Wang J, Connick TJ, et al. (CASL) perfusion MRI with an array coil and parallel imaging at 3T. Magn Reson Med 2005;54:732–7.

104. Lawrence KS, Wang J. Effects of the apparent transverse relaxation time on cerebral blood flow measurements obtained by arterial spin labeling. Magn Reson Med 2005;53:425–33.

105. Fernandez-Seara MA, Wang J, Wang Z, et al. Imaging mesial temporal lobe activation during scene encoding: comparison of fMRI using BOLD and ASL. Hum Brain Mapp 2007;8:1391–400.

106. Wu RH, Bruening R, Noachtar S, et al. MR measurement of regional relative cerebral blood volume in epilepsy. J Magn Reson Imaging 1999; 9:435–40.

107. Brickman AM, Schupf N, Manly JJ, et al. Brain morphology in older African Americans, Caribbean Hispanics, and whites from northern Manhattan. Arch Neurol 2008;65(8):1053–61.

108. Longstreth WT Jr, Manolio TA, Arnold A, et al. Clinical correlates of white matter findings on cranial magnetic resonance imaging of 3301 elderly people. The Cardiovascular Health Study. Stroke 1996;27(8):1274–82.

109. Hachinski VC, Potter P, Merskey H. Leuko-araiosis. Arch Neurol 1987;44(1):21–3.

110. Munoz DG, Hastak SM, Harper B, et al. Pathologic correlates of increased signals of the centrum ovale on magnetic resonance imaging. Arch Neurol 1993; 50(5):492–7.

111. Pantoni L, Garcia JH. Pathogenesis of leukoaraiosis: a review. Stroke 1997;28(3):652–9.

112. Fazekas F, Englund E. White matter lesions. In: Erkinjuntti T, Gauthier S, editors. Vascular cognitive impairment. London: Dunitz; 2002. p. 135–44.

113. Breteler MM, van Swieten JC, Bots ML, et al. Cerebral white matter lesions, vascular risk factors, and cognitive function in a population-based study: the Rotterdam Study. Neurology 1994;44(7):1246–52.

114. Young VG, Halliday GM, Kril JJ. Neuropathologic correlates of white matter hyperintensities. Neurology 2008;71(11):804–11.

115. Gurol ME, Irizarry MC, Smith EE, et al. Plasma beta-amyloid and white matter lesions in AD, MCI, and cerebral amyloid angiopathy. Neurology 2006;66(1):23–9.

116. Brickman AM, Zahra A, Muraskin J, et al. Reduction in cerebral blood flow in areas appearing as white matter hyperintensities on magnetic resonance imaging. Psychiatry Res 2009;172(2):117–20.

117. Marstrand JR, Garde E, Rostrup E, et al. Cerebral perfusion and cerebrovascular reactivity are reduced in white matter hyperintensities. Stroke 2002;33(4):972–6.

118. Sachdev P, Wen W, Shnier R, et al. Cerebral blood volume in T2-weighted white matter hyperintensities using exogenous contrast based perfusion MRI. J Neuropsychiatry Clin Neurosci 2004;16(1): 83–92.

119. Gerdes VE, Kwa VI, ten Cate H, et al. Cerebral white matter lesions predict both ischemic strokes and myocardial infarctions in patients with established atherosclerotic disease. Atherosclerosis 2006;186(1):166–72.

120. Naka H, Nomura E, Takahashi T, et al. Combinations of the presence or absence of cerebral microbleeds and advanced white matter hyperintensity as predictors of subsequent stroke types. AJNR Am J Neuroradiol 2006;27(4):830–5.

121. Roman GC, Erkinjuntti T, Wallin A, et al. Subcortical ischaemic vascular dementia. Lancet Neurol 2002; 1(7):426–36.

122. Kuller LH, Longstreth WT Jr, Arnold AM, et al. White matter hyperintensity on cranial magnetic resonance imaging: a predictor of stroke. Stroke 2004;35(8):1821–5.

123. Bowen BC, Barker WW, Loewenstein DA, et al. MR signal abnormalities in memory disorder and dementia. AJNR Am J Neuroradiol 1990;11(2): 283–90.

124. Kertesz A, Black SE, Tokar G, et al. Periventricular and subcortical hyperintensities on magnetic resonance imaging. 'Rims, caps, and unidentified bright objects'. Arch Neurol 1988;45(4):404–8.

125. Mirsen TR, Lee DH, Wong CJ, et al. Clinical correlates of white-matter changes on magnetic resonance imaging scans of the brain. Arch Neurol 1991;48(10):1015–21.

126. Fazekas F. Magnetic resonance signal abnormalities in asymptomatic individuals: their incidence and functional correlates. Eur Neurol 1989;29(3):164–8.

127. Lindgren A, Roijer A, Rudling O, et al. Cerebral lesions on magnetic resonance imaging, heart disease, and vascular risk factors in subjects without stroke. A population-based study. Stroke 1994;25(5):929–34.

128. Ylikoski A, Erkinjuntti T, Raininko R, et al. White matter hyperintensities on MRI in the neurologically nondiseased elderly. Analysis of cohorts of consecutive subjects aged 55 to 85 years living at home. Stroke 1995;26(7):1171–7.

129. Schmidt R, Fazekas F, Offenbacher H, et al. Neuropsychologic correlates of MRI white matter hyperintensities: a study of 150 normal volunteers. Neurology 1993;43(12):2490–4.

130. de Groot JC, de Leeuw FE, Oudkerk M, et al. Cerebral white matter lesions and cognitive function: the

Rotterdam Scan Study. Ann Neurol 2000;47(2): 145–51.

131. Vermeer SE, Hollander M, van Dijk EJ, et al. Silent brain infarcts and white matter lesions increase stroke risk in the general population: the Rotterdam Scan Study. Stroke 2003;34(5):1126–9.

132. Longstreth WT Jr, Arnold AM, Beauchamp NJ Jr, et al. Incidence, manifestations, and predictors of worsening white matter on serial cranial magnetic resonance imaging in the elderly: the Cardiovascular Health Study. Stroke 2005;36(1):56–61.

133. Yoshita M, Fletcher E, DeCarli C. Current concepts of analysis of cerebral white matter hyperintensities on magnetic resonance imaging. Top Magn Reson Imaging 2005;16(6):399–407.

134. Esiri MM, Nagy Z, Smith MZ, et al. Cerebrovascular disease and threshold for dementia in the early stages of Alzheimer's disease. Lancet 1999; 354(9182):919–20.

135. Gunning-Dixon FM, Raz N. The cognitive correlates of white matter abnormalities in normal aging: a quantitative review. Neuropsychology 2000; 14(2):224–32.

136. DeCarli C, Miller BL, Swan GE, et al. Cerebrovascular and brain morphologic correlates of mild cognitive impairment in the National Heart, Lung, and Blood Institute Twin Study. Arch Neurol 2001; 58(4):643–7.

137. Lopez OL, Jagust WJ, Dulberg C, et al. Risk factors for mild cognitive impairment in the Cardiovascular Health Study Cognition Study: part 2. Arch Neurol 2003;60(10):1394–9.

138. Nordahl CW, Ranganath C, Yonelinas AP, et al. Different mechanisms of episodic memory failure in mild cognitive impairment. Neuropsychologia 2005;43(11):1688–97.

139. Wolf H, Ecke GM, Bettin S, et al. Do white matter changes contribute to the subsequent development of dementia in patients with mild cognitive impairment? A longitudinal study. Int J Geriatr Psychiatry 2000;15(9):803–12.

140. Prins ND, van Dijk EJ, den Heijer T, et al. Cerebral white matter lesions and the risk of dementia. Arch Neurol 2004;61(10):1531–4.

141. Scheltens P, Barkhof F, Valk J, et al. White matter lesions on magnetic resonance imaging in clinically diagnosed Alzheimer's disease. Evidence for heterogeneity. Brain 1992;115(Pt 3):735–48.

142. Vermeer SE, Prins ND, den Heijer T, et al. Silent brain infarcts and the risk of dementia and cognitive decline. N Engl J Med 2003;348(13):1215–22.

143. Erkinjuntti T, Gao F, Lee DH, et al. Lack of difference in brain hyperintensities between patients with early Alzheimer's disease and control subjects. Arch Neurol 1994;51(3):260–8.

144. Leys D, Soetaert G, Petit H, et al. Periventricular and white matter magnetic resonance imaging hyperintensities do not differ between Alzheimer's disease and normal aging. Arch Neurol 1990; 47(5):524–7.

145. Pantoni L, Simoni M, Pracucci G, et al. Visual rating scales for age-related white matter changes (leukoaraiosis): can the heterogeneity be reduced? Stroke 2002;33(12):2827–33.

146. Wahlund LO, Barkhof F, Fazekas F, et al. A new rating scale for age-related white matter changes applicable to MRI and CT. Stroke 2001;32(6): 1318–22.

147. Fazekas F, Kleinert R, Offenbacher H, et al. Pathologic correlates of incidental MRI white matter signal hyperintensities. Neurology 1993;43(9): 1683–9.

148. Scheltens P, Barkhof F, Leys D, et al. A semiquantative rating scale for the assessment of signal hyperintensities on magnetic resonance imaging. J Neurol Sci 1993;114(1):7–12.

149. Scheltens P, Barkhof F, Leys D, et al. Histopathologic correlates of white matter changes on MRI in Alzheimer's disease and normal aging. Neurology 1995;45(5):883–8.

150. Kapeller P, Barber R, Vermeulen RJ, et al. Visual rating of age-related white matter changes on magnetic resonance imaging: scale comparison, interrater agreement, and correlations with quantitative measurements. Stroke 2003;34(2):441–5.

151. Mäntylä R, Erkinjuntti T, Salonen O, et al. Variable agreement between visual rating scales for white matter hyperintensities on MRI. Comparison of 13 rating scales in a poststroke cohort. Stroke 1997; 28(8):1614–23.

152. Scheltens P, Erkinjuntti T, Leys D, et al. White matter changes on CT and MRI: an overview of visual rating scales. European Task Force on Age-Related White Matter Changes. Eur Neurol 1998; 39(2):80–9.

153. van Straaten EC, Fazekas F, Rostrup E, et al. Impact of white matter hyperintensities scoring method on correlations with clinical data: the LADIS study. Stroke 2006;37(3):836–40.

154. Grimaud J, Lai M, Thorpe J, et al. Quantification of MRI lesion load in multiple sclerosis: a comparison of three computer-assisted techniques. Magn Reson Imaging 1996;14(5):495–505.

155. Guttmann CR, Kikinis R, Anderson MC, et al. Quantitative follow-up of patients with multiple sclerosis using MRI: reproducibility. J Magn Reson Imaging 1999;9(4):509–18.

156. Alfano B, Brunetti A, Larobina M, et al. Automated segmentation and measurement of global white matter lesion volume in patients with multiple sclerosis. J Magn Reson Imaging 2000;12(6):799–807.

157. Itti L, Chang L, Ernst T. Segmentation of progressive multifocal leukoencephalopathy lesions in fluid-attenuated inversion recovery magnetic

resonance imaging. J Neuroimaging 2001;11(4): 412–7.

158. Zijdenbos AP, Forghani R, Evans AC. Automatic "pipeline" analysis of 3-D MRI data for clinical trials: application to multiple sclerosis. IEEE Trans Med Imaging 2002;21(10):1280–91.

159. Anbeek P, Vincken KL, van Osch MJ, et al. Probabilistic segmentation of white matter lesions in MR imaging. Neuroimage 2004;21(3):1037–44.

160. Wen W, Sachdev P. The topography of white matter hyperintensities on brain MRI in healthy 60- to 64-year-old individuals. Neuroimage 2004; 22(1):144–54.

161. Admiraal-Behloul F, van den Heuvel DM, Olofsen H, et al. Fully automatic segmentation of white matter hyperintensities in MR images of the elderly. Neuroimage 2005;28(3):607–17.

162. DeCarli C, Murphy DG, Tranh M, et al. The effect of white matter hyperintensity volume on brain structure, cognitive performance, and cerebral metabolism of glucose in 51 healthy adults. Neurology 1995;45(11):2077–84.

163. Java Image (JIM). Available at: http://www.xinapse. com. Accessed July 28, 2011.

164. Altaf N, Daniels L, Morgan PS, et al. Cerebral white matter hyperintense lesions are associated with unstable carotid plaques. Eur J Vasc Endovasc Surg 2006;31(1):8–13.

165. Benedict RH, Weinstock-Guttman B, Fishman I, et al. Prediction of neuropsychological impairment in multiple sclerosis: comparison of conventional magnetic resonance imaging measures of atrophy and lesion burden. Arch Neurol 2004;61(2):226–30.

166. Dalaker TO, Larsen JP, Bergsland N, et al. Brain atrophy and white matter hyperintensities in early Parkinson's disease(a). Mov Disord 2009;24(15): 2233–41.

167. Murphy DG, DeCarli C, Schapiro MB, et al. Age-related differences in volumes of subcortical nuclei, brain matter, and cerebrospinal fluid in healthy men as measured with magnetic resonance imaging. Arch Neurol 1992;49(8):839–45.

168. Murphy DG, DeCarli CD, Daly E, et al. Volumetric magnetic resonance imaging in men with dementia of the Alzheimer type: correlations with disease severity. Biol Psychiatry 1993;34(9):612–21.

169. DeCarli C, Murphy DG, Teichberg D, et al. Local histogram correction of MRI spatially dependent image pixel intensity nonuniformity. J Magn Reson Imaging 1996;6(3):519–28.

170. DeCarli C, Fletcher E, Ramey V, et al. Anatomical mapping of white matter hyperintensities (WMH): exploring the relationships between periventricular WMH, deep WMH, and total WMH burden. Stroke 2005;36(1):50–5.

171. DeCarli C, Maisog J, Murphy DG, et al. Method for quantification of brain, ventricular, and subarachnoid CSF volumes from MR images. J Comput Assist Tomogr 1992;16(2):274–84.

172. Evans AC, Collins DL, Mills SR, et al. 3D Statistical neuroanatomical models from 305 MRI volumes. Nuclear Science Symposium and Medical Imaging Conference (1993 IEEE Conference Record) 1993;3:1813–7. DOI: 10.1109/NSSMIC. 1993.373602.

173. Grady L. Random walks for image segmentation. IEEE Trans Pattern Anal Mach Intell 2006;28(11): 1768.

174. Grady L. Random walker image segmentation algorithm. Available at: http://cns.bu.edu/~lgrady/ software.html. Accessed July 28, 2011.

175. Sachdev P, Wen W. Should we distinguish between periventricular and deep white matter hyperintensities? Stroke 2005;36(11):2342–3 [author reply: 2343–4].

176. Velikina JV, Johnson KM, Wu Y, et al. PC HYPR flow: a technique for rapid imaging of contrast dynamics. J Magn Reson Imaging 2010;31(2): 447–56.

177. Wu Y, Chang W, Johnson KM, et al. Fast whole-brain 4D contrast-enhanced MR angiography with velocity encoding using undersampled radial acquisition and highly constrained projection reconstruction: image-quality assessment in volunteer subjects. AJNR Am J Neuroradiol 2010;32(3):E47–50.

178. Barger AV, Block WF, Toropov Y, et al. Time-resolved contrast-enhanced imaging with isotropic resolution and broad coverage using an under-sampled 3D projection trajectory. Magn Reson Med 2002;48(2):297–305.

179. Mistretta CA, Wieben O, Velikina J, et al. Highly constrained backprojection for time-resolved MRI. Magn Reson Med 2006;55(1):30–40.

180. Johnson KM, Velikina J, Wu Y, et al. Improved waveform fidelity using local HYPR reconstruction (HYPR LR). Magn Reson Med 2008;59(3):456–62.

181. Johnson KM, Lum DP, Turski PA, et al. Improved 3D phase contrast MRI with off-resonance corrected dual echo VIPR. Magn Reson Med 2008;60(6): 1329–36.

Index

Note: Page numbers of article titles are in **boldface** type.

Neuroimag Clin N Am 22 (2012) 399–402
doi:10.1016/S1052-5149(12)00027-5
1052-5149/12/$ – see front matter © 2012 Elsevier Inc. All rights reserved.

Printed and bound by CPI Group (UK) Ltd, Croydon, CR0 4YY

03/10/2024

01040359-0006